WORLD HEALTH SYSTEMS

Challenges and Perspectives

WORLD
HEALTH
SYSTEMS

Challenges and Perspectives

Edited by Bruce J. Fried
and Laura M. Gaydos

Health Administration Press, Chicago, Illinois
AUPHA Press, Washington, D.C.

AUPHA
HAP

Your board, staff, or clients may also benefit from this book's insight. For more information on quantity discounts, contact the Health Administration Press Marketing Manager at (312) 424-9470.

06   05   04   03   02   5   4   3   2   1

Library of Congress Cataloging-in-Publication Data

Fried, Bruce, 1952-
    World health systems : challenges and perspectives / Bruce J. Fried and Laura M. Gaydos.
        p.   cm.
     ISBN 1-56793-182-0 (alk. paper)
     1. World health.   2.   Medical   care—Cross-cultural   studies.
3. Medicine—Cross-cultural studies.   I. Gaydos, Laura M.   II. Title.
RA441 .F754 2002
362.1—dc21   2002017236

The paper used in this publication meets the minimum requirements of American National Standard for Information Sciences—Permanence of Paper for Printed Library Materials, ANSI Z39.48-1984. ♾™

Acquisitions editor: Marcy McKay; Project manager: Joyce Sherman; Book and cover designer: Matt Avery

Health Administration Press
A division of the Foundation
   of the American College of
   Healthcare Executives
One North Franklin Street
Suite 1700
Chicago, IL 60606
(312) 424-2800

Association of University Programs
   in Health Administration
730 11th Street, NW
   4th Floor
Washington, DC 20001
(202) 638-1448

Dedication

To Dr. James Veney, who provided the inspiration and support for this project and has shown a lifetime of commitment to global health.

TABLE OF CONTENTS

PREFACE

Health systems in every country in the world, regardless of their level of economic development or wealth, are struggling to manage multiple demands and pressures. These demands are well-known even to the casual observer of the healthcare scene in virtually any country, and they include:

- ensuring access to care while operating within cost constraints,
- balancing the need for preventive and curative services,
- pressures to adopt new technologies versus allocating resources for primary care,
- ensuring that healthcare services reach difficult-to-serve populations,
- achieving an appropriate balance between public and private provision of services,
- maintaining a well-trained healthcare workforce,
- balancing the need for healthcare against other needs,
- responding to current and future epidemics and other threats to health, and
- ensuring consumer participation in how healthcare services are provided.

The manner and extent to which these pressures are experienced varies by country, but in discussions with authors, we found all health systems under stress. In large part, this book is about the pressures being exerted on health systems and the ways in which a variety of countries—through their health systems—have responded to and plan to cope with these pressures. The introduction and chapters 1 through 3 provide a summary of the current issues facing virtually all world health systems, and chapters 4 through 31 profile the health systems of 28 countries. Our intent in selecting these countries was to represent different regions of the world and countries in various stages of economic development. Several Eastern European countries, formerly in the Soviet bloc (including the Russian Federation) are discussed. We feel the reader will be struck by many of the similarities in the challenges facing different countries, but also enlightened by the country- and culture-specific responses to these challenges.

Specifically, part I is devoted to better understanding the overall challenges facing health services. Chapter 1, by Gaydos and Veney, seeks to summarize a wealth of epidemiologic and demographic literature about the state of health in the world today and the relationships between and among health status, economic development, poverty, and the variety of illnesses and causes of mortality and morbidity.

In chapter 2, Sanders addresses fundamental issues in how health systems are organized and financed. Among other questions is the central issue of how health systems obtain financing, and he draws on frameworks developed by Roemer and others in developing a conceptual understanding of the role of governments and private markets in financing health services. We felt this to be a critical issue to address because it focuses so intensely on the debate ensuing in so many countries about public versus private financing. The debate is ongoing, and evidence concerning the optimal public-private mix is complicated by economic conditions, health disparities, cultural and historical factors, and a host of other factors.

Zakus and Cortinois address in chapter 3 the issue of primary care and community participation in the design and delivery of health services. They review the history of the primary care and community participation movements, which have historically occurred hand-in-hand. Although community participation has been a desired characteristic in the design of health services in so many countries—and has been cited as such by a variety of national and international commissions and statements—it has repeatedly been impeded by national governments and other interests that have restricted its implementation. This chapter is a plea to learn from past mistakes and missteps, to move beyond the rhetoric of community participation, and to consider the concept as a centerpiece of health systems.

We then move into the second part of the book, which profiles health systems in 28 countries. Veney's critical "Introduction to the Countries" provides the rationale for our selection of countries for inclusion in the book. He suggests that the countries portrayed fall into seven categories that represent the key aspects of the countries or their health services systems. As he suggests, the key defining characteristic of all health systems is wealth, which comprises three main categories: the wealthy countries, the transitional countries, and the very poor countries. Within each of these three categories of wealth, countries have adopted somewhat different approaches to the design and financing of their systems.

The approach we took in profiling the 28 countries is unique among books that attempt to describe world health systems. In each country, we identified an individual who met certain characteristics, including having knowledge of the health system and its history; having an understanding of the country-specific and cultural factors affecting the system's evolution; and perhaps most important, not having a stake in its current arrangements. We felt this important because we were interested not simply in descriptions of the population, health status indicators, and health system characteristics, but also a critical appraisal of social and political trends and their implications for the health system.

For consistency among chapters, we as editors provided guidance to the authors about the content to be included, such as basic information about disease patterns and health system financing. However, we encouraged authors to describe in their own terms the history, present status, and future challenges of their health systems. Virtually every chapter is written by an individual from the respective country; in several cases, these authors were paired up with an individual from an English-speaking country to assist with editing and clarity. These coauthors also share an interest in the country and participated in research required for the country. We sought to provide essential information on each country's health status and health systems so that the reader could indeed compare countries. Given the difficulties involved in obtaining comparable data from so many countries, the reader will find that data from certain countries are more complete than others. We preferred to err on the side of excluding data that the authors felt were unreliable rather than include information that might be misleading.

This project was a multiple-year undertaking and involved truly global cooperation. Thanks go first and foremost to the authors who contributed their expertise and time to this project and were extremely patient with us as we faced our own time constraints.

Our editors at Health Administration Press, Marcy McKay and Audrey Kaufman, showed outstanding patience and encouraged us throughout the project. Joyce Sherman's wonderful editing showed remarkable sensitivity to the subject matter. We commend as well Matt Avery on his creative cover design.

Arnold Kaluzny, Jim Veney, Sagar Jain, and Tom Ricketts provided much help in developing the concept for this book and helped identify many of the contributors in the volume.

With manuscripts arriving from all over the world, a volume such as this requires considerable editing, and special thanks go to Diamanta Tornatore and MaryAnne Gobble. Both of these individuals worked tirelessly to preserve the writers' intent in their editorial work.

Donna Cooper in the Department of Health Policy & Administration at the University of North Carolina at Chapel Hill provided an extraordinary level of support for this project by helping to maintain contact with our authors and the editors at Health Administration Press. Kerry Kilpatrick and Laurel Files, chair and associate chair of the Department of Health Policy & Administration, encouraged us throughout the entire process of the project.

Acknowledgments

Bruce Fried: I thank my wife and children—Nancy, Shoshana, Noah, and Aaron—for their patience and encouragement. And special thanks to my parents—Pearl and George Fried—who have always supported me in my various endeavors.

Laura Gaydos: I thank my parents, Joan and Robbie, who are always there to help. Thanks to Jamie, Larry and Darlene, and Fred and Mel for unending support. And special thanks to my husband, Chris, who gives me more than I could ever express in words.

CURRENT ISSUES FACING GLOBAL HEALTH SYSTEMS

THE NATURE AND ETIOLOGY OF DISEASE

Laura Marti Dokson Gaydos and James E. Veney

The State of Health in the World

Global health conditions improved more in the past half-century than in all of the years before (World Bank 1993). Worldwide, life expectancy has risen to an average of 65 years, and death rates have declined, especially among young children (WHO 1996). In the wealthiest countries, average life expectancy climbed from roughly 67 years in 1950 to 77 years in 1995; in the developing countries, life expectancy jumped from 40 to 64 years. Even in the least developed regions, such as sub-Saharan Africa, average life expectancy has climbed from 36 to 52 years. The only exception to these positive regional trends occurred in the transitional economies of the former Soviet Union, where life expectancy for men declined to 1980 levels in all 12 republics, reaching a low of 57.7 years in the Russian Federation in 1994 (WHO 1996b). Major strides have also been made in reducing child mortality. As recently as 1950, 287 children out of every 1,000 born in the developing countries would die before reaching age five; by 1995, that number had dropped to 90 out of every 1,000 (WHO 1996).

Yet this incredible progress should not mask the fact that health conditions remain dismal in many parts of the world and that huge disparities exist between the richest and the poorest countries and, indeed, between the rich and the poor within the same country or even the same city. Today nearly one-fifth of all people in the developing countries are not expected to survive to age 40 (UNDP 1997).

Poverty and Health Status

Despite dramatic global economic growth, one-quarter of the world's population today is still affected by severe poverty, and the gaps between rich and poor continue to grow (UNDP 1994). For all developing countries, of a total population of 4 billion, 240 million, an estimated 1 billion, 314 million live in poverty (UNDP 1994).

Poverty not only increases the risk of poor health and the vulnerability of people, it also has serious implications for the delivery of effective healthcare, including reduced demand for services, lack of continuity or compliance in medical treatment, and increased transmission of infectious diseases.

Poverty is not just a lack of money. It generally includes the following elements: inadequate income; lack of education, knowledge, and skill; poor health status and lack of access to healthcare; poor housing; lack of access to safe water and sanitation; insufficient food and nutrition; and lack of control over the reproductive process.

In the least-developed countries (LDCs), a special effort is needed to enhance the health status of their populations and to reduce the gap with respect to the industrialized world and even to other developing countries. In the early 1990s, the average life expectancy at birth in the LDCs was only 50.1 years, and the average mortality rate for children under the age of five was 160 per 1,000 live births. Sierra Leone—a country that has been torn by civil war in recent years—has a life expectancy of roughly 38 years, which is the lowest in the world; it is less than half that of Japan, which boasts the highest life expectancy worldwide at nearly 80 years (UN 1996). These figures confirm a blatant inequality with the rest of the world. In fact, average life expectancy in the LDCs is about 67 percent of that in industrialized countries (Carrin and Politi 2000).

Similarly, although huge improvements in child survival have been made, it must be noted that more than 20 percent of children born in the LDCs will die before reaching age five (in Angola, nearly 30 percent of children will die); in the richest countries, less than one percent will. Average maternal mortality in the LDCs was 730 per 100,000 live births in 1990 (UNICEF 2000). An excessively large gap is observed with regard to children's and women's health in the LDCs: the average mortality rates of children under five and of mothers are at least ten and 30 times as high, respectively, as the corresponding rates in industrialized countries. A comparison with other developing countries shows that the average mortality rates of children under five and of mothers are 2.4 and 2.7 times as high, respectively (Carrin and Politi 2000).

Table 1.1 shows basic indicators for developing nations; Table 1.2 allows for these figures to be compared with those of the more developed, wealthier nations.

As expected, among those countries facing high levels of poverty, one can see higher infant and child mortality rates, substantially lower life expectancies, and other diminished health indicators. Most notable is the magnitude of the differences in health status between the wealthy and impoverished nations.

The United Nations Development Programme has devised a Human Poverty Index (HPI) that serves as a scale for its annual development report. A low HPI score is a positive indicator, showing that a low percentage of a nation's people live in poverty. The HPI accounts for the following:

TABLE 1.1
Basic Health Indicators for a Selection of the World's Most Impoverished Countries

Country	Gross national product per capita (U.S.$), 1997	Under-5 mortality rate (per 1,000), 1998	Infant mortality rate (under 1 year, per 1,000 live births), 1998	Total population (thousands), 1998	Annual number of births (thousands), 1998	Annual number of under-5 deaths (thousands), 1998	Life expectancy at birth (years), 1998	Total adult literacy rate (percent), 1995
Afghanistan	250	257	165	21,354	1,113	286	46	32
Angola	260	292	170	12,092	583	170	47	42
Burkina Faso	250	165	109	11,305	519	86	45	19
Chad	230	198	118	7,270	318	63	47	48
Congo, Democratic Republic of the	110	207	128	49,139	2,264	469	51	77
Ethiopia	110	173	110	59,649	2,652	459	43	33
Guinea-Bissau	230	205	130	1,161	48	10	45	31
Madagascar	250	157	95	15,057	600	94	58	46

TABLE 1.1 (continued)

Malawi	210	213	134	10,346	489	104	39	56
Mali	260	237	144	10,694	499	118	54	32
Mozambique	140	206	129	18,880	817	168	44	38
Myanmar	220	113	80	44,497	943	107	60	83
Nepal	220	100	72	22,847	779	78	58	36
Niger	200	280	166	10,078	488	137	49	13
Somalia	110	211	125	9,237	484	102	47	24
Yemen	270	121	87	16,887	807	98	58	40
Averages	211.7647	195.4118	122	25,111.882	1,030.4118	195.1765	49.47059	41.58824

SOURCE: World Health Organization (1998).

TABLE 1.2 Basic Health Indicators for a Selection of the World's Wealthiest Nations

Countries	Gross national product per capita (U.S.$), 1997	Under-5 mortality rate (per 1,000), 1998	Infant mortality rate (under 1 year, per 1,000 live births), 1998	Total population (thousands), 1998	Annual number of births (thousands), 1998	Annual number of under-5 deaths (thousands), 1998	Life expectancy at birth (years), 1998	Total adult literacy rate (percent), 1995
Australia	20,650	5	5	18,520	246	1	78	—
Belgium	26,730	6	6	10,141	106	1	77	—
Canada	19,640	6	6	30,563	344	2	79	97
Finland	24,790	5	4	5,154	57	0	77	—
France	26,300	5	5	58,683	713	4	78	—
Germany	28,280	5	5	82,133	749	4	77	—
Italy	20,170	6	6	57,369	512	3	78	98
Japan	38,160	4	4	126,281	1,261	5	80	—
Netherlands	25,830	5	5	15,678	179	1	78	—

TABLE 1.2 (continued)

Norway	36,100	4	4	4,419	57	0	78	—
Singapore	32,810	5	4	3,476	50	0	77	91
Spain	14,490	6	6	39,628	360	2	78	97
Sweden	26,210	4	4	8,875	86	0	79	—
Switzerland	43,060	5	5	7,299	80	0	79	—
United Kingdom	20,870	6	6	58,649	689	4	77	—
United States	29,080	8	7	274,028	3,788	30	77	99
Averages	$27,073.13	5.3125	5.125	50,056	579.8125	3.5625	77.9375	96.4

SOURCE: World Health Organization (1998).

- longevity (percent of population expected to die before age 40)
- knowledge (adult literacy rate)
- decent standard of living
- access to healthcare and safe water
- malnutrition in children under age 5

Developing nations, not surprisingly, have an overall high score on the HPI scale. Large portions of the populations of developing countries do not have access to necessities such as healthcare and safe water, and this leads to a plethora of diseases that, although they are not exclusive to developing nations, often define mortality in these countries. Ninety percent of the 1.3 billion people who live in absolute poverty live in South Asia, sub-Saharan Africa, and China.

Poverty and Disability

Despite all their benefits, mortality figures do not capture the huge burden of sickness and disability caused by diseases that do not result in death but that prevent adults from working, keep children out of school, and generally slow economic and social development. Statistics on morbidity, which is the measure of disease incidence, are even harder to come by than mortality numbers.

Over the years, various investigators have attempted to overcome these limitations by developing new metrics that factor in disability or quality of life along with mortality. One such measure recently developed is the disability-adjusted life year (DALY). DALYs combine losses from premature death (defined as the difference between the actual age of death and the life expectancy at that age in a low-mortality population) and loss of healthy life that results from disability. In simple terms, a DALY strives to tally the complete burden that a particular disease exacts. Key elements to consider include the age at which the disease or disability occurs, how long its effects linger, and its impact on quality of life. Losing one's sight at age 7, for instance, is a greater loss than losing one's sight at 67. Similarly, a bout of acute illness that is over quickly carries less weight in the DALY calculation than an illness that leaves lingering weakness, such as persistent worm infections (Murray and Lopez 1996).

Examined from this perspective—which considers not just premature death but disability as well—the huge toll of ill health in developing countries stands out even more starkly. Nearly nine-tenths of the global burden of disease occurs in developing regions where only one-tenth of global health expenditures occur (Murray and Lopez 1996). As Figure 1.1 illustrates, the burden of ill health in sub-Saharan Africa is twice the global average and nearly five times what is found in the richest countries.

When measured with DALYs, communicable diseases are the single most important cause of ill health globally, accounting for 44 percent of

FIGURE 1.1

Burden of
Disease by
Region of
the World

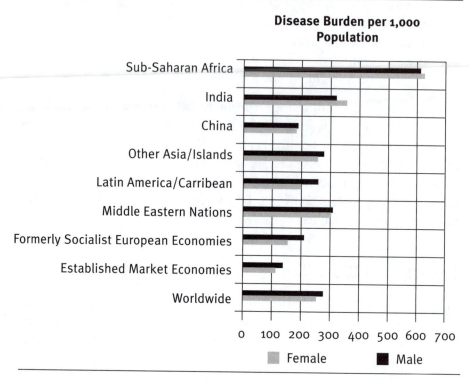

Disease Burden per 1,000 Population

SOURCE: Murray and Lopez (1996).

the total. This level of importance in large part reflects the early age at which many infectious diseases strike. Of the top ten causes of DALYs globally, seven are communicable diseases, with lower respiratory infections and diarrheal diseases heading the list (Muir 2000). DALYs also underscore the disproportionate burden of ill health borne by the world's children. Children under age 15 account for almost half of all DALYs worldwide. Figure 1.2 further illustrates comparisons between mortality and DALYs.

The Epidemiological Transition

Until recently, it was widely assumed that, with increasing economic growth, the developing countries would follow the same paths as Europe and North America and experience what has become known as the "epidemiologic transition"; this term refers to a change in the type of diseases and illnesses experienced within a society. Changes in mortality structure are the principle outcome indicator by which the epidemiological transition is assessed.

Mankind has undergone multiple epidemiological transitions, beginning with a cultural shift from a foraging to an agricultural society that led to the development of new diseases, including zoonotic infections that resulted from the domestication of animals.

The first modern epidemiologic transition resulted from the development of urban centers. Early in their history, large urban settlements

FIGURE 1.2

Death versus

DALYs

Comparing Causes of Death Worldwide with DALYs

Top 10 causes of DALYs, 2000	Top 10 causes of death, 2000
1. Lower respiratory infections	Ischemic heart disease
2. Perinatal conditions	Cerebrovascular disease
3. Human immunodeficiency virus/ acquired immunodeficiency syndrome	Lower respiratory infections
4. Unipolar depressive disorders	Human immunodeficiency virus/acquired immunodeficiency syndrome
5. Diarrheal diseases	Chronic obstructive pulmonary disease
6. Ischemic heart disease	Perinatal conditions
7. Cerebrovascular disease	Diarrheal diseases
8. Road traffic accidents	Tuberculosis
9. Malaria	Road traffic accidents
10. Tuberculosis	Trachea, bronchus, and lung cancers

SOURCE: Data extracted from "The World Health Report 2001—Mental Health: New Understanding, New Health." Figure 2.2, Annex Table 2. Retrieved 10 October 2001 from http://www.who.int/whr/2001.

began to experience problems involving waste disposal and contaminated water and food sources. Communicable diseases such as cholera, which is transmitted by contaminated water, became problematic. Viral diseases such as measles, mumps, and smallpox threatened epidemic proportions as the close urban living quarters allowed for repeated and multiple exposures.

With industrialization came an even greater environmental and social transformation. City dwellers were forced to contend with industrial waste and polluted water and air. Slums arose in industrial cities and became focal points for poverty and the spread of disease. Epidemics of smallpox, typhus, diphtheria, measles, and yellow fever were well-documented. Tuberculosis and respiratory diseases such as pneumonia and bronchitis were even more serious problems, and they were exacerbated by harsh working situations and crowded living conditions.

The next part of this chapter will focus on the second epidemiological transition, which involved the rise of chronic and degenerative diseases, and the third transition, which was a reemergence of infectious diseases with antibiotic resistance.

The Second Epidemiological Transition: The Rise of Chronic and Degenerative Diseases

The second epidemiological transition was the shift from acute infectious diseases to chronic, noninfectious, degenerative diseases. The increasing prevalence of these diseases is related to an increase in longevity. Cultural advances result in a larger percentage of individuals reaching the oldest age segment of the population. Simultaneously, the technological advances that have allowed for increased longevity can also cause an increase in environmental degradation, and these advances arguably lead to new chronic diagnoses. Interestingly, within developing countries, many of the chronic diseases first appear in the wealthier segments of the population or in those segments with greater access to Western products and practices.

With increasing developments in technology, medicine, and science, a better understanding of the source of infectious disease arose and was followed by an increased ability to control these diseases. The development of immunizations resulted in the control of many infections and the eradication of diseases such as smallpox. The decrease in infectious diseases and the subsequent reduction in infant mortality have resulted in greater life expectancy at birth. In addition, longevity has increased for adults, and this has resulted in an increase in chronic and degenerative diseases.

Many of the diseases of the second transition share common factors related to human adaptation, including diet, activity level, mental stress, behavioral practices, and environmental pollution. For example, the industrialization and commercialization of food often results in malnutrition. Obesity, which is another form of malnutrition, is a direct result of an increasingly sedentary lifestyle in conjunction with increasing caloric intakes.

Chronic diseases are a relatively recent factor in human morbidity, and this is indicative of a strong environmental factor in disease etiology. Although biological factors such as genetics are clearly important in determining who succumbs to disease, genetics alone cannot explain the widespread changes seen in the second epidemiological transition.

The Third Epidemiological Transition: Reemergence of Infectious Diseases

The third epidemiological transition is a reemergence of infectious diseases with antibiotic resistance; this reemergence has the potential for a global impact. This transition is a result of an interaction of social, demographic, and environmental changes that have resulted in the adaptation and genetic mutation of the microbe; this change has been influenced by international commerce and travel, technological change, the breakdown of public health measures, and other factors. Ecological changes such as agricultural development projects, dams, deforestation, floods, droughts, and climatic changes have resulted in the emergence of diseases such as Hantavirus and possibly HIV and AIDS.

The catalyst driving the reemergence of many diseases is ecological change that brings humans into contact with pathogens. The development of antibiotic resistance in any pathogen is the result of medical and agricultural practices. Antibiotics have been used indiscriminately and inappropriately, resulting in hospitals that are the source of multidrug-resistant strains of bacteria that infect a large number of patients. Similarly, agricultural uses of antibiotics such as supplementation of animal feed have become more prevalent.

The Demographic Transition

The demographic transition model seeks to explain the transformation of countries from agricultural to industrial societies. The model approximates occurrences in Western Europe and to some extent the experience of most developed nations. In developed countries, this transition began in the eighteenth century and continues today; LDCs are still in the midst of earlier stages in the model.

As countries become developed and industrialized, they experience declines in death rates followed by declines in birth rates. As a result, nations move from rapid population growth to slow growth, then to zero growth, and finally to a reduction in population; this is the essence of the demographic transition model. Demographers have observed that this transition takes place in four distinct stages, as described below.

1. *Preindustrial Stage.* In this first stage, when the economy is under-developed, both birth and death rates will be very high. High birth rates are attributed to such factors as early marriages and religious and social customs; death rates are high due to poor diet, ill health, and the absence of medical facilities. As a result, population growth is slow in the preindustrial stage.
2. *Transitional Stage.* In this second stage, which typically occurs shortly after industrialization, national and per capita incomes rise due to the implementation of developmental programs. The standard of living will be high, health and sanitary conditions will be improved, and diseases are controlled. Consequently, the death rate falls, but the birth rate continues to be high. As a result, population growth will be high, and a population explosion will result.
3. *Industrial Stage.* The third stage of the transition occurs as industrialization becomes widespread. When development reaches an advanced stage, many changes occur in the economic as well as in the social structure. People understand the benefits of family planning, and they deliberately restrict the size of their families. Restriction of family size is equated with higher standards of living, so birth and death rates will be low at this stage. The advanced countries of the world are now in this stage.
4. *Postindustrial Stage.* The fourth and final stage occurs when birth rates decline even further to equal the death rate, thus causing the rate of population growth to reach zero. The birth rate falls below the death rate, and total population size slowly decreases. By 1991,

18 European countries had reached or were approaching zero population growth, and Hungary and Germany were experiencing population declines (Muir 2000).

Figure 1.3 provides a graphical representation of the demographic transition.

Developing Nations and the Demographic Transition

Many developing nations are currently in the transitional stage. This is sometimes referred to as the "demographic trap," because it is a dangerous stage from the perspective of population growth. An estimated 17 percent of the world's current population—more than 67 nations—are in this stage (WHO 1998); this has led to record increases in population size.

One example of a region of the world that is in this demographic trap is sub-Saharan Africa, which has experienced nearly constant fertility rates coupled with a decrease in death rates due to longer life expectancy. Mortality has decreased without a corresponding change in fertility, which has led to a population explosion in this region that is mirrored worldwide.

It is important to note that, although the demographic transition is widely accepted in scholarly examinations of developing nations with regard to healthcare, a vast body of literature refutes the idea that all developing nations will converge to reach the same status as developed nations such as the United States and certain Western European nations. Such literature discusses numerous examples (especially within Latin America and Africa) that are showing trends of divergence (e.g., increased poverty and underdevelopment) rather than convergence and progression in accordance with the demographic transition model. Therefore, although the demographic transition model is a useful tool for analysis, it should not be viewed as the set path of progression for all developing nations.

Diseases of Poverty

The diseases of poverty are typically acute ailments caused by poor nutrition, environment, and lack of access to appropriate care. Whereas wealthier nations typically treat and prevent these diseases with ease, in impoverished nations these diseases often present issues of life and death.

In the poorest nations, child health is of primary concern, because children's less-developed bodies are more prone to both the diseases themselves and the underlying causes of these diseases that keep children from developing fully functional immune systems and other natural defenses.

Infant and Child Mortality

In 1955, 21 million deaths occurred worldwide of children under five; in 1997, about 10 million occurred. This number is expected to drop to 5 million for 2025, when the world population is projected to reach 8 bil-

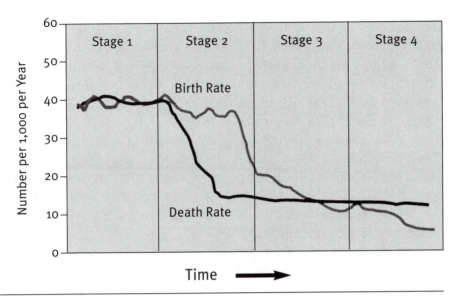

SOURCE: Muir (1998).

FIGURE 1.3
The Demographic Transition

lion. Under-five mortality rates per thousand live births for the aforementioned years are 210, 78, and 37, respectively (WHO 2000c). Infant mortality is linked to several predictive correlates, including the following:

- birth order
- economic conditions
- ethnicity and culture
- low birth weight (often resulting from premature birth)
- maternal age
- maternal education
- sex

The factors listed above have a large impact in the prenatal period, during which a fetus may not receive the proper medical care and nutrition needed to develop fully. In fact, more than half of all infant deaths take place within the first few days of life, largely because of inadequate care for the mother during pregnancy and childbirth (WHO 2000). An entire international body of literature exists that discusses correlations among maternal education, age, and external cultural factors with regard to prenatal care and proper nutrition.

Malnutrition

Each year, more than 11 million children die from the effects of disease and inadequate nutrition. In some countries, more than one in five children die before they reach their fifth birthday, and many of those who do survive are unable to grow and develop to their full potential.

In 1995, malnutrition was responsible for 6.6 million of the 12.2 million deaths in the under-five age group; this represents 54 percent of young-child mortality in developing countries. During the same year, the growth of more than 200 million children was stunted by malnutrition. These children are more likely to have poor cognitive development and neurological impairment; in adulthood, they are at an increased risk for cardiovascular disease, high blood pressure, obstructed lung disease, diabetes, high cholesterol concentrations, and renal damage (WHO 2000a).

Protein energy malnutrition (PEM) affects more than one-third of the world's children, with a range of underweight children from 8 percent in the region with the least PEM (South America) to 60 percent in the poorest region (Southeast Asia). PEM is caused by a combination of insufficient food intake and infectious diseases, and it is closely related to insufficient knowledge, poor sanitation, poverty, and insufficient access to medical care. PEM and other dietary deficiencies of vitamins and minerals can lead to learning disabilities, mental retardation, poor health, low work capacity, blindness, and premature death.

Micronutrient malnutrition, which affects at least two billion people of all ages, has come to refer primarily to an insufficient dietary intake of iodine, iron, and vitamin A. Some functional consequences of the micronutrient deficiencies are described in Figure 1.4.

Infection—particularly frequent or persistent diarrhea, pneumonia, measles, or malaria—undermines nutritional status. Poor feeding practices including inadequate breastfeeding, offering the wrong foods, giving food in insufficient quantities, and not ensuring that a child eats his or her share contribute to malnutrition. For these and other reasons, malnourished children are more vulnerable to disease.

Food Safety

In addition to malnutrition, food contamination is one of the most widespread health problems today, and it is an important cause of reduced economic productivity. Hundreds of millions of people, particularly infants and children, suffer from diseases caused by contaminated food and water sources; such contamination constitutes a particular problem in developing countries (WHO 1996).

Acute Respiratory Infections

Acute respiratory infections are estimated to be the primary cause of mortality for all ages in developing nations (WHO 1996). According to the World Health Organization, most young children worldwide have from four to eight episodes of respiratory infections per year, and most of these episodes are self-limiting infections of the upper respiratory tract. However, the incidence of acute lower respiratory infections, particularly pneumonia, is very high in developing countries because of the many individual and environmental factors that significantly heighten the risk of developing these conditions, especially low birth weight, poor nutrition, low income,

FIGURE 1.4

Consequences
of Selected
Micronutrient
Deficiencies

Problem	Functional Consequences	Economic Implications
Iodine deficiency (pregnancy and early childhood)	Mental retardation, stunted growth, delayed growth and maturation	Diminished productivity due to increased difficulty in training and education
Vitamin A deficiency (early childhood)	Blindness, increased severity and frequency of infections, pediatric mortality	Diminished productivity, increased healthcare costs
Iron deficiency (anemia)	Learning disabilities, lowered work capacity, low birth weight, maternal mortality	Diminished educability, diminished productivity, increased healthcare costs

SOURCE: Adapted from Basch (1999).

and indoor air pollution. About four million children die from these infections each year, mostly as a result of pneumonia (WHO 2000b).

Control of acute respiratory infections is difficult because many of the causal agents are airborne. Some disease-causing agents such as measles can be reduced through immunization. Immunization against pneumonia, however, is difficult because 83 different serotypes are known, and each is immunologically unique.

Beyond specific disease-causing agents, exposure to certain ambient air pollutants (e.g., sulfur dioxide and particulate matter) causes severe respiratory problems throughout the world. Road traffic emissions of lead and nitrogen oxides and episodes of air pollutants from localized sources are also often encountered. In the indoor environment, exposure to nitrogen oxides, volatile organic compounds, and environmental tobacco smoke have significant effects on human health and comfort (WHO 2000b).

Diarrheal Disease

Another two million children in developing countries die each year from diarrheal diseases, making these diseases the second highest killer of children under five worldwide. Diarrhea can, in most cases, be prevented and treated; correct management of diarrhea could save the lives of up to 90 percent of children who currently die from the effects of the disease (WHO 1996a). Basic causes of diarrheas include toxins, allergies, lactose intolerance, and malaria. However, by far the most common causes of diarrheas in children are pathogens ingested through contaminated food or water intake, particularly in developing countries.

The immediate result of acute diarrheal disease is dehydration. Loss of approximately 5 percent of body weight through dehydration can typically be tolerated, although this may be accompanied by symptoms such as lightheadedness from a drop in blood pressure. A loss of 10 percent of bodyweight, as is often seen in children in developing countries, can produce real danger with possibilities of shock, kidney failure, and death.

The introduction of oral rehydration therapy (ORT) in recent years has proved very effective, is relatively simple and inexpensive, and has saved perhaps millions of pediatric lives. ORT replaces lost fluids orally rather than intravenously, and it works regardless of which agent caused the episode because it counteracts the resulting dehydration rather than the cause.

However, no treatment, including ORT, is perfect. In addition to relatively minor side effects such as increased stool production, ORT does require access to certain resources such as clean, safe water. Although water may seem like a feasible resource, in many nations clean, safe water is costly and out of reach of those most in need. Consequently, many children in need of ORT do not truly have access.

Adult Illness and Poverty

The standard international health framework discusses illness in poorer countries in terms of communicable and reproductive diseases. As with child health, adults in developing and impoverished nations have long been believed to suffer most often from the following diseases:

- diarrheal disease
- tuberculosis
- malaria
- venereal diseases
- respiratory infections
- maternal and perinatal illness

The causal factors associated with these illnesses are the same for adults as for children, including a lack of safe drinking water and food, poor sanitation, poor housing conditions, malnutrition, chronic parasitic infections, and lack of effective curative measures.

Higher mortality rates among the poor may also result from non-communicable diseases. The specific determinants of these differences are not always evident, but poor nutrition, stress, indoor air pollution (in select countries), smoking, and workplace hazards are also important factors for consideration. Access to effective medical care is also likely to have a significant impact on mortality from noncommunicable diseases.

Health Problems of Affluence

In contrast with developing and poor nations, the more affluent, developed nations of the world have largely conquered communicable and reproductive diseases with medical science. That is not to say that no communicable and reproductive diseases exist in wealthier nations, but these health problems are secondary causes of morbidity and mortality, with rates that lag far behind chronic and noncommunicable diseases.

In wealthy nations, major sources of morbidity and mortality result from chronic and noncommunicable diseases. Many of these diseases are related to lifestyle, such as increased lung cancer due to smoking or high rates of cardiovascular disease that result from obesity and lack of exercise.

Common diseases among wealthy, developed nations include the following:

- arthritis
- cancer
- cardiovascular disease
- diabetes
- hypertension

Note that these are not diseases that result from malnutrition or lack of access to health services; they may be related to excesses in personal lifestyle or they may simply be due to increased longevity, which causes the body to become more susceptible to such conditions.

Similarly, because these diseases are not caused by a single contaminant or pathogen, medical treatment often focuses on management of these diseases rather than cure. Consequently, the wealthy nations of the world have populations with substantial chronic disease prevalence and, therefore, continual healthcare needs. These needs may seem less extreme than those present in the poorer countries, but the resources required to treat diseases of affluence are also significant.

The Changing World Scene

As epidemiological transitions progress on a more global level, similar changes are also observed among specific nations and societies. Among developing nations in the late twentieth century, the more traditional frameworks for evaluating health needs in poverty-stricken nations such as those discussed above have been observed to no longer hold strictly true to form. Although impoverished nations have not largely improved their economic standing, the people of these nations are beginning to develop the diseases of affluence in addition to the diseases of poverty.

Most low- and middle-income countries are already facing a double burden of disease. They suffer an unacceptable backlog of common infections, malnutrition, and reproductive health problems. At the same time, without having addressed these challenges, they have to cope with the emerging problems represented by noncommunicable diseases, heart disease, cancer, new infections, and injuries.

What is causing this addition of new diseases in less-wealthy nations? Development seems to be the primary factor involved. Economic development, as touted by organizations such as the World Bank and the United Nations Development Programme, has many positive consequences. However, economic development also brings to less-developed nations the modern determinants of health, which arise primarily from changes in behavior and from the hazards of new and imperfectly understood technology. As the wealthier nations of the world reach out to help developing nations grow and become "civilized," both positive and negative influences are introduced. Among the negative influences involved is the introduction of unhealthy habits.

Tobacco Use

The causal relationships between tobacco usage and several noncommunicable diseases such as lung cancer and emphysema are well-established. Smoking may also have an impact on cardiac health, premature and complicated births, and many other health problems. Although tobacco consumption in developed nations has been on the decline (largely because of increased public health efforts designed to inform people about the dangers of the drug), the reverse is true in developing nations.

Several reasons explain this. First, antismoking campaigns essentially do not exist in less-wealthy countries, so the public health effects of public awareness are virtually nonexistent. Similarly, in developing nations, few if any restrictions are placed on advertising, and this results in unchecked, widespread campaigns that target the entire population. Finally, developing nations typically have no controls on the content of tobacco products. Therefore, although the percentage of tar used in cigarettes in developed nations has been consistently on the decline, tar levels in cigarettes in poorer nations remain very high. As a consequence of all these factors, the wealthier nations have introduced a vice to developing nations that is not coupled with any of the controls that are often taken for granted in the more-developed countries.

Alcohol Use

Ethyl alcohol, the active ingredient in all alcoholic drinks, is a toxic compound with addictive properties. Alcohol consumption may lead to a number of acute and chronic health problems in addition to possible mental health concerns. Alcohol can cause alcohol poisoning, acute gastritis, and suicidal behavior, and it may contribute to accidents. Long-term exposure to alcohol can also cause cirrhosis of the liver, stomach ulcers, diabetes, and fetal alcohol syndrome. Alcohol dependency may also lead to a series of social and economic problems.

Average alcohol consumption is increasing in most nations of the world. However, this increase is substantially larger among developing and less-wealthy nations. Alcohol consumption has led to numerous socioeconomic consequences in impoverished nations, and one of the primary results is a decreased workforce due to chronic intoxication.

Intentional Violence: Suicides, Homicides, and Warfare

Suicide is a major cause of mortality in both developed and developing countries. Worldwide, about a million suicides occur each year. Several psychological factors have an impact on suicidal tendencies, including social isolation, crises, depression, and alcoholism.

Suicide is a complex issue, and very few effective preventive methods have been discovered. However, high socioeconomic status and community support seem to be highly correlated with the success of suicide prevention.

As with suicide, homicide is also related to a variety of social factors. However, homicide rates vary to a much larger degree across nations, possibly as a reflection of variances in culture and laws. Homicide rates are higher in most developing nations than in their developed counterparts. Within developing countries, homicide rates also vary by numerous factors including gender (males have higher rates), income (the poor have higher rates), place of residence (rates are higher in urban areas), and ethnicity.

In addition, warfare kills and disables substantial portions of the populations of many developing countries, especially in the Middle East, southern Africa, Central America, and Southeast Asia. Although accurate data are often difficult to obtain because of the nature of war and the less-developed tracking systems in developing nations, warfare mortality is often caused by conflicts between criminal gangs and police agencies as well as conflicts among gangs themselves. Warfare of this sort is often tied to the ever-increasing presence of illicit drug trafficking.

Dietary Imbalance

As noted earlier, the major dietary problem in the developing world is lack of food. However, as nations develop, food supplies often increase, and diets change. Whereas the old diets of many less-developed nations, when adequate, typically included large amounts carbohydrates (e.g., rice, polenta), soy or lentils, and perhaps some fish or meat, newer diets consist of more processed foods. These new diets are typically much higher in saturated fat and sodium and lower in simple fiber. Although the exact impact of diet on disease manifestation is still up for debate, a considerable amount of evidence links this more "westernized" diet with a number of chronic diseases including hypertension and certain forms of cancer.

Changes in Physical Activity

It is well-established that regular physical activity promotes greater health. The effects of regular activity, whether occupational or recreational, lead to decreases in coronary heart disease and possibly decreased risk for stroke, cancer, and other diseases. In less-developed countries, most people have enough activity in their daily lives to maintain a health benefit. In developed countries, however, levels of activity have been on a steady decline due to conveniences such as automobiles and many other labor-saving devices. As less-developed countries mature and adopt many of these conveniences, the populations of these countries begin to face the same deficit of physical activity as is seen in developed nations.

Mortality and Automobiles

Automobile collisions are one of the major causes of adult mortality in the developing world, and about half a million deaths each year result from these types of accidents. Injuries from motor vehicle collisions affect 10 to 25 times more people, with as many as half of these injuries requiring hospitalization (Basch 1999). As the number of automobiles increases in developing countries, the levels of associated morbidity and mortality have grown at alarming rates. Similarly, countries with high proportions of motorcycles and other unprotected vehicles (e.g., many counties in Southeast Asia) have even higher risks of driver and passenger injury from motor vehicle collisions.

Whereas in developed nations the majority of accidents occur to people between the ages of 15 and 24, in developing nations, the majority of accidents occur to those over age 25. As vehicle ownership becomes more widespread, these demographics will likely be altered to mirror those found in wealthier nations.

The Environment

As discussed previously in this chapter, contaminated drinking water, food, and indoor air are major causal factors of ill health in impoverished nations. Industrialization and modernization of many developing countries have created new sources of clean water and food, but they have simultaneously produced increased pollution that may add to rather than decrease health problems unless adequate preventive measures are taken.

Air pollution is a growing problem in many poorer countries. The main sources of pollution vary among nations, but in general they result from motor vehicles, power plants, industry, and residential heating and cooking devices. Pollution given off from these sources can damage the lungs and other organs. Such pollution likely also contributes to chronic diseases of the lungs, such as asthma.

Chemical contamination of food and water sources is also of growing concern in poorer nations. As with air pollution, many industries in developing nations contaminate water through various production processes. When polluted waterways are used for drinking water, cooking, irrigation, or as a source of fish, these contaminants can cause severe health problems.

Food contamination is largely a problem of biological contamination, but chemical contamination is also an issue. Poisoning outbreaks have occurred from contamination during food processing.

Depletion of the ozone layer and the "greenhouse effect" are also problems that affect low-income nations. As industry develops, these nations are adding to the causes of ozone depletion by using manufactured products. Ozone depletion affects all nations of the world, not just those responsible for causing the depletion.

Workplace Injuries

Deaths from workplace injuries are approximately ten times more likely in low-income, developing nations than in wealthier nations. Injuries are common in agriculture, construction, transport, and the primary industries such as mining; all of these industries constitute important sources of employment in poorer countries.

Unlike the more-developed nations, the poorer nations of the world do not yet have organizations and regulatory agencies dedicated to improving workplace safety (e.g., the Occupational Safety and Health Administration [OSHA] in the United States). Without these types of guidelines, especially within more physical areas of employment, accidents are more likely to occur. The effects of workplace hazards are substantial. Worldwide, at least 33 million occupational injuries occur each year, 145 thousand of which are fatal (Basch 1999), and these numbers are likely underestimated because of poor data reporting in many countries. Many of these accidents occur in poorer countries and result in increased healthcare costs, decreased productivity, and substantial morbidity and mortality.

Conclusion

What is the state of health in the world today? Clearly no definitive answer to this question exists. Although global health conditions improved more in the past half-century than in all of the years before, it is evident that there is still a very long way to go. The dramatic poverty and illness that face such a large proportion of the world's population reach far beyond acceptable limits. Even in the developed nations of the world, illness—albeit chronic rather than acute—is still very much present at substantially high levels.

How should these mounting challenges be handled? As health and healthcare systems continue to evolve around the world, existing paradigms face many challenges that they are unable to answer, and many problems continue to increase in severity. Perhaps health professionals need to reevaluate approaches to healthcare around the world; perhaps new paradigms are needed. Regardless of the theoretical constructs, healthcare professionals must continue to fight against the growing inequalities and deficiencies in health systems around the world.

REFERENCES

Basch, P. F. 1999. *Textbook of International Health*. New York: Oxford University Press.

Carrin, G., and Politi, C. 2000. "Exploring the Health Impact of Economic Growth, Poverty Reduction and Public Health Expenditure." Retrieved January 2001 from www.who.int/ico/articles/mesd18.html.

Murray, C. J. L., and Lopez, A. D. (eds.) 1996. *The Global Burden of Disease: Volume 1*. Geneva: World Health Organization, Harvard School of Public Health, and The World Bank.

Feachem, R., and Kjellstrom, T. 1992. *The Health of Adults in the Developing World*. Washington, DC: The International Bank for Reconstruction and Development.

Muir, P. 1998. "The Demographic Transition." Retrieved 16 May 2000 from www.orst.edu.

UNICEF. 2000. "The State of the World's Children 2000." Retrieved 05 June 2000 from www.unicef.org.

United Nations Development Programme. 1997. *Human Development Report 1997*. New York: United Nations Development Programme.

United Nations Population Division. 1996. *World Population Prospects, 1950–2050 (The 1996 Revision)*. New York: United Nations.

The World Bank. 1993. *World Development Report 1993: Investing in Health*. Washington, DC: The World Bank.

World Health Organization. 2000. "About WHO: Safe Motherhood." Retrieved 20 May 2000 from www.who.org.

———. 2000a. "About WHO: Nutrition." Retrieved 20 May 2000 from www.who.org.

———. 2000b. "About WHO: Acute Respiratory Infections." Retrieved 20 May 2000 from www.who.org.

———. 2000c. "Reducing Mortality from Major Killers of Children." Retrieved 20 May 2000 from www.who.org.

———. 1998. *World Health Report*. Retrieved 01 March 2001 from www.who.org.

———. 1996. "Evaluating the Implementation of the Strategy for Health for All By the Year 2000." Retrieved 01 March 2001 from www.who.org.

———. 1996a. *The World Health Report 1996: Fighting Disease, Fostering Development*. Geneva: World Health Organization.

———. 1996b. "World Health Statistics Annual 1995." Geneva: World Health Organization Press.

World Resources Institute. "Global Health Patterns." Retrieved March 2001 from www.igc.apc.org/wri/wri/wr-98-99/001-ptns.htm.

FINANCING AND ORGANIZATION OF NATIONAL HEALTH SYSTEMS

Jeffrey Sanders

The organization and financing of healthcare are different for each country described in this book. Each country's political culture, history, and wealth affect the design of health services and the means by which these services are financed. In this chapter, a framework is developed to help compare healthcare systems in a meaningful manner.

To better understand trends and patterns in national health systems, analysts have created models to explain these systems. Most notable is the work of Odin Anderson and Milton Roemer. Anderson developed the concept of the "uneasy equilibrium" between the public and private healthcare sectors, and he organized health systems on a continuum based on the level of government involvement in the financing and organization of health services. Anderson noted that "the degree to which a state centralizes financing and planning and the relative size of its public sector determine its position in the continuum, as does the extent to which it intervenes in the operations of the economy itself" (Craig 1999). The diagram in Figure 2.1 illustrates Anderson's market-minimized/market-maximized continuum.

The market-maximized end of the continuum draws on the concept of change through the private market with limited government involvement. According to Anderson, "Such change may be fast or slow, but it is organic to the system and its pace is natural: it is incremental, not revolutionary" (Anderson 1989). Anderson places the United States at the far end of the market-maximized end of the spectrum. The market-minimized end of the spectrum, in Anderson's words, "draws on the socialistic doctrine of planned economies and government programs for distributive justice and aspires to change with deliberate speed and at a scheduled pace" (Anderson 1989). Anderson places the United Kingdom, with its National Health Services, at the far end of the market-minimized end of the continuum.

In his seminal work, *National Health Systems of the World,* Milton Roemer identified economic output, political culture, and history as key determinants of a country's health system. In that study, Roemer organized national health systems by wealth and by the degree of government involvement in the organization and financing of health services. He categorized health systems in the following three categories:

FIGURE 2.1
Role of
Government

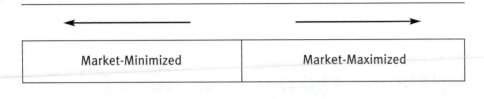

Market-Minimized	Market-Maximized

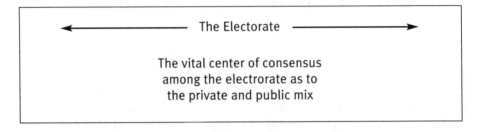

The Electorate

The vital center of consensus
among the electrorate as to
the private and public mix

SOURCE: Reprinted from Anderson (1972, 27).

1. *The entrepreneurial model.* The entrepreneurial model is character-
    ized by employment-based or individual purchase of private health
    insurance coverage financed by individual and/or employer contri-
    butions and mainly private ownership of the factors of production.
    This model has contributed greatly to the scientific advancement of
    medical technology and research. The cost-conscious behavior of
    private employers in the United States has also led to the prolifera-
    tion of cost-saving practices; of these practices, utilization review
    and disease management have been most effective. The biggest
    drawback of the entrepreneurial model is the inequitable distribu-
    tion of healthcare resources. The most glaring example is the
    United States, where the number of uninsured has surpassed 40 mil-
    lion.
2. *The mandated insurance model.* The mandated insurance model is
    characterized by compulsory universal coverage that is generally
    within the framework of social security and financed by the
    employer, includes individual contributions through nonprofit
    insurance funds, and allows for public and/or private ownership of
    factors of production. An advantage of this model is the participa-
    tion in the financing of healthcare by employers and employees
    and the risk-sharing nature of the insurance pools. The German
    sickness funds are the most well known example of the mandated
    insurance model. The Clinton administration borrowed heavily
    from the German insurance model in its effort to reform the U.S.
    healthcare system in the early 1990s. A key disadvantage of this
    model is its inability to adopt the cost-saving measures of managed
    care because of legal restrictions against buyers contracting with
    providers that were put in place in the 1930s.

3. *The national health service model.* The national health service model is characterized by universal coverage, general tax-based financing, and national ownership and/or control of the factors of production (Craig 1999).

   In this chapter, the Roemer model is used to compare the organization and financing of health services. Because elements of each model are present in nearly all of the healthcare systems included in this book, a "proxy measure" is used to determine the appropriate model for each country. For purposes of this analysis, the percentage of healthcare expenditures that are government funded is used to determine the model that best fits the country's healthcare system. Figure 2.2 illustrates where the health services for selected countries fall along the continuum.

   The economic levels of the countries were determined by the gross domestic product (GDP) per capita. Following is the GDP per capita for each category:

- Very poor countries: U.S.$98 to $1,153
- Transitional countries: U.S.$1,211 to $6,956
- Wealthy countries: U.S.$8,257 to $33,085

   Further organization of the coutries into one of the health system categories was based on the level of government financial support for health services as a proportion of the total support required for health services. As noted later in this chapter, the level of overall financial support and government support for healthcare services is directly related to the wealth of the country. As such, no standard level or percentage of government support is given for each of the aforementioned categories (entrepreneurial,

Economic Level (GDP per capita)	Entrepreneurial Model	Mandated Insurance Model	National Health Service Model
Wealthy countries	Argentina South Korea United States	Germany Italy Spain	Canada Japan United Kingdom
Transitional countries	China Mexico	Botswana Brazil Jamaica South Africa	Costa Rica Cuba Poland Russia Turkey
Very poor countries	Congo India Nigeria		

FIGURE 2.2
Typology of Health Systems

SOURCE: Roemer (1991).

mandated, or national); instead, countries were organized into these categories on the basis of the level of government support relative to the GDP of the country.

Financing Health Services

Substantial variation is found among countries in the modes of financing health services. The common financing mechanisms are described in the following paragraphs.

The use of *general tax revenue* to finance healthcare is most common in industrial Western countries and is most closely associated with the comprehensive national insurance systems in Canada and England. Financing from general tax revenue is prevalent in established market democracies that can afford to develop, sustain, and administer a government bureaucracy to collect and manage tax revenues. This type of system is least likely to be used in poorer countries, where personal income is low and other public goods (e.g., roads, education, military) must compete for scarce government resources.

Social insurance, or social security, systems are associated with mandatory insurance systems. Germany was the first country to develop and implement a social health insurance system in the nineteenth century under Chancellor Bismarck. The German system and other social insurance systems rely on contributions from workers and employers to finance health services.

The *voluntary insurance* market is most closely identified with the United States, where employment-based health insurance is purchased from private companies. This approach is seen to a lesser degree in countries like Germany, which permit wealthier individuals to purchase private insurance in lieu of participating in the mandatory health insurance system.

Charitable donations are present in every health system model. The share of charitable donations can reach 40 percent (Uganda in 1993) or may even be as high as 84 percent (Gambia in 1994) (WHO 2000). However, charitable donations in the form of multilateral and bilateral donations are the predominant means of financing in some of the poorer countries. Sources of multilateral support include the United Nations Development Programme, the World Bank, and the United Nations Fund for Population Activities. Bilateral support includes direct foreign aid from one country to another country.

Individual or out-of-pocket payment for services is present in every type of health system in one form or another. Individual payments range from different types of cost sharing (e.g., coinsurance, copayments) to payment in full for services.

The sources of financial support for healthcare and the government funding available tend to be related to a country's wealth. Figure 2.3 illustrates the linear relationship between GDP and expenditures on health for the countries included in this book. The global income elasticity of per capita health spending relative to per capita GDP is estimated at 1.13. This means that a 10 percent increase in per capita GDP is associated with 13 percent higher health spending (Schieber 1999). A further illustration of the disparity of health spending between rich and poor countries is demonstrated by the fact that the countries that belong to the OECD spend 100 times the amount spent in low-income countries and 10 times that spent in middle-income countries (Schieber 1999).

The amount of government spending on health services is also related to the per capita GDP of the country. Figure 2.4 shows the relationship between a country's GDP and government expenditures on health. The relationship indicates that government expenditures increase by .928 percent for every dollar increase in GDP per capita. This relationship accounts for nearly 45 percent of the variation in government expenditures on health. The weaker relationship between GDP per capita and share of government expenditures on health suggests that many other factors (e.g., culture, political ethos) influence the degree of government involvement in healthcare. However, the income elasticity for the public component of health spending is 1.21, which indicates that government spending on health services increases by 21 percent for every 10 percent increase in per capita GDP.

The following sections of this chapter describe significant trends in healthcare expenditure among the different country groupings.

The Wealthy Countries

Among wealthy countries, government expenditures as a percentage of total healthcare expenditures range from 38 percent in South Korea to 97 percent in the United Kingdom. In addition, the share of GDP allocated

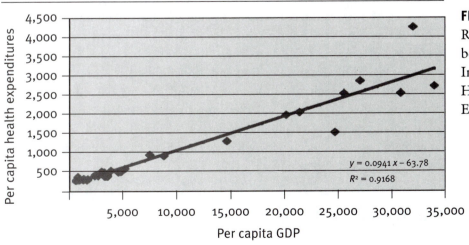

FIGURE 2.3
Relationship between Income and Health Expenditures

$y = 0.0941 x - 63.78$

$R^2 = 0.9168$

SOURCE: Roemer (1991).

FIGURE 2.4

Government
Financing of
Healthcare

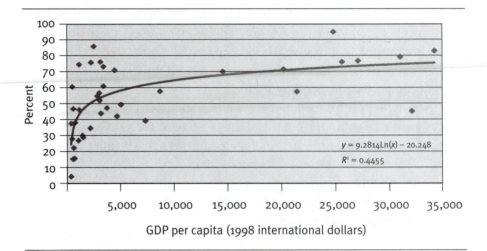

$y = 9.2814\text{Ln}(x) - 20.248$

$R^2 = 0.4455$

GDP per capita (1998 international dollars)

SOURCE: Statistics Division of the UN Secretariat and International Labour Office (2002).

to healthcare ranges from 4 percent in Argentina to 6.7 percent in Denmark. Figure 2.5 shows the level of government support for healthcare for the wealthy countries included in this study.

With the exception of the United States, all of the countries in this group guarantee all citizens' health insurance coverage (Anderson and Poullier 1999). The manner by which the countries raise revenue to fund the government portion of the health expenditures mirrors the health system model. The two primary revenue-generating mechanisms are direct taxation and social security programs. Although both forms of revenue generation appear in nearly all of the countries in this category, direct taxation is more prevalent in countries that have embraced a national health insurance model, whereas social security is more common in countries with mandatory and entrepreneurial health system models (Roemer 1991). Figure 2.6 shows sources of government funding.

All of the wealthy countries are struggling to contain healthcare costs while at the same time improving access to care. In Western Europe, countries have attempted to address these problems through a multitude of reforms, including decentralization and infusing market incentives into the healthcare system (Saltman and Figueras 1998). In the United States, government, insurers, and patients continue to seek a balance between market mechanisms and government regulation. Although private sector efforts to contain costs have been widely hailed, they have created widespread concern about access and adequate levels of care.

The Transitional Countries

Among this group of countries, the government share of healthcare expenditures ranges from 25 percent in China to nearly 88 percent in Cuba. The

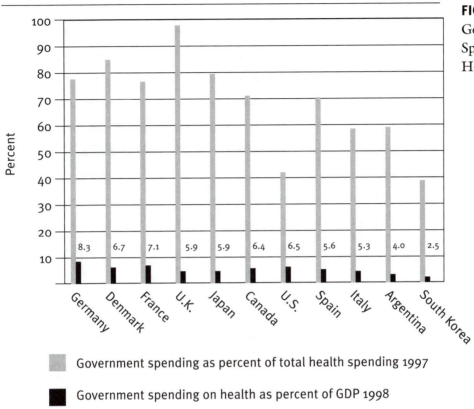

SOURCE: WHO (2000); The International Bank for Reconstruction and Development and the World Bank (2000).

FIGURE 2.5

Government Spending on Healthcare

Government spending as percent of total health spending 1997

Government spending on health as percent of GDP 1998

share of the GDP allocated to healthcare ranges from just .1 percent in Belize[1] to 8.2 percent in Cuba. Figure 2.7 shows government support in each of the countries in this category.

With the exception of Cuba and Costa Rica, the transitional countries devote a smaller proportion of their GDP to healthcare than do the wealthier countries. This is due in part to the countries' per capita incomes, which have an impact on both private and public spending on healthcare. In addition, governments in transitional countries are less able to raise revenue for government-run programs than are the wealthier countries. Among the countries in this study, only a few governments in the transitional group are able to generate revenue equal to 31 percent of their entire GDP for their healthcare sector. Although this figure is nearly 9 percent greater than the amount generated by very poor countries, it is much lower than the 42 percent raised by wealthy countries (Schieber 1999). In addition, transitional countries rely less on social welfare programs to fund healthcare services. As indicated in Figure 2.8, only two transitional countries collect more than 50 percent of their revenue through a social security system.

FIGURE 2.6

Source of Government Funding as a Percentage

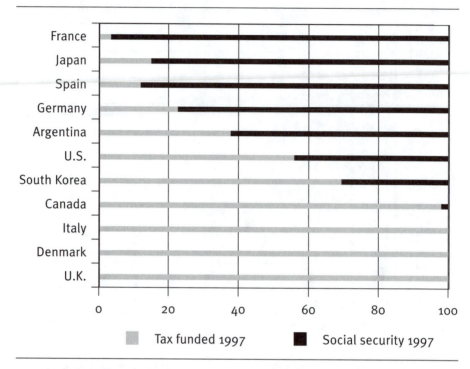

SOURCE: WHO (2000).

The Very Poor Countries

Among the very poor countries, only Tanzania[2] finances a majority of the total healthcare spending through public resources. Figure 2.9 shows the government commitment to healthcare in these countries.

In addition, all of the countries in this category finance public health expenditures through direct taxation. Following are some of the general characteristics of healthcare in low-income countries (World Bank 1993):

- private out-of-pocket payments account for more than half of total health spending per person
- nongovernment organizations, including multilateral and religious organizations, make significant contributions to the provision of healthcare services
- little private insurance is available

Not surprisingly, these trends result in significant health differentials between the poorest countries and other nations throughout the world.

Organization of Health Resources

As illustrated by the three models highlighted earlier in this chapter (entrepreneurial, mandated, and national), the degree of government ownership

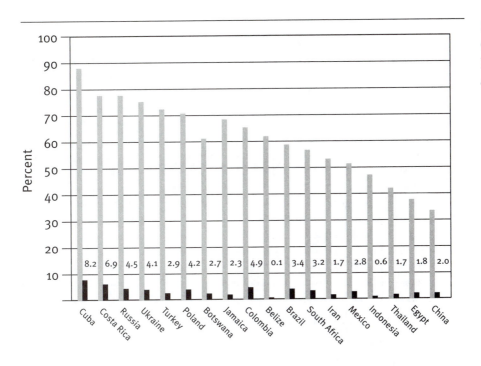

FIGURE 2.7
Government
Expenditures
on Health

Public expenditures as percent of total health expenditures 1997

Public health expenditures as percent of GDP 1998

SOURCE: WHO (2000).

and management of health resources is related to the extent of public financing of health services. As such, countries that operate a national heath insurance system are more likely to own the health resources and employ the healthcare staff. In contrast, countries that fall within the entrepreneurial model are more likely to rely on private ownership of facilities and private employment of clinicians. *The World Health Report 2000* highlights three distinct organizational forms: a hierarchical structure, long-term contractual arrangements, and market-based interactions.

The *hierarchical structure* is synonymous with the rigid bureaucratic organization of healthcare services. This form is most common in government-sponsored national health insurance models such as that found in Turkey. This organizational framework is also common in strict managed care plans in the United States, such as Kaiser Permanente. The key feature of the hierarchical model is government ownership of facilities and employment of clinical personnel.

Long-term contractual arrangements include contractual arrangements between government and private practice clinicians. Such contracts might include treatment for certain health problems such as diabetes, and this arrangement can be found in any of the three organization models.

FIGURE 2.8

Source of
Government
Funding

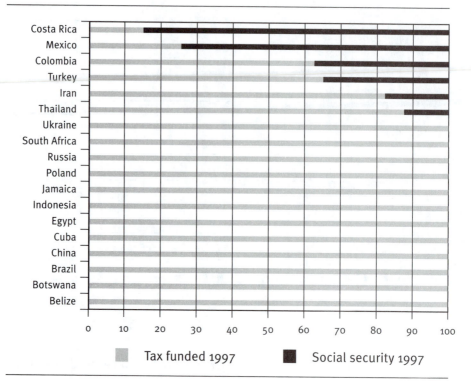

SOURCE: WHO (2000).

Because many countries are now focusing on providing health insurance for basic services in times of resource constraint, this practice has grown tremendously, especially in emerging market economies such as those in Eastern Europe.

Market-based interactions are associated with the direct interaction between providers and the population. Market-based interactions account for 80 percent of healthcare spending.

Roemer (1991) developed a framework that illustrates the relationships between the financing and organization of healthcare resources. Figure 2.10 indicates that no pure system of financing or organization of resources exists; each system includes elements of both government and private financing and control. Cells A and B show that *public* financing can be used to finance both government-employed providers and private practice providers. Likewise, cells C and D indicate that *private* financing can be used to support both government-employed providers and providers in private practice.

Much like the availability of financial support for health spending, physician supply and the supply of hospital beds are largely dependent on a country's per capita GDP. Figure 2.11 indicates that every unit increase in per capita GDP results in an increase of .42 physicians for every 1,000 people. Furthermore, the GDP of a country accounts for only 26 percent of the variation in physician supply among countries. Clearly other factors

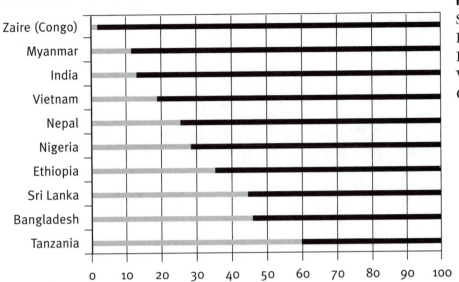

FIGURE 2.9

Source of Healthcare Expenditures, Very Poor Countries

Public expenditures as percent of total health expenditures 1997

Private expenditures as percent of total health expenditures 1997

SOURCE: WHO (2000).

such as culture, history, and government regulation contribute to physician supply. An illustration of the noneconomic factors that contribute to physician supply is the large supply of physicians in some of the poorer countries. The supply of physicians is not associated with better access to care in these countries; instead, it speaks to the weak regulation and oversight of medicine in many of the poorer countries.

The supply of hospital beds is also associated with a country's wealth. Figure 2.12 shows a linear relationship between GDP per capita and the supply of hospital beds. Every U.S.$5,000 increase in GDP per capita results in an increase of one hospital bed per 1,000 people. This relationship accounts for nearly 24 percent of the variation in hospital beds among the countries in this study. As is the case with physician supply, many other factors affect the supply of hospital beds.

Source of Funding	Healthcare Provider	
Public	A	B
Private	C	D

FIGURE 2.10

Public and Private Provision of Health Services

SOURCE: Roemer (1991).

FIGURE 2.11

Impact of
GDP on
Physician
Supply

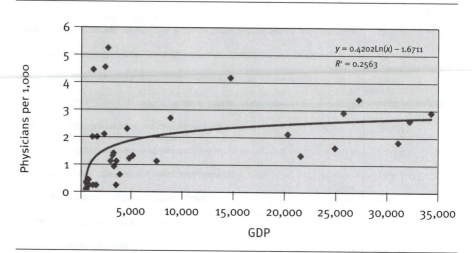

SOURCE: The International Bank for Reconstruction and Development and the World Bank (2000).

FIGURE 2.12

Impact of
GDP on
Supply of
Hospital Beds

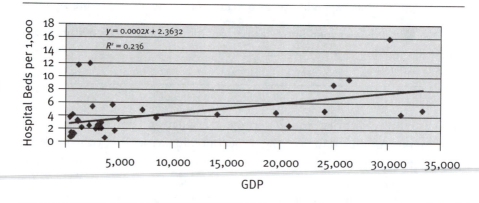

SOURCE: The International Bank for Reconstruction and Development and the World Bank (2000).

Conclusion

As indicated earlier in this chapter, the financing and organization of health-care services are dependent on many factors. Although a strong association exists between national wealth and health spending, several other factors determine the role of the private and public sectors in the financing and organization of health services. Paramount among these other variables is the political culture of the country.

The effect of culture and history on the financing and organization of healthcare services is most evident among the wealthy countries in this study. The contrast between the countries of Western Europe and the United States illustrates the magnitude of the difference. The governments of the wealthy European countries finance a large proportion of healthcare services and play a direct role in the ownership of healthcare facilities. In contrast, the U.S. government finances only 45 percent of healthcare services, and the overwhelming majority of health facilities are privately owned, either on a not-for-profit or a for-profit basis. The difference in funding and organization among countries of similar wealth points to the overarching importance of national character in determining the balance between public and private sectors in health services organization and financing. Canadian economist Robert Evans highlighted the importance of national character (political ethos) in determining the most appropriate healthcare system (Craig 1999):

> Nations do not borrow other nations' institutions. The Canadian system may be "better" than the American. . . . Even if it is better, I am not trying to sell it to you. You cannot have it. It would not "fit" because you do not see the world, or the individual, or the state, as we do. . . . The point is that by examining other people's experience you can extend your range of perception of what is possible.

Notes

1. The healthcare system of Belize is not profiled in this book.
2. The healthcare system of Tanzania is not profiled in this book.

REFERENCES

Anderson, G. F., and Poullier, J.-P. 1999. "Health Spending, Access, and Outcomes: Trends in Industrialized Countries." *Health Affairs* May/June: 178–92.

Craig, A. 1999. *Health of Nations: An International Perspective on Health Care Reform*. Washington, DC: Congressional Quarterly, Inc.

Creese, A. "Global Trends in Health Care Reform." *World Health Report* 15: 317–22.

Donelan, K., Blendon, R. J., Schoen, C., et al. 1999. "The Cost of Health System Change: Public Discontent in Five Nations." *Health Affairs* May/June: 206–27.

Kaddar, M. 1996. "Health Systems and Structures," pp. 26–30. World Health Organization internal working document (unpublished).

Roemer, M. I. 1991. *National Health System of the World Volume 1: The Countries*. New York: Oxford University Press.

Saltman, R. B., and Figueras, J. 1998. "Analyzing the Evidence on European Health Care Reforms." *Health Affairs* March/April: 85–108.

Schieber, G. 1999. "Health Care Financing and Delivery in Developing Countries." *Health Affairs* May/June: 193–205.

Statistics Division of the UN Secretariat and International Labour Office. Retrieved March 2002 from www.un.org/depts/unsd/social/inc-econ.htm.

The International Bank for Reconstruction and Development and the World Bank. 1993. *World Development Report 1993: Investing in Health*. New York: Oxford University Press.

————. 2000. *World Development Indicators*. New York: Oxford University Press.

World Health Organization. 2000. *The World Health Report 2000. Health Systems: Improving Performance*. New York: Oxford University Press.

3

PRIMARY HEALTHCARE AND COMMUNITY PARTICIPATION: ORIGINS, IMPLEMENTATION, AND THE FUTURE

David Zakus and Andrea A. Cortinois

Introduction

Population health status and the protection and improvement of personal health continue to be of concern at both national and international levels. However, in spite of a growing recognition of health and access to health services as fundamental individual rights (Fuenzalida-Puelma and Scholle Connor 1989), the ideal of universal access to health services is frequently not realized, especially in less-developed regions of the world, where preventable infectious diseases, malnutrition, illiteracy, and poverty are endemic. Third World and developing populations generally have neither the access to services and resources nor the knowledge required to lead healthy and fulfilling lives within their difficult environments.

Responses to these issues challenge traditional approaches to health and health policy. New systems and technologies have been developed to save lives, increase life expectancies, and hopefully, improve quality of life. Primary healthcare and community participation in health planning systems have come to be widely recognized as necessary components of a successful health strategy. International acceptance of a goal of Health for All by the Year 2000 coupled with widespread recognition of the central role of primary healthcare and community participation in any health system marked an enormous step forward in the struggle for universal health. Adoption of the goal led to formalization of the primary-healthcare-centered model in the late 1970s and early 1980s, although many governments had adopted primary healthcare policies before this time.

The fundamental principles of a primary-healthcare-centered strategy (health as a basic human right, community self-reliance and self-determination, social control over health services, and the need for locally and nationally sustainable basic health interventions) reveal the critical role of community participation. In fact, community participation has been considered a sine qua non for the implementation of a successful primary healthcare strategy. Community participation is understood to yield numerous benefits, including more adequate and sustainable health services; improved use of financial, human, and material resources; positive changes in health behaviors; a more equitable relationship between healthcare users and providers; individual empowerment; greater diffusion of health knowledge; and increased use of indigenous expertise (Rifkin 1996; Zakus and Lysack 1998). These benefits are also implied in a commonly accepted definition of community participation as the process by which community members, individually or collectively, commit to the following:

- developing the capability to assume greater responsibility for assessing their health needs and problems
- planning and then acting to implement solutions
- creating and maintaining organizations to support these efforts
- evaluating the effects and bringing about necessary adjustments of goals and programs on an ongoing basis (Zakus and Lysack 1998)

The concepts of primary healthcare and community participation in health did not just suddenly appear. This chapter explores the development of these concepts both within international bodies (mainly the World Health Organization) and within society at large. The final two sections attempt to outline the extent to which community participation has been put into practice and to describe the continuing challenges encountered as this strategy is implemented.

Early History

The recognition of health as an international concern was officially marked by the convening of the first International Sanitary Conference in Paris in 1851. The conference was organized in response to severe and repeated outbreaks of pestilent diseases whose spread throughout Europe was facilitated by improvements in transportation systems (Goel 1977). A prime issue at the conference was the discussion of quarantine measures for the Mediterranean area as an instrument of economic protection (Pannenborg 1979). The economic imperative has retained its prominence in the justification of health services since that time.

The 1850s saw a number of significant developments in medicine and public health: John Snow (1936) investigated and published his conclusions about the cholera epidemics in London, and Robert Koch informed the world about disease and its causation (Evans 1976; Oatley 1998). These are but a few examples that, along with the rise of public health and the growing recognition of the importance of sanitation and hygiene, led to a new way of thinking about health (Lyons and Petrucelli 1987; Sagan 1987).

A more holistic view of health began to take hold during the early twentieth century. The first attempt to integrate primary care services was formulated in England in the Dawson report of 1920, and similar actions took place in the United States later in the decade (Pannenborg 1979). However, these were isolated, country-specific cases, and international efforts were slow to follow. The two world wars impeded international exchanges, but the establishment of the United Nations (UN) in 1946 paved the way for international developments in health policy.

The creation of the UN offered the opportunity for international cooperation in a number of areas, including healthcare. Health was quickly recognized as a field of operations for a new organization; the World Health Organization (WHO) was established as a unit of the UN by the end of 1946. China and the United Kingdom were the first members, and most of the rest of the world soon followed. The WHO Constitution, which defined health as a state of complete physical, mental, and social well-being and not merely the absence of disease or infirmity, together with the Universal Declaration of Human Rights in 1949, gave new institutional and legal impetus to the development of public health systems by declaring health to be a right of all people. Health was now firmly established as an issue of concern at the international level.

The First Two Decades of WHO

During its first two decades, WHO made great strides in developing a decentralized organizational structure, with six administrative regions that cover the entire world: the Americas (represented by the Pan-American Health Organization [PAHO]), Europe, the Eastern Mediterranean, Africa, Southeast Asia, and the South Pacific. Although much of WHO's focus during the first years was on medical care, the late 1950s and 1960s saw a pronounced shift toward preventive medicine (WHO 1968) and a growing emphasis on the development of local health services, particularly for the world's poor. The UN Third Expert Committee on Public Health Administration (1959) discussed the organization and development of local-level health services for rural areas (WHO 1968). Increasing attention was given to providing essential preventive and curative health services to all people but especially to poor inhabitants of remote areas, where formal health services were often nonexistent. The Fifteenth World Health Assembly in May 1962 stated that "the creation of a network of minimum basic health services must be regarded as an essential pre-investment operation, without which agricultural and industrial development would be hazardous, slow and uneconomic" (WHO 1968). Much of the credit for the initial shift in the general approach to providing healthcare services should be given to the poorer countries themselves. Taking their membership status in the UN and WHO seriously, these nations asserted themselves, demanding help to develop and reorganize their health systems according to their own priorities.

In an evolving response to the needs of the less-wealthy nations, the fourth session of the WHO Advisory Committee on Medical Research in

June 1962 endorsed studies to establish broad guiding principles for the development of basic health services in developing countries (WHO 1964). The Committee also supported the need for comparative studies to evaluate health services where curative and preventive functions had been integrated at the local level. Upon reviewing the second decade of WHO's operations, the Director-General predicted that the development of basic health services in the developing countries would be of great importance in the future (WHO 1968); however, he made no mention of primary healthcare or community participation.

The Third Decade of WHO

During the 1970s, the separation between public health specialists and social scientists began to fade as WHO increasingly recognized that social scientists had an important role to play in formulating curative and preventive health policies and programs (Goel 1977). The 27th World Health Assembly of 1974 recognized sanitation, safe water, nutrition, local health services, and citizen and community participation in health systems as important factors in public health and passed a resolution calling on WHO to initiate programs addressing the impact of psychosocial factors on health. Emphasis was also given to the development of preventive medicine, the use of nonmedical solutions to health problems, the encouragement of multidisciplinary approaches, and the integration of health services.

In his address to the 27th World Health Assembly, Dr. T. A. Lambo, the WHO Deputy Director-General, said the following (WHO 1975a):

> It has been made painfully clear in recent years that health services too frequently lack relevance to the total needs of people. In highly developed countries increasingly complex and costly medical interventions yield decreasing returns in terms of relief of human suffering, and in many developing countries even the most basic elements of health care are not available to many people. . . . Faced with these failures, it is tempting to concentrate attention on the resources and technologies available to health care services and their distribution, hoping that some formula can be found to "solve the problem" in technical and material terms.

The stage was set for the emergence of such a formula. Signs of an impending breakthrough were evident throughout international institutional levels. In addition to the encouraging signals from WHO and the heralding of the various UN Development Decades, other sectors of human endeavor had gained increasing acceptance and credibility. Attempts to create a more just world order began with the recognition of inequities and the subsequent movement for a new international economic order (Pannenborg 1979). This was followed by world conferences on the environment, food, population, trade, women, habitat, and water. By the late 1970s, the UN was well-prepared for revolutionary change to spread to the health sector.

Other International Developments

Other factors outside the UN framework were also shaping thinking about development during this period. In the 1950s and 1960s, development thinking was dominated by economics, and the main strategy for development was capital accumulation (Leisinger 1984). Priorities focused on industrialization, urbanization, high-level technology, and capital-intensive projects. Development strategy was dictated by high-level decision makers working with the philosophy that benefits would eventually "trickle down" to the most disadvantaged (Rostow 1960). The trickle-down theory lost credence in the late 1960s and early 1970s, the failure of its explanatory and predictive powers vividly illustrated by a minimal per capita increase in income of only one or two dollars per year between 1950 and 1975 for the poorest 40 percent of the world, in spite of rapid and sustained economic growth (Leisinger 1984).

New theories of neocolonialism and dependence replaced the discredited trickle-down philosophy. Most of the remaining colonial states broke away from their imperial overseers during this period and established themselves as independent nations with the desire to set their own priorities. The newly founded nations, along with others in similar socioeconomic situations, exerted new influence over world affairs. The formation of the Organization of the Petroleum Exporting Countries (OPEC) oil cartel and the subsequent 1973 oil crisis is only the best-remembered of many such skirmishes that occurred as smaller, poorer nations demanded equity in the international arena. Several other movements echoed developing-world demands for equity. Feminism, the growth of the peace movement, the casting off of Cold War attitudes, the renaissance of ecology, and the birth of a new environmental movement in response to pending environmental crises all called for a more inclusive and participative world order (Carson 1962; Commoner 1971; Ward and Dubos 1972).

It was becoming increasingly clear that the achievement of true equity would require focused attention on the poor. It was also becoming clear that human quality of life is determined by exchange and interaction with the environment (PAHO 1973). This point received strong empirical support from industrial and environmental disasters like the London Fog in 1952, the fallout from the 1960s Aswan Dam project in Egypt, and repeated oil spills blanketing the world's shores and destroying vast quantities of marine life. On a similar note, the Club of Rome Report on human population growth in relation to the resource base predicted dire consequences unless drastic measures were implemented to control such growth (Meadows, Randers, and Behrens 1972).

Oddly enough, even as this kind of growth was being castigated, growth in income and material wealth had become overriding principles for success in more developed societies (Lock Land 1973), in spite of internal resistance (Schumacher 1975). Growth had become "the secular religion of Western society, providing a social goal, a basis for political solidarity, and a source of individual motivation; the pursuit of happiness [had] come to be defined almost exclusively in material terms, and the entire society—individuals, enterprises, the government itself—[had] an enormous vested interest in the continuation of growth" (Ophuls 1977).

Considering growth as a primary goal had many ramifications, particularly the increase of a belief among the dominant powers that their lifestyles, ideologies, and supporting technologies were the proper developmental prescription for all. This led to many confusing and inappropriate technology transfers to developing countries. As Hafdan Mahler, then Director-General of WHO, stated while addressing the Ad Hoc Committee on the Restructuring of the UN in the Economic and Social Sectors in February 1976, "I think we were, to put it briefly, suffering from tunnel vision. In the early days of WHO, if vertical support of a medical care system, a teaching hospital, or a research laboratory seemed a productive way of raising health care standards in developed countries, we simply tried to export the same approach to the developing world" (Mahler 1976 in Pannenborg 1979).

Although many were enjoying the benefits of this kind of growth, many more were being left out. The specter of vast sections of humanity living on the brink of death was communicated to millions through radio and television. By the mid-1970s, approximately 50 percent of those living in underdeveloped countries subsisted in a condition of absolute poverty, "a condition of life so limited by malnutrition, disease, illiteracy, low life expectancy, and high infant mortality as to be beneath any rational definition of human decency" (McNamara 1980 in Leisinger 1984). This translated into almost 800 million desperately poverty-stricken people (excluding China), a figure that continued to expand alongside population growth trends.

In response to this calamity in the developing world and to strong internal pressures within industrialized nations, governments assumed an increased role in health service delivery. Health had gradually come to be viewed as a yardstick of equity as well as an instrument of equity and development planning (Pannenborg 1979). The growing conviction that healthcare is a fundamental right accompanied by the perception that governments should create conditions for universal healthcare access led to increased government intervention in the health field. Social security and health insurance schemes grew in most Western nations as the concept of the welfare state became institutionalized (Gough 1978).

At the same time, contemporary health interventions were increasingly recognized as insufficient to solve the health problems of the developing world, which were largely the result of a vast array of preventable infectious and parasitic diseases. "To all these threats, health care has not been able to come up with anything effective in practice" (WHO 1975). Institutional health systems were failing to meet the healthcare needs of entire populations for a wide array of reasons rooted in entrenched institutional structures as well as in social and developmental philosophies. It was becoming increasingly evident that morbidity was rooted in sociopsychological factors at least as much as in medical etiology. It was also clear that "many of the causes of common health problems derive from parts of society itself and that a strict health sectoral approach is ineffective, [with] other actions outside the field of health perhaps having greater health effects than strictly health interventions" (Newell 1975).

Primary Healthcare and Community Participation as Concepts in Health

Following earlier proposals that focused on local healthcare and the growing recognition of the need for a community-based approach, the concept of "a basic set of needs" gained acceptance among many health planners and policymakers. Such a community-based approach was also taking root in other sectors of society, as was seen with the U.S. Government's "war on poverty" in the 1960s, in which community action based on maximum feasible participation by the poor became the key policy (Lemann 1988). Innovations in health service delivery proliferated, including a rural-based, community-oriented system in South Africa (Kark 1952 in Tollman 1991); community health centers in Canada (Hastings 1973) and the United States (Folsom 1966); and the "barefoot doctor" movement in China (Sidel and Sidel 1974). The Chinese experiment in particular generated much interest as an intriguing model for meeting basic health needs among poorer populations. Sometime during the 1970s, a term was adopted to describe this approach to health challenges, especially in the developing world: *primary healthcare*.

Precisely when "primary healthcare" entered into the consciousness of the international health and development communities is difficult to identify. Apparently, however, the concept evolved into its present form simultaneously with or a short time before the development of the "health for all" concept, which developed in the mid- to late 1970s. The primary healthcare movement received its first impetus at the meeting of the UNICEF-WHO Joint Committee on Health Policy in February 1975, which recommended that the two organizations seek ways to extend primary healthcare to underprivileged populations in developing countries (UNICEF-WHO 1975). In May of the same year, the 28th World Health Assembly endorsed the joint recommendation, thereby giving further direction to the primary healthcare movement, which during the preceding few years had been making its way slowly into the awareness of development planners (WHO 1975a). However, it was not until two years later that the truly momentous events developed.

By mid-1977, plans were underway to implement the UNICEF-WHO recommendation. In May 1977, the 30th World Health Assembly decided that "the main social target of governments and of WHO should be the attainment by all the people of the world by the year 2000 of a level of health that will permit them to lead a socially and economically productive life" (WHO 1981). Christened Health for All by the Year 2000, the statement was hailed by Dr. Mahler as an international social revolution (Bankowshi and Bryant 1984), and it became a truly international health goal. Although its evident failure has resulted in cynicism, it has evolved into the hopeful Health for All in the 21st Century.

The Alma-Ata Conference

The primary healthcare movement culminated in the Alma-Ata Conference in September 1978. The WHO-UNICEF International Conference on Primary Health Care, held in Alma-Ata, which is the capital city of Kazakhstan (at that time a Soviet republic), brought official representatives from virtually every nation in the world, all of the UN agencies, and a large number of nongovernmental organizations (NGOs) to formalize the ideas generated during the previous decade. The conference defined primary healthcare and community participation, passed 22 specific recommendations, and produced a full report on primary healthcare (WHO-UNICEF 1978). However, the most important document produced by the conference was the Declaration of Alma-Ata, which still serves as the foundation of international public health philosophies. The Declaration reaffirmed health and healthcare as fundamental human rights and health for all as a critically important worldwide social goal; furthermore, it insisted on primary healthcare as the key to attaining health for all by the year 2000.

The Declaration of Alma-Ata, together with the report, broadly defined primary healthcare and outlined several essential features of primary healthcare and of health systems based on it. The representatives defined primary healthcare in the Declaration as follows (WHO-UNICEF 1978):

> . . . the essential health care based on practical, scientifically sound and socially acceptable methods and technology made universally acceptable to individuals and families in the community through their full participation and at a cost that the community and country can afford to maintain at every stage of their development in the spirit of self-reliance and self-determination. It forms an integral part both of the country's health system, of which it is the

central function and main focus, and of the overall social and economic development of the community. It is the first level of contact of individuals, the family and community with the national health system bringing health care as close as possible to where people live and work, and constitutes the first element of a continuing health care process.

As a complement to the Declaration, the report emphasized the necessity of health development for social and economic development and, consequently, argued that health development and socioeconomic development initiatives should be regarded as mutually supportive rather than competitive. The report went on to describe more specifically the features of a primary-care-focused health system and to indicate how primary healthcare might be organized as part of a comprehensive health system.

The Declaration of Alma-Ata was the culmination of years of progress toward a new model for health policy; a paradigm shift was in the making. Many individuals who participated in the Declaration's development (including Dr. Mahler, who continually supported the movement toward primary healthcare [Smith 1978]) and the participants and organizers had, according to Dr. Tejada, then WHO Assistant Director-General, the foresight and courage to make the conference a "political rather than a medical" one (Pannenborg 1979). Still, much remains to be accomplished.

Health for All by the Year 2000

The Declaration of Alma-Ata and its report quickly won the support of the international community. In 1979, the 32nd World Health Assembly launched its Global Strategy for Health for All by the Year 2000, which was based on the Alma-Ata Declaration and Report and the WHO Executive Board's guiding principles for strategy formulation (WHO 1979). In November of that same year, the UN General Assembly adopted a resolution that identified health as an integral part of development. The General Assembly "endorsed the Declaration of Alma-Ata, welcomed the efforts of WHO and UNICEF to attain Health for All by the Year 2000, and called upon the relevant bodies of the UN system to coordinate with and support the efforts of WHO by appropriate actions within their respective spheres of competence" (WHO 1981).

The Global Strategy, which was finally adopted by the 34th World Health Assembly in 1981, is based on a set of principles very similar to those set out in the Declaration of Alma-Ata and emphasizes the following:

- health as a human right
- the right and duty of all people to participate both individually and collectively in the planning and implementation of their healthcare

- the responsibilities of governments and the push for them to become more self-reliant in health matters
- the need for a multisectoral approach, which requires coordinated efforts from all social and economic sectors, including agriculture, animal husbandry, food, industry, education, housing, public works, and communications (WHO 1981)

According to WHO (1981):

> The main thrusts of the Strategy are the development of the health system infrastructure, starting with primary health care for the delivery of country-wide programs that reach the whole population. These programs include measures for health promotion, disease prevention, diagnosis, therapy and rehabilitation. The Strategy involves specifying measures to be taken by individuals and families in their homes, by communities, by the health service at the primary and supporting levels, and by other sectors. It also involves selecting technology that is appropriate for the country concerned in that it is scientifically sound, adaptable to various local circumstances, acceptable to those for whom it is used and to those who use it, and maintainable with resources the country can afford. Crucial to the Strategy is making sure of social control of the health infrastructure and technology through a high degree of community involvement.

The Strategy also articulates the international and national (political) actions required to promote and support it (specific targets were set in many areas [WHO 1981]), to generate and mobilize resources (especially human ones), and to monitor and evaluate levels. The role of WHO in the execution of the Strategy is also described.

Twenty Years of Experience

The development of primary healthcare concepts continued at the international level. Throughout the 1980s, WHO and other organizations worked to define the apparatus needed to implement the Strategy by developing health indicators, carrying out evaluations, redefining priorities as necessary, and further developing and promoting the concepts of primary healthcare and community participation and the mechanisms for their implementation (WHO 1981, 1982, 1983, 1985, 1986, 1987). In 1988, at an international conference in Riga, Latvia, WHO reaffirmed the work accomplished at Alma-Ata and passed the effort on to the nations of the world (WHO 1988). "The WHO, representing the collective will of its Member States, now assumes that the individual Member States will stand by the agreement made on common policies in the World Health Assemblies, Executive Boards and Regional Committees, as well as what has been decided, for example, in the WHO/UNICEF Alma-Ata Conference on Primary Health Care" (Kaprio 1985).

Primary healthcare and community participation are now accepted policy elements in more than 150 nations (Rifkin 1989), making them the most widely accepted concepts in health service delivery today. Since the 1980s, countless health projects have been developed around the world on the basis of the principles of primary healthcare and community participation; a large number of these projects have successfully applied those principles and achieved predefined objectives. In 1997, Sukati described a significant and steady decline in the infant mortality rate observed in Swaziland between 1983 and 1995 that was almost certainly related to the improved coverage of the immunization program. In 1999, Perry and colleagues described the successful experience of a project in Bolivia, where local priorities and resource allocation were determined jointly by health professionals and the community on the basis of locally acquired epidemiological information. Also in 1999, Eliason described a very successful initiative in Cameroon, where a primary healthcare project was successfully implemented thanks to the community's direct and continuous involvement in managing village health programs and human and financial resources. Examples such as these are numerous.

In most cases, however, such projects have met with mixed success. In fact, the same positive examples reported above also illustrate the limitations of community participation strategies. In Swaziland, although the infant mortality rate went down, little effort was expended to encourage community involvement in health and health services. Intersectoral collaboration was not aggressively pursued, and universal coverage was still considered a utopian ideal rather than an achievable goal (Sukati 1997). The Bolivian experience (Perry et al. 1999) was a pilot project limited to small geographic areas and supported by international financial resources, and its long-term sustainability was far from certain. The lessons learned could very well be applied to the rest of the country, but the situation of local health systems in Bolivia is still problematic, as other authors report (Darras 1997). Finally, although the community contribution to the Cameroon primary healthcare project was surely important, other factors may have been equally important. As the author recognizes (Eliason 1999), the project benefited from continuing education programs for all health workers, adequate staffing, strong support by the local staff, a close working relationship with government health authorities, and financial support from both the central government and international donors. In fact, the lack of most of these resources is one of the main factors hindering successful implementation of primary healthcare projects around the world.

Some of the problems related to the practical implementation of primary healthcare and community participation strategies are rooted in the lack of clear-cut, shared definitions. The Declaration of Alma-Ata purposely left these concepts vague and flexible (Rifkin 1996); achieving a shared definition is difficult, and agreeing on practical objectives derived from the definitions may be even more difficult. van der Geest and colleagues (1990) suggested that Alma-Ata needed to ignore the specific views and interests of participants to transform primary healthcare into a global movement. The lack of clarity led to different interpretations of these concepts at different levels in the political hierarchy responsible for designing and implementing health strategies at international and national levels. According to van der Geest and colleagues, the concept of community participation is understood at the international level as springing from the community's faith in its powers to improve lives locally through its own initiative, which reflects a Western notion of self-reliance and equity. However, for rural communities in poorer nations, the notion of participation may mean something very different. As Rifkin (1989) reports from a study in Nepal, rural people in that country do not see self-reliance as the central feature of participation but instead place a high value on interdependence and exchange. Comparable differences may also be found in other cultures (van der Geest, Speckmann, and Streefland 1990).

In addition, in many countries, the existing centralized, urban-based, bureaucratic structure of the health sector fails to promote an enabling environment for community participation; this is particularly evident in Ethiopia (Kloos 1998). Also, the health sector is often not culturally prepared to understand and support the complex mechanisms of community involvement and frequently maintains old, ineffective strategies (Sukati 1997).

Additional problems in the implementation of primary healthcare and community participation strategies originate at the national level, where powerful interest groups are not always willing to embrace these principles. Primary healthcare and community participation are often not attractive to politicians because these interventions are often directed at rural areas, where political visibility is low and where it may take considerable time for measurable results to be evident. As a result, many governments of nonindustrialized countries have adopted the primary healthcare concept in form only, hoping to economize at the local level and, at the same time, acquire more international financial aid at the top level (van der Geest 1990; Krogstad and Ruebush 1996).

Into a New Century: Old and New Challenges

Since the Declaration of Alma-Ata, primary healthcare and community participation—both as principles and as implemented strategies—have faced numerous, powerful challenges. Most of these challenges remain even as new ones emerge with the new century. The last two decades have seen the emergence of regressive forces alongside the development of primary healthcare and community participation strategies (Berlinguer 1999). Public health services and healthcare for all have come to be seen by some as obstacles to development and acquisition, thereby triggering a reduction in health expenditures by some governments. WHO has lost its leadership, with a shift of power and influence in health policy to the World Bank and the International Monetary Fund. The primary healthcare model has been abandoned by many countries, and often this abandonment is coupled with a trend toward dismantling the machinery of public health, replacing community services with private insurance rather than focusing on vertical disease-control programs, and making the state responsible only for the poor. World health is no longer seen as a single issue for all nations. The vision of world health has been supplanted in North America and Europe by the belief that rich countries can enjoy the best possible healthcare without regard for the suffering of other people.

The emphasis on economic issues in health policy, which was already present at the first International Sanitary Conference in Paris in 1851, is stronger than ever. Economic globalization has reduced national and local control of infrastructure and technology distribution while inequities among and within countries continue to grow (Navarro 1999). The power of transnational corporations is often as great as or greater than that of independent states. Some UN agencies, such as the United Nations Development Programme (UNDP), have been criticized for soliciting funds from global corporations with poor records in the arena of human rights (Karliner, Srivastava, and Bruno 1999).

Numerous new and not-so-new global phenomena also threaten the health of the world population and the goal of Health for All in the 21st Century: (1) the exacerbation of old infections and the emergence of new ones, most obviously the HIV/AIDS pandemic; (2) increasing environmental devastation; (3) the continuous lowering of occupational and environmental safety standards, especially in underprivileged countries; (4) drug trafficking on a global scale; and (5) widespread destruction and self-destructive violence.

Those who advocate and practice primary healthcare and community participation must continue to confront these problems. These concepts have evolved during the past 25 to 30 years through various stages of definition and acceptance, and they have now been endorsed by many of the highest-level decision-making bodies in all nations. However, as the gap between rich and poor continues to widen and health remains an elusive state for untold millions, care must be taken not to get distracted from the realization of the Goal and the Strategy. If the vision and energy exercised at Alma-Ata and in other forums since is not to dissipate, those committed to these concepts must continue refining them through critical analysis, practice, and praxis to make them more relevant and acceptable (Freire 1974). Their acceptance and implementation must be continually advocated for whenever the opportunity arises.

REFERENCES

Berlinguer, G. 1999. "Globalization and Global Health." *International Journal of Health Services* 29 (3): 579–95.

Carson, R. 1962. *Silent Spring*. Boston: Houghton Mifflin Co.

Commoner, B. 1971. *The Closing Circle*. New York: Alfred A. Knopf.

Darras, C. 1997. "Local Health Services: Some Lessons from their Evolution in Bolivia." *Tropical Medicine and International Health* 2 (4): 356–62.

Eliason, R. N. 1999. "Towards Sustainability in Village Health Care in Rural Cameroon." *Health Promotion International* 14 (4): 301–06.

Evans, A. A. 1976. "Causation and Disease: The Henle-Koch Postulates Revisited." *The Yale Journal of Biology and Medicine* 49: 175–95.

Folsom, M. B. (chair). 1966. "Health Is a Community Affair." Report of the National Commission on Community Health Services. Cambridge: Harvard University Press.

Goel, S. L. 1977. *International Administration—WHO South-East Regional Office*. New Delhi, India: Sterling Publishers Pvt. Ltd.

Gough, I. 1978. "Theories of the Welfare State: A Critique." *International Journal of Health Services* 8 (1): 27–40.

Hastings, J. E. F. 1973. *The Community Health Centre in Canada: The Report of the Community Health Centre Project to the Conference of Health Ministers*. Ottawa: Information Canada.

Kaprio, L. A. 1985. "Introductory Remarks," pp. 5–6. In *Health Policy, Ethics and Human Values—An International dialogue*, edited by Z. Bankowshi and J. H. Bryant. Proceedings of the XVIIIth CIOMS Round Table Conference, Athens, Greece, 29 October–2 November, 1984. Geneva: Council for International Organizations of Medical Sciences.

Karliner, J., Srivastava, A., and Bruno, K. 1999. "United Nations Development Program Solicits Funds from Corporations." *International Journal of Health Services* 29 (4): 813–19.

Kloos, H. 1998. "Primary Health Care in Ethiopia under Three Political Systems: Community Participation in a War-Torn Society. *Social Science & Medicine* 46 (4–5): 505–22.

Krogstad, D. J., and Ruebush II, T. K. 1996. "Community Participation in the Control of Tropical Diseases." *Acta Tropica* 61: 77–78.

Leisinger, K. M. 1984. *Health Policy for Least Developed Countries*. Monographs on Sociology and Social Policy, Volume 16. Basel: Social Strategies Publishers Co-operative Society.

Lemann, N. 1988. "The Unfinished War." *The Atlantic Monthly* 262 (6): 37–56.

Lock Land, G. T. 1973. *Grow or Die—The Unifying Principle of Transformation*. New York: Dell Publishing Co., Inc.

Lyons, A. S., and Petrucelli, R. J. 1987. *Medicine: An Illustrated History*. New York: Abrams.

Mahler, H. 1979. "World Health Is Indivisible." Address to the 31st World Health Assembly, 5–9, pp. 393–404. In *A New International Order—An Inquiry into the International Relations of World Health and Medical Care* by C. O. Pannenborg. Alphen aan den Rijn, The Netherlands: Sijthoff & Noordhoff.

Meadows, D. L., Randers, J., and Behrens III, W. W. 1972. "The Limits To Growth." A Report for the Club of Rome's Project on the Predicament of Mankind. New York: New American Library.

Navarro, V. 1999. "Health and Equity in the World in the Era of 'Globalization.'" *International Journal of Health Services* 29 (2): 215–26.

Newell, K. W., ed. 1975. *Health By the People.* Geneva: World Health Organization.

Oatley, K. 1998. *A Natural History.* Middlesex, England: Viking, Penguin Books.

Ophuls, W. 1977. *Ecology and the Politics of Scarcity.* San Francisco: W. H. Freeman and Company.

Pan-American Health Organization. 1973. *Ten-Year Health Plan for the Americas—Final Report of the III Special Meeting of Ministers of Health of the Americas.* Official Document No. 118. Washington, DC: Pan-American Health Organization.

Pannenborg, C. O. 1979. *A New International Order—An Inquiry into the International Relations of World Health and Medical Care.* Alphen aan den Rijn, The Netherlands: Sijthoff & Noordhoff.

Perry, H., Robison, N., Chavez, D., Taja, O., Hilari, C., Shanklin, D., et al. 1999. "Attaining Health for All through Community Partnerships: Principles of the Census-Based, Impact-Oriented (CBIO) Approach to Primary Health Care Developed in Bolivia, South America." *Social Science & Medicine* 48 (8): 1053–67.

Rifkin, S. B. 1989. "Cultural Crossroads of Community Participation in Development: A Case from Nepal." *Human Organization* 48: 206–13.

———. 1996. "Paradigms Lost: Toward a New Understanding of Community Participation in Health Programmes." *Acta Tropica* 61: 79–92.

Rostow, W. W. 1960. *The Stages of Economic Growth.* Cambridge, U.K.: University Press.

Sagan, L. A. 1987. *The Health of Nations: True Causes of Sickness and Well-being.* New York: Basic Books, Inc.

Schumacher, E. F. 1975. *Small Is Beautiful: Economics As If People Mattered.* New York: Harper & Row.

Smith, R. A. (ed.) 1978. *Manpower and Primary Health Care—Guidelines for Improving/Expanding Health Service Coverage in Developing Countries.* Honolulu, HI: The University Press of Hawaii.

Snow, J. 1936. *On the Mode of Communication of Cholera.* 2d ed. New York: The Commonwealth Fund.

Soberon, G., and Narro, J. 1985. "Equity and Health Care in Latin America: Principles and Dilemmas," pp. 124–29. In *Health Policy, Ethics and Human Values—An International Dialogue,* edited by Z. Bankowshi and J. H. Bryant. Proceedings of the XVIIIth CIOMS Round Table Conference, Athens, Greece, 29 October–2 November, 1984. Geneva: Council for International Organizations of Medical Sciences.

Sukati, N. A. 1997. "Primary Health Care in Swaziland: Is It Working?" *Journal of Advanced Nursing* 25 (4): 760–66.

Tollman, S. 1991. "Community Oriented Primary Care: Origins, Evolution, Applications," *Social Sciences & Medicine* 32 (6): 633–42.

United Nations Children's Fund (UNICEF)–World Health Organization (WHO). 1975. Report of the Twentieth Session Held at the Headquarters of the World Health Organization, UNICEF-WHO Joint Committee on Health Policy, Geneva, 4–6 February, 1975.

van der Geest, S., Speckmann, J. D., and Streefland, P. H. 1990. "Primary Health Care in a Multi-Level Perspective: Towards a Research Agenda." *Social Science & Medicine* 30 (9): 1025–34.

Ward, B., and Dubos, R. 1972. *Only One Earth*. New York: W. W. Norton & Company.

World Health Organization (WHO). 1964. *The Medical Research Programme of the World Health Organization—Report by the Director-General, 1958–1963*. Geneva: World Health Organization.

———. 1968. *The Second Ten Years of the World Health Organization, 1958–1967*. Geneva: World Health Organization.

——— 1975. *Promoting Health in the Human Environment, a Review Based on the Technical Discussions Held during the Twenty-seventh World Health Assembly, 1974*. Geneva: World Health Organization.

———. 1975a. Twenty-eighth World Health Assembly, Geneva, 13–30 May, 1975. *Official Records of the World Health Organization, No. 227*. Geneva: World Health Organization.

———. 1979. *Formulating Strategies for Health for All by the Year 2000*. Health For All Series, No. 2. Geneva: World Health Organization.

———. 1981. *Global Strategy for Health for All by the Year 2000*. Health for All Series, No. 3. Geneva: World Health Organization.

———. 1982. *Review of Primary Health Care Development*. Geneva: World Health Organization.

———. 1983. *Activities of the WHO in Promoting Community Involvement for Health Development*. Geneva: World Health Organization.

———. 1985. *Community Involvement for Health Development—Report of the Interregional Meeting, Brioni, Yugoslavia, 9–14 June, 1985*. Geneva: World Health Organization.

———. 1987. *Report on Mechanisms For Community Involvement*. Copenhagen: World Health Organization Regional Office for Europe.

———. 1988. "Alma-Ata Reaffirmed at Riga—A Statement of Renewed and Strengthened Commitment to Health For All by the Year 2000 and Beyond." Adopted at WHO meeting, From Alma-Ata to the Year 2000: A Midpoint Perspective, Riga, USSR, 22–25 March, 1988.

World Health Organization Global Program Committee. 1986. *District Health Systems Based on Primary Health Care*. Geneva: World Health Organization.

World Health Organization–United Nations Children's Fund. 1978. *Primary Health Care*. A Joint Report by the Director-General of the WHO and the Executive Director of the United Nations Children's Fund on the International Conference on Primary Health Care in Alma-Ata, USSR, 6–12 September, 1978. Geneva and New York: World Health Organization.

Zakus, J. D. L., and Lysack, C. L. 1998. "Revisiting Community Participation." *Health Policy and Planning* 13 (1): 1–12.

PART

PROFILED COUNTRIES

The Wealthy Countries

The Transitional Countries

The Very Poor Countries

INTRODUCTION TO THE COUNTRIES

James Veney

The health systems of 28 countries of the world are discussed in this book. The countries are grouped into seven categories that represent salient aspects of the countries or their health services systems. These seven categories are themselves contained within three other broad categories that are emblematic of the single most important health-determining characteristic for countries of the world today: wealth. The first three sets of countries discussed are grouped into what the book calls the *wealthy countries;* these are countries in which the gross national product (GNP) per capita is in excess of U.S.$8,000 per year. The second three sets of countries are classified as *transitional countries,* in which the GNP per capita ranges from about U.S.$800 per year to a little more than U.S.$5,000 per year. These countries are not really wealthy, but they are not really poor, either. The last section of the book deals with the *poor countries.* The three countries included in this section have annual GNP per capita of less than U.S.$400.

The distinction in wealth—GNP per capita—among these countries is quite astounding if one is not familiar with the differential distribution of wealth in the world. The wealthiest country discussed in the book is Japan. With a GNP per capita of about U.S.$38,000 (UNICEF 2000), Japan is nearly 350 times as wealthy as the poorest country discussed, the Democratic Republic of Congo, which has a GNP per capita of about U.S.$110. The first three sections of the portion of the book that deals with specific countries discuss the health systems of the wealthy countries. These 12 countries have a per country (as opposed to per person) average GNP per capita of more than U.S.$20,000. The transitional countries discussed in the three subsequent sections (13 countries total) have a per country GNP per capita of just a little more than U.S.$3,100. This difference gives the wealthy countries an average GNP that is six and one-half times larger than the average GNP for the transitional countries. The three poor countries discussed in the book have an average GNP per country of just over U.S.$250. This makes the transitional countries, on average, a little more than 12 times as rich as the poor countries; the wealthy countries are a little more than 80 times as rich as the poor countries.

Perhaps too obvious to mention, this difference in GNP per capita, which translates very closely to both personal and societal wealth, has a profound and continuing effect on the opportunities, lifestyles, and health of the people living in the various countries. For most people living in the poorest countries, and even for people in many of the transitional countries, owning a personal automobile would be unimaginable; owning a bicycle or motorcycle may be possible for some. For people in most of the wealthy countries of the world, a personal automobile is nearly a necessity of daily life. In the wealthy countries, people can expect to have piped, potable water coming to their houses, uninterrupted electrical power (except in California), and the constant availability of multiple television channels. In the transitional countries, and particularly in the poor countries, piped water, whether potable or not, is much less likely. In many of the poor countries and in some of the transitional countries, the need to carry water over long distances still exists and is still the responsibility of women and girls. Electricity is also questionable in the transitional and poor countries; even in the capital cities of the poor countries, electricity may not be available many hours during a day and must be supplied, if it is even available, by local generators. Television—where electrical power is available—has probably made greater inroads in the poor countries than many other amenities that are taken for granted in the wealthy countries. But even there, the programs will probably be limited to one or two government channels and (sometimes bootleg) satellite TV.

Health problems faced by the people of the various countries reflect the disparities in wealth. In the wealthy nations, the major health problems are the chronic and degenerative diseases such as heart disease, circulatory system problems, and cancer; this pattern is reflected in the transitional countries. In the poorest countries, however, diseases like malaria, schistosomiasis, leishmaniasis, and trypanosomiasis (which are all but unheard of in the wealthy countries) are commonplace. These diseases are accompanied in many transitional countries and in the poorest countries by the steady rise of the wealthy-nation diseases of heart disease and cancer, which is due in large part to the growing smoking rate in the transitional and poorest countries.

Health services systems in the three groups of countries also reflect the disparities in wealth. The demand for medical services will almost always outstrip the financial resources available to supply them. However, wealthy countries are able to provide nearly all of their citizens with whatever medical services are required—or in the case of the entrepreneurial countries, whatever medical services they are able to purchase—from open heart surgery to AIDS medication. In the transitional countries, such services are much less likely to be available and much more likely to be subject to the ability to use personal wealth to move outside the mainstream healthcare system and acquire services in a fee-for-service medical care system. In the poor countries the same is true except for the fact that the personal resources available to move outside the mainstream system are so scarce that most people cannot do it. Instead, the citizens of these countries must rely on

low-quality services provided by poorly trained and unmotivated personnel who work in poorly equipped facilities, provided that the facilities are
accessible at all.

The financial difference between the wealthy countries and poor
countries may be said to be not as great in reality as it seems when GNP
figures are cited. However, this argument is weighted by the importance
of in-kind exchanges and differentials in the costs of goods and services.
At certain levels, this argument is important. Currently, living for a day in
rural India is cheaper than living for a day in Paris. However, with the
increasing importance of the global economy, these differences between
countries are rapidly disappearing, and U.S.\$100 in Kinshasa is becoming
increasingly to be worth as much as U.S.\$100 in Tokyo. To the extent that
this happens, those living in places like Kinshasa, where acquiring U.S.\$100
requires the work of an entire year, will be much worse off than those living in Japan, where acquiring U.S.\$100 may be the result of four or five
hours of work.

The 12 wealthy countries discussed in this book are divided into
three categories on the basis of the nature of their health services systems:
entrepreneurial systems, mandated health insurance systems, and social welfare systems. This classification scheme was the centerpiece of the tour de
force *Health Systems of the World* by Milton Roemer (1993). These three
categories mark significant differences in the way in which health services
are organized, financed, and provided. The three categories of transitional
countries are based not on types of health service systems but rather on
geographical considerations. The three poor countries are representative
of Africa and Asia, the primary places where very poor countries are found
in the world today.

The Wealthy Countries: Entrepreneurial Systems

Roemer pointed out that only two wealthy countries in the entire world,
the United States and South Korea (The Republic of Korea), maintained
an entrepreneurial system for providing health services to the majority of
their populations. Since Roemer's work was published, a third country;
Argentina, may be said to have moved into a financial position where it has
been able to earn the dubious (in Roemer's view) distinction of being a
wealthy nation with an entrepreneurial health services system.

The basis of an entrepreneurial system is the fee-for-service concept.
Service providers are private practitioners who offer their services to the
public for what is considered by the parties on each side of the transaction
to be a fair price. Hospitals, as the site at which the more complex and difficult services are provided, are also private and for the most part not-for-
profit, but they are also frequently and increasingly for profit. As a health
services researcher from Denmark said, the basic underlying theme of the
U.S. health services system, which is the leading example of the entrepreneurial system, is that "everyone is entitled to whatever services they can

afford." The basic entrepreneurial system is not restrictive in the services people receive except to the extent that it is restricted by what individuals are willing or able to purchase. As such, services like breast implants and other cosmetic surgery comprise a not insignificant portion of medical services dispensed under an entrepreneurial system. An entrepreneurial system is the true vision of capitalism at both its best and its worst.

However, probably no system in the world is a pure type. For example, in practice, the entrepreneurial system in the United States has been eroded through numerous public and private initiatives. The first major chink in the fee-for-service armor was the founding of the Blue Cross system. Blue Cross came about not because of a concern for the ability of people in a depression-ridden nation to pay for their medical expenses but because of a concern on the part of hospitals that, if people could not pay, hospitals could not remain open. Hospitals organized in their own interest made the first significant inroads into the strict entrepreneurial model as far as the average citizen was concerned; private hospital insurance and Blue Shield to pay physician expenses soon followed. It became clear by the mid-1960s, however, that these funding mechanisms could not keep up with the growing medical expenses of the elderly and the bad debt of the very poor. As a result, Medicare and Medicaid came into existence over the strong opposition of organized medicine. In addition, many people get their care through wholly government-sponsored systems such as the Veteran's Administration health system and the military health system.

As shown here, even in the most entrepreneurial of societies, much medical service is dispensed through means other than fee-for-service mechanisms. Also, during Democratic administrations, the idea of a national health insurance system is still discussed. However, the basis of the entrepreneurial system is the idea that people will find their own means, independent of the government or other organizing forces, to identify, access, and finance necessary healthcare services.

The Wealthy Countries: Mandated Insurance Systems

Among the wealthy countries of the world, most have discovered a way to ensure that their populations have a certain means for financing healthcare services. One mechanism for this, which is widespread in continental Western Europe, is mandated health insurance. In the section of this book about wealthy countries with mandated health insurance, the health services systems in the European countries of Germany, Italy, France, Spain, and Portugal are discussed, and one country in the Middle East, Israel, is also described. Although the nature of the mandated system differs from country to country, the basic structure is the same: health insurance coverage is required for most members of the countries' population and is typically tied to employment. This mandated insurance is usually available from a limited number of providers certified by the state. In general, the insurance is financed through a combination of worker and employer contributions and can represent a significant expense for both groups. Within all of the mandated systems, government funding mechanisms provide health insurance for people who are unable, either because of lack of employment or low income, to finance it through their own means.

Some of the mandated systems have roots deep in history. The system in Germany traces its beginnings to the rule of Otto von Bismark. According to Roemer (1993), Bismark launched the first German statutory health insurance laws in the 1880s to "steal the thunder" of the socialists in the country. In Israel, the mandated system has its roots in mutual assistance societies established well before the existence of the State of Israel itself. In other countries, the systems are more recent; in Spain, the mandated health insurance system arose with the demise of Franco in 1975.

In many ways the mandated health insurance systems have the best of the entrepreneurial model without the strain the entrepreneurial model puts on personal finances and access to medical services. Generally, in the mandated systems, physicians and many hospitals remain private entrepreneurs and are available to provide whatever care is desired or needed as long as it is covered by the mandated health insurance. Furthermore, both preventive and maintenance care are more likely to be covered under the mandated systems than under the system patches that have been developed within the context of the entrepreneurial systems. A comparison between New York City and Paris found that childhood asthma in New York was treated primarily as an emergent problem in the emergency rooms of the city, whereas in Paris the condition almost never found its way to the emergency room. The latter was attributed to the treatment of childhood asthma in Paris as a matter of routine medical maintenance. Women who have recently given birth in France are provided home-visit nurses to monitor the progress of both the newborn and the mother. This would occur in countries such as the United States only in circumstances in which the mother was confined to a bed, and even then it might not occur.

The Wealthy Countries: Social Welfare Systems

The third basic system for financing health services among the wealthy countries is what Roemer calls the *social welfare system*. Three countries of the world that use this system are presented in chapters in this book: Canada, Japan, and the United Kingdom.

The classification as a social welfare system indicates that the financing of health services has been taken over by institutions of government. In the entrepreneurial system, the financing of health services has largely moved from the individual recipient of services to large not-for-profit or for-profit corporations without a government mandate. In the mandated systems, financing is in the hands of large, generally not-for-profit, often quasi-governmental organizations through which services are required to be financed for the vast majority of people. In the social welfare systems, the financing of services is directly in the hands of the government.

The health systems of both Canada and the United Kingdom have often been held up as outstanding models of health systems and have been proposed as models that should be seriously considered for adoption by the United States. The health system in Japan is less well known, but it serves a country that has the highest life expectancy of any country in the world. That fact alone would seem to recommend the Japanese health system model as one that should be examined carefully by countries wishing to improve their health systems. However, wealth, rather than an outstanding healthcare-financing system, has probably produced the long life enjoyed in Japan. About 60 percent of the variance in life expectancy at birth across the countries of the world can be explained with information about GNP per capita. In an analysis of this relationship, one finds that Japan, with its very high GNP per capita, actually does a little worse in overall life expectancy, even with the highest in the world, than would be expected on the basis of GNP per capita alone.

The Transitional Countries: Former Soviet Block Countries

The four former Soviet Block countries discussed in this book are Poland, Russia, the Czech Republic, and Hungary; these countries are classified as transitional countries. The average per country GNP per capita for all countries classified as transitional in this book is U.S.$3,109; the average per country GNP per capita for the former Soviet Block countries is U.S.$4,005, which makes these countries richer on average than the rest of the transitional countries. In fact, the Czech Republic, at U.S.$5,240, has the highest GNP per capita of any of the transitional countries.

Optimistically, those countries in the position between the poor countries and the wealthy countries are naturally thought to be transitioning up. For the former Soviet Block countries, however, this is not necessarily a given. In fact, substantial evidence shows these countries have already transitioned downward, at least as far as wealth is concerned, and probably in health services as well. Before the collapse of the Soviet Union, the ruble was more or less on par—at least officially—with the U.S. dollar. The exchange rate now is about 29 rubles to the dollar, making the ruble worth a little more than 3 percent of its former Soviet Union value. This is a marked drop in buying power, at least on paper, and is being reflected in the lifestyles of people living in Russia. The paper wealth in the other three countries has been affected similarly.

In terms of health services, the transition may be just as marked. Before the collapse of the Soviet Union, these countries all had centrally owned, financed, and controlled health services systems. In these systems, all services, from nursing service through physician service to hospital facilities, were owned by the government and provided to those in need free of charge or at nominal cost. With the transition from the Soviet Union, the state health services systems also collapsed. Now these systems are being restructured along the lines of Western systems but without the Western experiences of voluntarism and voluntary health insurance available for assistance. The result, as the chapters in this section will show, is a system in every country that is struggling against many difficulties to provide necessary medical care services.

The Transitional Countries in Asia and Africa

The transitional countries in Asia and Africa are something of a hodge-podge and come together only by geographic location. The four countries discussed in this book (China, Turkey, South Africa, and Botswana) represent very different situations, histories, and future paths. China, the most populous country in the world (but being rapidly pursued by India—a third of all of the people in the world live either in China or India), until very recently would have been considered among the poor countries. With a GNP per capita of U.S.$860, it remains well below the U.S.$3,109 average for transitional countries discussed in this book, yet it is still far beyond the poor countries in GNP per capita. China has traditionally had a health services system that is much like the Soviet model, but recently it has been experimenting with the introduction of voluntary health insurance. How well that experiment will work remains to be seen. On the other hand, China's one-child policy has been extremely effective in reducing the country's birth rate.

Although China is relatively poor among the transitional countries, Turkey is just at the average in GNP per capita, and so are South Africa and Botswana. The South African health services system has been in some ways among the best in the world, but it has also been among the worst. Before the collapse of apartheid, South African whites enjoyed excellent healthcare services, including cutting-edge services like heart transplants. Blacks, on the other hand, were relegated to health services, when available, that were no better than most of the rest of Africa. With the collapse of apartheid, the South African service system has been opened up, but total resources and distribution remain significant problems. In addition, the burden of HIV/AIDS has hit South Africa very hard; more people are HIV positive in South Africa than in any other country of the world. Botswana has enjoyed extreme good fortune both economically and socially among African countries for a number of years. As recently as the early 1990s, the life expectancy in Botswana was near 60 years. However, Botswana, too, has been hit hard by HIV/AIDS. At the present time, the HIV/AIDS prevalence is an estimated 40 percent. By 1995, this situation had brought a decline in life expectancy to 47 years. The life expectancy in Botswana is expected to drop below 40 years as a consequence of the HIV/AIDS epidemic. This epidemic is putting increasing strain on the health services systems of all the countries of Southern Africa as well as those of many other countries of the world.

The Transitional Countries in Latin America and the Caribbean

Like the transitional countries of Africa and Asia, the transitional countries of Latin America and the Caribbean are held together more by geography than by their mechanisms for financing or ensuring the availability of health-care services. The countries discussed in this section of the book are Brazil, Mexico, Cuba, Costa Rica, and Jamaica.

Brazil enjoys the dubious distinction of having one of the highest Gini indexes in the world. The Gini index is a number assigned to represent the disparity in income within a country; it reflects the extent to which income is unequally distributed. To have a higher Gini index means that a larger proportion of wealth is in the hands of a smaller proportion of people. Although data necessary to calculate an exact Gini index are difficult to obtain, the United Nations estimates that 64 percent of the wealth in Brazil is in the hands of the richest 20 percent of the population; this is the highest percentage found in any country for which such data are available. The wealth in the hands of the richest 20 percent of the people in the United States is about 45 percent, and in Sweden it is about 35 percent. Higher Gini indexes are greatly speculated to be associated with poorer health status in a country. Verifying that Brazil does much worse than would be expected with regard to indicators as child mortality and life expectancy at birth considering its GNP per capita of U.S.$4,790 is relatively easy.

Cuba, Costa Rica, and Jamaica, on the other hand, are countries that do much better than would be expected considering their GNPs per capita on measures of health such as life expectancy at birth and child survival. Despite the fact that they have different health services systems (the Cuban system is quite similar to the former Soviet model, whereas the systems in Jamaica and Costa Rica are more similar to Western European models), each of these three countries seems to provide well for the health of its people. Mexico, with a GNP per capita second only to Brazil of the countries in this group, also has 55 percent of its wealth in the hands of the wealthiest 20 percent of the population; this probably contributes to Mexico's relatively poor showing on society-wide measures of health.

The Very Poor Countries

The health systems of three countries of the world are discussed in this book under the heading of Very Poor Countries: India, Nigeria, and the Democratic Republic of the Congo (formerly Zaire). The United Nations has recently listed more than 40 countries as being among the poorest in the world; this number is up from a few more than 20 only two decades ago. Interestingly, two of the countries discussed in this section, India and Nigeria, are not among the poorest according to the United Nations. Still, the three countries discussed have a GNP per capita at or below U.S.$1 per day, which is the criteria used by the United Nations to determine the poorest countries.

In many ways, all of these countries are anomalous as very poor countries go. Each one has tremendous natural and human resources available, but circumstances in each have conspired either to keep the GNP per capita low or to draw the country back into the realm of very poor countries.

India, with a GNP per capita of U.S.$370 per year, is the most well-off of these poor countries. With a population now nearly one billion people strong, it is also the second largest country in the world. In many ways, India is a developed country lost within an undeveloped country, a wealthy nation within a very poor nation. India boasts the atom bomb and missiles to deliver it, but thousands of homeless sleep each night on the streets and byways of its greatest cities. It has been said that in India a population as large as that of France (56 million) live as well as do the people in France; however, the other 940 million people live in conditions that characterize the poorest people of the world.

To understand the health services systems in India, one must understand that, although the government health services are nominally free and available to all, they are widely scattered and poorly staffed and equipped. Most people who can afford no better cannot always access these modest services. Those who can afford better services opt out of the government system and receive their healthcare from a wide variety of practitioners, some with excellent Western-style training and others practicing a variety of traditional medicines.

Nigeria, like India, is also unique as a very poor country. Nigeria has extensive reserves of oil, and before 1974, it was self-sufficient in agriculture. With the oil boom of the mid-1970s, however, many schemes were started that, due to mismanagement and outright graft, never came to fruition. The all-out shift to oil drew people from the farms, and Nigeria soon needed to begin to import food; oil revenue has never reached expectations. These factors, in combination with a history since independence of bad government, have left Nigeria, the most populous nation in Africa, on a long downhill slide. As recently as the mid-1980s, the Naira (Nigeria's currency) was worth more than a dollar at the official exchange rate; today the value of the Naira has fallen to about 120 to 130 to the dollar. The resulting inflation has generated massive problems for health services in Nigeria.

The country that is now called the Republic of the Congo is another country that does not fit easily into the category of the poorest countries, even though it certainly can be classified that way with regard to GNP. The country that is now called the Republic of the Congo has a long history as Zaire. Before independence, this nation was the sole property of the Belgian crown, and the abuses of colonialism are documented by both Conrad (*Heart of Darkness*) and Hochschild (*King Leopold's Ghost*). The Republic of the Congo was born out of civil war that continues today and that is wreaking havoc both on the economy and on the health and health services systems of the country.

The remainder of this book discusses each of the above-mentioned nations and their health systems in great detail. To understand these health systems, the context and economic realities of the nations in which they are housed must also be recognized and understood.

REFERENCES

Roemer, M. 1993. *Health Systems of the World*. New York: Oxford University Press.

UNICEF. 2000. "State of the World's Children 2001." www.unicef.org.

THE UNITED STATES OF AMERICA

Vaughn Mamlin Upshaw and Kelly Matthews Deal

Background Information

When Europeans settled in North America, little was known of how to effectively prevent or treat disease. Post–Revolutionary War medical schools in the United States initially distanced themselves from their European counterparts and throughout the late eighteenth, nineteenth, and early twentieth centuries promoted various medical theories, including herbal and homeopathic remedies, bloodletting, and rudimentary scientific approaches. Only in the 1920s was a curriculum of medical education standardized and adopted by U.S. colleges and universities.

Health insurance in the United States began as a private program in the early 1900s, and to this day most health insurance is provided by the private sector. Many observers see the wide array of private and public medical programs and insurance products that form today's U.S. health system as a strength. However, despite the variety of choices available, more than 43 million Americans are uninsured, making public responsibility for health services an important national issue (U.S. Census Bureau 1999).

As in most other industrialized nations, the current health policy environment in the United States is heavily influenced by macroeconomic factors. Growing concerns about the aging labor market, future economic growth, reducing national debt, and competing within the global market influence how political leaders view decisions about healthcare and health insurance.

The Economy

This chapter can only scratch the surface of the complex elements comprising the population and personal healthcare systems operating in the United States. To understand the context of healthcare in the United States, a discussion of employment, economics, education, and demographics will be presented, followed by a more detailed description of the health system.

Macroeconomic and political factors have brought substantial change to U.S. healthcare systems over the past 10 to 15 years, and these factors are likely to contribute to additional changes in the future. Both the structure and regulation of healthcare have been affected by changes in private and public financing and insurance systems. The primary challenge facing the U.S. health system is the same as that facing most other nations: how to meet healthcare needs with finite resources.

Changes in the structure of healthcare have been driven principally by employer demands. Because most working adults in the United States are insured through their employers, the unemployment rate and the cost of health insurance affect population insurance levels. As shown in Table 4.1, the total U.S. labor force in 1999 was more than 139 million workers, 4.2 percent of whom were unemployed.

Disposable personal income in the United States in 1998 was $21,633 a year per person, and the median was $46,737 for a family of four. More than 34 million people (12.7 percent of the total population) lived below the poverty level in 1998. The federal poverty limit for an individual is $8,350 a year and $17,050 for a family of four (*Federal Register* 2000). The average healthcare expenditure per person in 1997 was $3,925.

Demographics and Education

The United States is the third largest nation in the world, covering more than 3,787,425 square miles. It was also the third most populous nation in 1998, with more than 270 million residents, 49 percent of whom were male and 51 percent female. Just less than 10 percent of Americans were younger than 18 years old in 1998, with more than 4 percent in the 65-year-old or older age group. The population in the United States is aging

TABLE 4.1
Selected
Employment
and Economic
Indicators,
United States,
1999

Total civilian labor force in millions	139.4
Unemployment rate (percent)	4.2
Weekly earnings (U.S.$), 1982	271
Gross domestic product	
Total, billions of U.S.$	9,256
Per person, U.S.$	32,448
Consumer price index (percent change from immediate prior year [1982–84 = 100])	
All items	2.2
Food	2.1
Shelter	2.9
Medical care	3.5
Health spending	1,149
As a percent of GDP	13.5
Per capita health expenditures (U.S.$)	3,925
Consumers	535.6
Government (billions)	507.1
People without health insurance (percent)	16.1

SOURCE: U.S. Census Bureau (2000); *Health Care Financing Review* (1999).

as the baby boom generation (those born between 1940 and 1960) grows into later adulthood. A major health policy issue for the United States is to determine how to pay for healthcare for these adults as they get older and consume more healthcare resources.

The U.S. population is racially and ethnically diverse. In 1998, Caucasians comprised 71.3 percent of the population; African Americans accounted for 12.7 percent, Hispanics 11.2 percent, Asian or Pacific Islanders 3.9 percent, and Native Americans 0.9 percent. Demographic trends indicate that the nation is becoming even more racially and ethnically diverse, with more rapid growth among groups other than Caucasians. Despite the increasing number of ethnic groups using health services in the United States, inequalities in access to health services and disparities in health outcomes persist among these groups. A summary of U.S. demographics is presented in Table 4.2.

In 1995, the adult literacy rate in the United States was 99 percent. An assessment of adult literacy in the United States and other countries found that the United States had one of the highest percentage of adults reading at the lowest literacy level as well as one of the highest concentrations of adults reading at the highest literacy level (National Center for Education Statistics 2000). In 1998, almost 83 percent of people 25 years old and older had completed high school, and more than 24 percent were college graduates. In 1998, total spending (by all sources) in the United States was $372 billion on elementary and secondary education and $247 billion on higher education (U.S. Census Bureau 2000).

Population	1990	1995	1996	1997	1998
Resident population in millions	248.8	262.8	265.2	267.7	270.3
Male	121.3	128.3	129.5	130.8	132.0
Female	127.5	134.5	135.7	137.0	138.3
Percentage of population					
18 years old or younger	25.7	26.1	26.1	26.0	25.8
65 years old or older	12.5	12.8	12.8	12.8	12.7
Demographics					
White	83.9	83.0	82.8	82.7	82.5
Black	12.3	12.6	12.6	12.7	12.7
Asian and Pacific Islander	3.0	3.6	3.7	3.8	3.9
American Indian, Eskimo, Aleut	0.8	0.9	0.9	0.9	0.9
Hispanic	9.0	10.3	10.6	10.9	11.2

TABLE 4.2
Selected Demographic Data

SOURCE: U.S. Census Bureau (1999).

Context: Health Needs

The leading cause of death in the United States in 1997 was cardiovascular disease, which was responsible for 31.4 percent of all deaths. In 1997, 23.3 percent of all deaths in the United States were attributed to cancer, 6.9 percent were due to stroke, 4.7 percent were caused by chronic obstructive pulmonary disease (COPD), and 4.1 percent were as a result of unintentional injuries. Figure 4.1 details the ten leading causes of death in the United States. The infant mortality rate in the United States is 7.2 per 1,000 live births (U.S. Census Bureau 2000). Average life expectancy in the United States in 1997 was 73.6 years for men and 79.4 years for women. Life expectancy differs significantly among population groups. White women have the longest life expectancy, followed by African American women and white males. Economic status is also linked to longer life expectancies, with individuals living in households that have annual incomes above $25,000 living three to seven years longer than those in households earning less than $10,000 a year.

FIGURE 4.1

Ten Leading Causes of Death, 1997

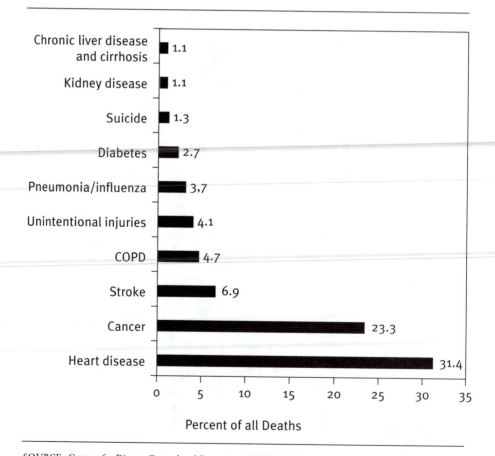

Percent of all Deaths

SOURCE: Centers for Disease Control and Prevention (1997); U.S. Department of Health and Human Services (2000).

"Healthy People 2010: Understanding and Improving Health" (U.S. Department of Health and Human Services 2000) is a national effort to focus attention on factors that influence health in the United States. The Healthy People 2010 document highlights ten leading health indicators:

1. physical activity
2. overweight and obesity
3. tobacco use
4. substance abuse
5. responsible sexual behavior
6. mental health
7. injury and violence
8. environmental quality
9. immunization
10. access to healthcare

These factors were chosen because they were thought to motivate people to action, data were available to assess their progress, and they were relevant to public health. The leading health indicators are intended to assist people in understanding health promotion and disease prevention and to encourage participation in improving health over the next decade.

Organization and Management of the Health System

Figure 4.2 shows the components of the United States healthcare system. The figure represents the dynamic interaction among the sources of funding, financing structures, and reimbursement mechanisms that provide resources to facilities and professionals who deliver services to individuals and populations. Funding sources include employers, governments, individuals, and other charitable sources. Financing structures are types of insurance and coverage options available to individuals. Reimbursement mechanisms vary depending on how the insurance product and contracts with healthcare facilities and health professionals are negotiated. A continuum of healthcare services is provided directly to individuals or delivered at a population level in the United States.

Financing

Healthcare consumed 14 percent of the U.S. gross domestic product in 1998. The price of medical care increased 14 percent between 1990 and 1998 (U.S. Census Bureau 1999), and estimates indicate that it will rise another 16 percent by 2010. Revenues for health services come from both private and public sources. Figure 4.3 shows that private health insurance paid for by employers and employees and out-of-pocket payments paid by

FIGURE 4.2

Components
of the United
States'
Healthcare
System

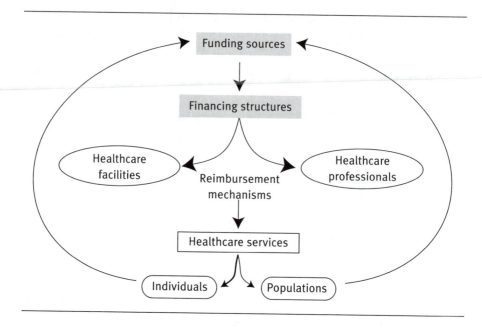

individuals made up more than 54 percent of healthcare payments in 1998.

Public revenues for health services are generated through taxes. Individual and employer-based taxes are collected at federal, state, and local levels to support government healthcare spending. Government-financed health insurance includes the following programs:

- Medicare
- Medicaid
- the Veterans Health Administration
- workers' compensation

Medicare is a national health insurance program for any citizen 65 years old or older who has contributed to the social security system. Between 1997 and 1999, 11 percent of the population was insured under Medicare (Kaiser Family Foundation 2001). Medicare has two parts. Part A, which covers some hospitalization and home health costs, is provided to every enrollee at no cost. On a voluntary basis, enrollees pay a premium ($45.50 per month in 2000) for Medicare Part B, which covers some outpatient physician services and medical equipment costs. *Medicaid* is a government-sponsored health insurance program financed by federal and state contributions to provide basic healthcare for low-income Americans. Participating states must provide a mandatory set of preventive, acute, and long-term healthcare services and may voluntarily add other services, such as dental coverage and medical devices. Medicaid provided coverage for 10 percent of the population between 1997 and 1999 (Kaiser Family Foundation 2001) *The Veterans Health Administration* administers the largest healthcare system in the world. It employs more than 191,000 people to provide health

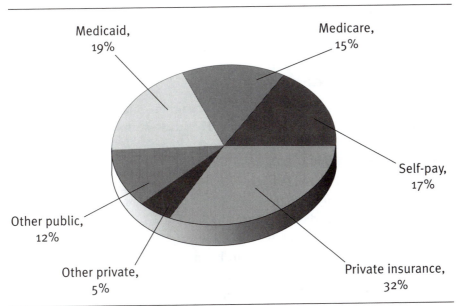

FIGURE 4.3

Where the Money Came From: Healthcare Dollars in the United States (1998)

Medicaid, 19%

Medicare, 15%

Self-pay, 17%

Other public, 12%

Other private, 5%

Private insurance, 32%

SOURCE: Health Care Financing Administration (2000).

services and preventive education to veterans and to be leaders in health research. Some type of *workers' compensation* is available in all 50 states. Workers' compensation provides payments to individuals for wages lost because of work-related disability and pays for all or part of necessary medical care related to the disability.

Individuals or employers may purchase private health insurance. Approximately 63 percent of Americans had private health insurance between 1997 and 1999 (Kaiser Family Foundation 2001). Of those with private insurance, 58 percent obtained health insurance through their employer, and 5 percent purchased insurance individually. Employers may elect to purchase health insurance for their employees or share the cost of health insurance with employees. An employer may also allow employees to purchase insurance independently (but usually at a higher payment rate than that which the employee could purchase individually, apart from the employer-based group).

Private health insurance companies may operate as for-profit or not-for-profit organizations. For-profit companies such as Aetna, United HealthCare, and Prudential sell shares or stocks to shareholders and must produce a profit for investors. Not-for-profit companies such as Blue Cross–Blue Shield and Group Health Cooperative are charitable organizations operated privately on the public's behalf. Another source of private funding for healthcare is charitable foundations. Charitable foundations contribute to healthcare research, demonstration programs, and direct services. Examples of charitable foundations include the W. K. Kellogg Foundation, which provides resources supporting community-based public health activities, and the Robert Wood Johnson Foundation, which gives grants to universities, state health agencies, and other healthcare organizations to finance health policy initiatives.

Financing Structures

In 2001, 65 percent of employers offered health insurance benefits to their employees (Kaiser Family Foundation/Health Research and Educational Trust Survey of Employer Sponsored Health Benefits 2001). Of Americans with employer-based health insurance in 2001, the majority (48 percent) are insured through preferred-provider organizations (Gabel et al. 2001). Preferred-provider organizations are a type of managed care in which the plan contracts with medical care providers and offers incentives (e.g., lower copayments) to individuals who use these providers. A breakdown of employer insurance types is shown in Figure 4.4.

Twenty-three percent of Americans are enrolled in health maintenance organizations (HMOs) (Gabel et al. 2001). Individuals enrolled in HMOs pay a monthly premium and a small copayment, usually around $10, for each visit and prescription. Most HMOs provide members a wide range of preventive and primary healthcare services that emphasize behaviors and services that will reduce disease and disability and avoid more costly care.

Point-of-service plans allow a person to choose to receive services from participating or nonparticipating providers, but benefits are usually more limited if a nonparticipating provider is used. Of those with employer-based health insurance, 22 percent had point-of-service plans in 2001 (Gabel et al. 2001).

Only 7 percent of Americans with employer-based health insurance had conventional health insurance plans, known as fee-for-service or indemnity plans, in 2001 (Gabel et al. 2001). Fee-for-service or indemnity health insurance plans are those in which the employer, individual, or both pay a monthly premium for health insurance, and the insurance plan pays for services as the individual uses them. In a typical indemnity plan, the user first must meet a deductible by paying a predetermined amount out of pocket (generally $250 to $500 or more, depending on the plan) before the insurance plan begins to pay. Once the deductible is met, the individual usually continues to pay a percentage of costs (usually 20 percent), and the insurance company pays the remaining percentage up to a given ceiling. For example, many indemnity plans pay 100 percent of a person's healthcare costs above a previously determined amount but not more than a total of $250,000.

In 1998, the U.S. Census Bureau estimated that 16.3 percent of all Americans are uninsured and that, among poor people, 32.3 percent have no health insurance (U.S. Census Bureau 1999). The number of uninsured Americans grew during the last decade as costs for healthcare services increased. Key factors associated with a lack of health insurance include age

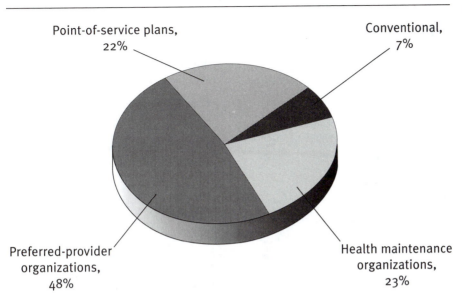

FIGURE 4.4

Employer-Based Health Insurance Enrollment in 2001

Point-of-service plans, 22%

Conventional, 7%

Preferred-provider organizations, 48%

Health maintenance organizations, 23%

SOURCE: Kaiser Family Foundation/Health Research and Educational Trust (2001).

(young adults between the ages of 18 and 24 years were less likely to have health insurance); race and ethnic origin; educational attainment (lower educational attainment is associated with a lack of insurance); and employment level (part-time workers were most likely to be uninsured).

The largest employers, usually those with more than 500 employees that operate in several states or internationally, often decide to provide their own insurance coverage with standard health benefits for all employees; these plans are referred to as self-funded plans. To protect large employers operating in many states, self-funded plans are covered under the federal Employer Retirement Insurance Security Act (ERISA). Under ERISA, a large employer can self-fund its health insurance program and thereby guarantee that all employees pay into a common pool and receive common benefits. With protection from ERISA, self-funded plans are exempt from varying state requirements that regulate health insurance benefits, solvency, and enrollment.

Reimbursement Mechanisms

Public and private health insurance programs may be indemnity or managed care plans, and these plans may pay providers and facilities in one or more of the ways described below and detailed in Figure 4.5.

The most commonly used reimbursement mechanisms in the United States are fee for service, capitation, and prospective payment. Indemnity plans are most likely to reimburse providers or facilities using fee-for-service mechanisms that pay after a service is delivered. The plan may pay the charge in full or at the usual, customary, and reasonable rate. If the plan

FIGURE 4.5
Payment
Pathways

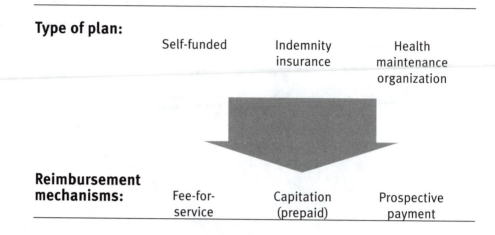

Type of plan:

| Self-funded | Indemnity insurance | Health maintenance organization |

Reimbursement mechanisms:

| Fee-for-service | Capitation (prepaid) | Prospective payment |

pays less than the full amount, the provider or facility may accept this as payment in full or seek to recover the remaining amount from the individual. Payments for less than the full amount may be a function of discounts awarded for volume or simply a result of market pressures.

Under a capitated payment system, an insurance plan negotiates a monthly rate that it will pay in advance to the provider or facility. Managed care insurance plans are the most likely to use capitation. In return for capitation, the provider or facility provides covered services to individuals enrolled in the managed care plan. Any unspent money at the end of the month belongs to the provider or facility, but the provider or facility is liable for any costs above the monthly capitation. Prospective payment systems function by estimating what the cost of services will be for a particular group and paying in advance for these individuals to receive those services. Actual usage is monitored, and if it is different from the anticipated use, providers and facilities can recover costs above the prospective payment.

For every dollar spent on health services in the United States, more than 33 percent goes to hospital care, 20 percent goes to physician services, and long-term care and prescription drugs each receive more than 7.5 percent. Five percent of healthcare dollars was spent on administration and net cost; more than 26 percent of healthcare costs was related to personal health and other purposes (Figure 4.6).

Health Resources

Healthcare service delivery in the United States is accomplished through multiple components. Healthcare professionals include clinical, administrative, technical, and scientific personnel. Facilities may offer inpatient, outpatient, community-based, or support services to the population. Healthcare technologies apply scientific knowledge acquired through research

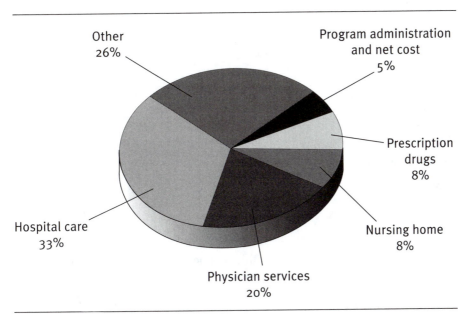

FIGURE 4.6
U.S. Healthcare Expenditures, 1998

Other
26%

Program administration and net cost
5%

Prescription drugs
8%

Hospital care
33%

Nursing home
8%

Physician services
20%

SOURCE: Health Care Financing Administration (2000).

to the organization, delivery, and evaluation of health services. This continuum of healthcare begins before birth and continues through the end of life.

Traditional modern healthcare in the United States consists of physicians and nurses delivering care in hospitals or clinics. Massive changes in the healthcare system over the past 10 to 15 years have altered and expanded this model considerably. As shown in Table 4.3, the overall number of healthcare professionals has increased. Additionally, the field of allied and auxiliary healthcare professionals has grown to include licensed midwives, physician assistants, nurses with varying degrees and graduated licenses (some of whom can prescribe drugs), physical and occupational therapists, and aides of all sorts to perform nonclinical duties. Although certain specialties have an oversupply of physicians, many parts of the United States are classified as "medically underserved areas." In fact, more than 46 million people live in areas with shortages of primary health professionals, and 25 million live in areas with shortages of dental health professionals (Health Resources and Services Administration 2000). Figure 4.7 details the distribution of health professionals among the various health-related occupations.

Healthcare is one of the largest industries in the United States. Health facilities are provided by both the government (federal, state, and local) and the private sector. Hospitals employ approximately 75 percent of healthcare personnel and consume 38 percent of healthcare expenditures. The private system includes the expected human resources as well as hospitals and clinics of all sorts: primary care, urgent care, outpatient care, specialty clinic care, mental health, and family planning. Private entities also

TABLE 4.3

Estimated Supply of Selected Health Personnel and Practitioner-to-Population Ratios

Health Occupation	Number, 1996	Percent Change, 1970–96
Physicians	701,200	116.6
Allopathic (M.D.)	663,900	113.3
Osteopathic (D.O.)	37,300	196.0
Dentists	154,900	61.4
Optometrists	29,500	60.3
Pharmacists	185,000	64.3
Veterinarians	56,700	118.9
Registered nurses	2,161,700	188.2
	Practitioners per 1,000 population	Percent change, 1970–96
Physicians	260	67.1
Allopathic (M.D.)	246.1	64.5
Osteopathic (D.O.)	13.8	126.2
Dentists	58.1	24.9
Optometrists	11.1	24.7
Pharmacists	69.4	27.3
Veterinarians	21.3	70.4
Registered nurses	808	120.8

SOURCE: Health Resources and Services Administration (2000).

operate long-term-care facilities, including skilled nursing facilities, rehabilitation facilities, mental treatment facilities, hospices, and nursing homes, as shown in Figure 4.7. The government provides a military and veteran health system, public hospitals, mental hospitals, public health service, Indian health service, and other services that fall under its mission, as well as ensuring service to underserved and rural populations.

One of the causes and results of drastic changes in American healthcare is technological innovation. Advances in medical research have led to technique changes, equipment changes, new drug therapies, and interesting prospects for the future. In addition to technological changes, healthcare managers—prodded by high expenses—have implemented structural innovations. The most common way is through integration, either vertical or horizontal. In vertical integration, one firm produces the products that either suppliers or customers could produce (e.g., integrating primary care practices). Horizontal integration is acquiring a firm that produces similar goods and services (e.g., two hospitals in a market).

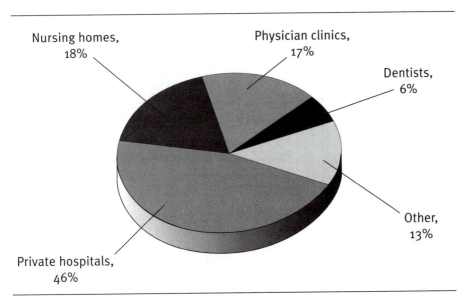

FIGURE 4.7
Health
Services
Employment

SOURCE: *Health Care Financing Review* (1991).

Delivering Health Services in the United States

Americans receive healthcare at many levels in many locations. This continuum, shown graphically in Figure 4.8, takes place at both the population and individual level.

Access to care generally depends on insurance coverage, although government-funded hospitals are legally obligated to provide certain types of care (e.g., emergency care) to anyone, regardless of their ability to pay. Most people obtain insurance through their employer. Government programs like Medicaid and Medicare cover special populations. The insurance plan dictates where a patient may go for care and what types of procedures will be paid for by the plan.

Prospects for the Future

National healthcare policy in the United States has evolved incrementally. Congress passed laws in the mid-1960s creating two national health insurance programs, Medicare and Medicaid, which guaranteed medical services for elderly and poor Americans, respectively. Since that time, U.S. lawmakers have adopted healthcare policies on a piecemeal basis, resulting in a complex set of regulations that often varies by state, by type of insurance, and by purchaser.

Although Americans spend more per capita on medical care than any other country, about 16 percent of the population does not have health insurance coverage. Rising health insurance costs and high numbers of uninsured citizens have prompted greater public interest in national laws

FIGURE 4.8

Continuum of
Health
Services in the
United States

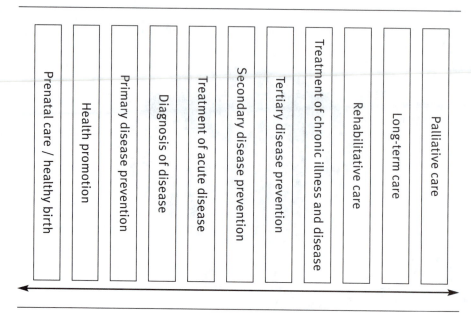

SOURCE: Barton, P. L. (1990). *Understanding the U.S. Health Services System,* Health Administration Press, Chicago.

that would guarantee universal access to healthcare. President Clinton's attempt to pass a national healthcare program in 1994 failed to overcome opposition charges that Americans would witness an increase in costs and lose the ability to select their own physicians, choose their health services, or obtain care in an efficient and timely manner. Despite the defeat of universal access, President Clinton and Congress later passed the Children's Health Insurance Program, which expanded federal funding to assist low-income working families in procuring health insurance for their children.

Rationing and cost-containment measures continue to be major health policy issues. In the absence of a national health policy, states have taken responsibility for many policy innovations. Oregon, for example, received attention in the 1980s for priority-ranking Medicaid-covered health procedures and then eliminating funding for services low on the list. Competitive market structures have been considered the preferred cost-containment methods; however, although competition has yielded many benefits, costs for healthcare continue to increase at rates exceeding inflation. States have employed various administrative, financial, and clinical policies to control healthcare costs.

Other significant policy issues include questions about the health impact of emerging technologies, particularly the mapping of the human genome and certain biotechnologies. How these technologies will affect health and medical services in the future is still being determined, but the implications for improving health and preventing disease are substantial. How technologies will be paid for and who will have access to them also remains unclear. In addition, questions remain concerning patient rights, provider responsibilities, and the responsibilities of insurance companies for determining appropriateness, cost, and quality of care in the context of these new technologies.

REFERENCES

Barton, P. L. 1999. *Understanding the U.S. Health System*. Chicago: Health Administration Press.

Centers for Disease Control and Prevention. 1997. National Center for Health Statistics, National Vital Statistics System, and unpublished data. Retrieved 01 March 2000 from http://www.cdc.gov/nchs/products/pubs/pubd/nvsr/47-pre/47-pre.htm.

Donham, C. S., Letsch, S. W., Maple, B. T., Singer, N., and Cowan, C. A. 1991. "Health Care Indicators." *Health Care Financing Review* 12 (4): 141–70, 150.

Federal Register. 2000. Vol. 65, No. 31, February 15, 7555–57. Retrieved 29 February 2000 from http://www.aspe.hhs.gov/poverty/figures-fed-reg.htm.

Gabel, J., Levitt, L., Pikereign, J., et al. 2001. "Job-Based Health Insurance in 2001: Inflation Hits Double Digits, Managed Care Retreats." *Health Affairs* 20 (5): 180–86.

Health Care Financing Administration. 2000. "The Nation's Health Dollar 2000." Retrieved March 2000 from http://www.hcfa.gov/stats/nhe-oact/tables/chart.htm.

———. 2002. "CMS Data and Statistics." Washington, DC: Health Care Financing Administration. Retrieved March 2002 from http://www.hcfa.gov/stats/stats.htm.

———. 1999. Vol. 20, No. 1, HCFA Pub. No. 03412. Washington, DC: Health Care Financing Administration.

Health Resources and Services Administration. 2000. "Bureau of Health Professions." Retrieved 14 March 2000 from www.hrsa.gov/bhpr/ORP/wiaa.htm.

Huber, M. 1999. "Health Expenditure Trends in OECD Countries, 1970–1997." *Health Care Financing Review* 21 (2): 99–117.

Kaiser Family Foundation/Health Research and Educational Trust. 2001. "Survey of Employer Sponsored Health Benefits." Retrieved 02 November 2001 from http://www.kff.org/content/2001/20010906a.

Kaiser Family Foundation. 2001. "State Health Facts Online." Retrieved 31 October 2001 from http://www.statehealthfacts.kff.org/cgi-bin/health-facts.cgi?.

National Center for Education Statistics. 2000. "NCES Fast Facts." Retrieved 29 February 2000 from http://www.nces.ed.gov/fastfacts/display.asp.

U.S. Census Bureau. 2000. "Statistical Abstract of the United States." Retrieved 02 August 2000 from http://www.census.gov/statab.

———. 1999. "Health Insurance Coverage." Retrieved 04 October 1999 from www.census.gov/statab.

———. 1999. "Statistical Abstract of the United States." Retrieved 10 November 1999a from http://www.census.gov/statab.

U.S. Department of Health and Human Services. 2000. *Healthy People 2010: Understanding and Improving Health*. Washington, DC: Government Printing Office.

Williams, S., and Torrens, P. 1999. *Introduction to Health Services*, 5th ed. Albany, NY: Delmar Publishers.

ARGENTINA

Peter Lloyd-Sherlock

Background Information

Although its economic success has not been fully sustained, Argentina was among the wealthiest nations of the world in 1947, and the current demographic structure is a consequence of its relative prosperity over the last century. With an estimated population of 37 million people in 2000, Argentina is geographically the second largest country in Latin America, and its per capita gross domestic product remains considerably higher than that of most of its geographic neighbors (U.S.$8,970 in 1999 as compared with a regional average of U.S.$3,940). Table 5.1 summarizes Argentina's key demographics.

Life expectancy in Argentina, estimated at 73 years, is high by Latin American standards, and this partly accounts for an aged population structure. In 1995, 13 percent of the population was 60 years or older and, because of a small number of young children, the demographic dependency ratio is relatively low. In addition, structural adjustment, rigorous exchange rate controls, and neoliberal policies led to a rapid economic growth of 5 percent annually between 1991 and 1997. However, this rediscovered prosperity has been achieved at a major social cost (Lloyd-Sherlock 1997). Unemployment and underemployment reached historic levels with open unemployment of 18 percent in the capital city by late 1995. In contrast, rapid expansion of the informal sector accounted for 34 percent of urban employment in 1992 and has since risen. Consequently, Argentina's health-care system faces a number of challenges, including the demands of a rapidly aging population and the exclusion of increasing numbers of workers from the salaried formal labor force. These figures are summarized in Table 5.2.

Context: Health Needs

Argentina's aged population structure (with its concomitant health needs), coupled with its incomplete epidemiological transition, makes it a unique case. Unlike richer, industrialized countries, Argentina has yet to complete the process of epidemiological transition, and large sections of the population, particularly in the poorer northern provinces, are exposed to mortal-

TABLE 5.1
Estimated
Demographic
Indicators for
Argentina in
the Late 1990s

Indicator		Year(s)
Sex ratio (percent female)	51.0	1999
Percent urbanized	89.3	1999
Percent 60 years old or older	13.5	1999
Life expectancy at birth (years)	73.1	1995–2000
Total fertility rate (per woman)	2.60	1995–2000
Population growth rate (percent)	1.26	1995–2000

SOURCE: INDEC (1999).

ity and morbidity risks no longer found in more prosperous countries.

Infant mortality rates are persistently high and stood at around 23 per 1,000 live births during the 1980s and early 1990s. Argentina has since seen some reduction in these numbers (21 per 1,000 in 1996), but they are still higher than those of several other Latin American countries with lower levels of income and healthcare expenditures such as Chile, Costa Rica, and Venezuela. In fact, an estimated two-thirds of infant deaths in Argentina are officially classified as "avoidable." The gap in regional disparities in infant mortality widened during the 1990s, ranging from 13 per 1,000 live births in Buenos Aires to 34 per 1,000 live births in the poorer northern region, with significant increases in some provinces (INDEC 1998).

The three most important causes of death by age group are presented in Table 5.3 and indicate a high level of concentration. That is, in the section of the population that is less than 1 year old, the three leading causes of death, perinatal, congenital, and pneumonia/influenza, account for 70 percent of deaths. For those 50 years old or older, the three primary causes of death, heart disease, cancer, and stroke, constitute 66 percent of cases. Note that the high rate of heart disease is likely attributable in part to very high levels of red meat consumption.

Other diseases afflicting Argentines include HIV/AIDS, cholera, tuberculosis, leprosy, malaria, and Chagas' disease. By 1995, 5,303 cases of HIV/AIDS had been reported, with a ratio of 4.7 men for every woman infected. As elsewhere, the main cause of infection has shifted from unprotected homosexual activity, which comprised 58 percent of cases between 1982 and 1987, to a wider range of risk factors. In 1994, intravenous drug use accounted for the highest proportion of new infections at 41 percent.

In addition, considerable attention has been given to the regional cholera epidemic, especially in northern Argentina. However, this has been much less significant than a range of other infectious diseases (PAHO 1995). The total number of reported cholera cases peaked at 2,080 in 1993, but

	1980	1999
Open urban unemployment (percent)	2.6	14.5
Open urban underemployment (percent)	4.5	13.7
Per capita GDP (U.S.$)	4,023	8,970

SOURCE: INDEC (1999); IADB (1994).

TABLE 5.2
Socioeconomic Indicators, 1980 and 1999

this number has since declined. In contrast, 13,000 new cases of tuberculosis are diagnosed each year, which lead to 1,500 deaths, and approximately 20,000 cases of leprosy still exist in Argentina. Malaria had been eliminated, but it reemerged in the late 1980s. Moreover, Chagas' disease clearly remains the leading public health problem in Argentina. An estimated 8 percent of the population is infected, with particularly high concentrations among impoverished districts to the north (Stillwaggon 1998).

Organization and Management of the Health System

As is the case in other Latin American countries, Argentina's health system is highly fragmented, and it consists of three main subsystems: the publicly funded sector, social insurance funds, and private healthcare.

The publicly funded health sector is highly decentralized. The Federal Ministry of Health and Social Action remains, theoretically, the policy-making, normative, and regulatory authority, with the responsibilities for provision and financing having been given to provincial ministries of health and sometimes to municipal agencies. However, the division of authority between these levels is often unclear and therefore undermines administration, referral, financing, and planning procedures. The situation is further disjointed because the internal organization of healthcare provision and financing varies considerably among the different provinces. Recent reform initiatives have sought to promote the model of managerially autonomous public hospitals, but no evaluations of this program are available.

The social insurance segment consists of more than 200 different funds (obras sociales), most of which are administered by trade unions. These usually contract with private sector providers and mainly serve urban formal sector workers (Belmartino and Bloch 1998). The coverage provided by the obras sociales and private health plans is detailed in Table 5.4. Overall, the level of insurance coverage is high by Latin American standards. However, with rising unemployment, social insurance coverage fell from around 18 million to 16 million between 1990 and 1995. More recent comparable data are not available, but the trend has continued downward since 1995.

TABLE 5.3

Leading
Causes of
Mortality by
Age Group,
1993

	Under 1 Year	1 to 4 Years	5 to 14 Years	15 to 49 Years	50 Years and Older
First cause	49.4% perinatal causes	21.3% accidents	32.4% accidents	18.5% heart disease	35.6% heart disease
Second cause	16.4% congenital anomalies	9.2% congenital anomalies	13.4% cancers	17.2% accidents	19.6% cancers
Third cause	4.5% pneumonia and influenza	8.8% heart disease	7.5% heart disease	15.4% cancers	10.8% stroke

SOURCE: INDEC (1995).

In theory, social insurance funds operate within a fairly strict regulatory framework, but in practice, regulation has been virtually absent, and the responsible state agency has been unable to obtain even basic information about affiliation rates. Until recently, each union fund had a monopolistic entitlement to a particular occupation group. This arrangement was criticized for stifling competition and reducing efficiency, and a series of major organizational reforms was implemented between 1992 and 1996 (World Bank 1997). These reforms, which received substantial financial support from the World Bank, obligated all funds to provide a minimum package of health services and enabled affiliates to choose their social insurance fund. The next stage of this reform is to open up the funds to competition from private insurers, but when this will occur is unclear (Barrientos and Lloyd-Sherlock 2000).

Argentina has a separate social insurance fund for older people, the Programa de Atención Médica Integral (PAMI), which was established in 1971 and structured along lines similar to the Medicare system in the United States. PAMI provides a range of healthcare and other social services to nearly 4 million affiliates, but those older people without social insurance protection (approximately 25 percent) are largely denied these services. Like the union funds, PAMI primarily contracts with private providers. The program had been considered a pioneering success story until it experienced a major financial crisis in the mid-1990s, incurring debts of several billion U.S. dollars (Lloyd-Sherlock 1997a). PAMI is now in the process of substantial restructuring, and its future remains uncertain.

The private healthcare sector encompasses both financing and provision. Private insurance has enjoyed rapid expansion over the past decade, fueled by higher incomes among richer groups and general dissatisfaction

	Health Insurance Plan					TABLE 5.4
	No Plan	Obras Sociales	Other Private	Obras Sociales Plus Other Private	Other	Total
Population coverage (percent)	37.4	48.8	8.6	3.8	1.3	100
By age group (percent)						
0 to 1 year	52.1	37.4	8.1	1.6	0.9	100
1 to 4 years	47.5	41.9	6.8	2.8	9.9	100
5 to 14 years	43.2	46.0	7.5	2.3	1.1	100
15 to 24 years	45.8	41.7	8.2	2.7	1.7	100
25 to 49 years	38.7	46.1	10.4	3.4	1.4	100
50 to 64 years	27.9	54.3	11.2	4.9	1.7	100
65 years and older	7.3	78.0	4.1	9.7	0.9	100

TABLE 5.4
Health Insurance Coverage by Type (1996–97)

SOURCE: Barrientos and Lloyd-Sherlock (2000).

with the quality of services provided by social insurance funds. By 1991, slightly more than one-fifth of Argentines were estimated to have private coverage. The private insurance industry consists of approximately 200 private for-profit companies (pre-pagas) and more than 1,000 mutual insurance funds (mutuales). Overseas health insurance firms, particularly Institutos de Salud Previsional (ISAPREs) from Chile and health maintenance organizations from the United States, have become important players in this market. Several cases of private firms illegally taking over the operation of social insurance funds have arisen. This has been possible because the private insurance sector is completely unregulated. Not surprisingly, recent proposals to change this state of affairs were strongly resisted by the industry.

Argentina's health system is plagued by several problems in the interactions among the different subsystems. For example, publicly funded services intended for uninsured groups are widely used by the population in general without reimbursement from insurers. Private insurers have largely succeeded in taking high-income, low-risk individuals away from the social funds. Current reforms do little to address these problems of fragmentation and equity.

Financing

In 1993, Argentina spent 7.2 percent of its GDP on healthcare, which was broken down as follows:

- 22 percent spent in the publicly funded sector
- 24 percent funneled to the social insurance funds
- 12 percent spent for PAMI
- 42 percent sent directly to the private sector

More recent data are not available, but the share of social insurance will likely have fallen and private spending will have risen. Overall levels of spending have risen slightly over the past decade and are typical of higher-income Latin American countries.

Historically, the financing of publicly financed health services has faced many problems. First, decentralization has given rise to large regional disparities in per capita expenditures in this sector. By the mid-1990s, provincial governments accounted for almost three-quarters of public health spending, and the remainder was shared evenly between the municipal and federal levels. In theory, this mechanism of transferring funds among the provinces and the federal government and back again should reduce the impact of geographical variations in tax revenue on health budgets, but figures from 1980 show a ratio of nearly six to one between the highest- and lowest-spending provinces. Generally speaking, per capita spending in the poorer provinces (where, incidentally, insurance programs are also less well developed) has historically been lower than in richer ones.

A second problem has been short-term fluctuations in public sector spending allocations. These were particularly severe during the 1980s, when Argentina experienced considerable macroeconomic instability. Since the 1990s, spending has been more consistent and has increased slightly. Nevertheless, a very large historical allocation backlog remains, and this is reflected by the poor state of building structures and a sharp fall in perceived quality of service.

Consequently, public sector hospitals in Buenos Aires and other parts of the country are now entitled to levy user charges. Such charges are, technically, voluntary, and they are managed through locally based foundations known as *cooperadoras*. Voluntary fees can be an important source of extra-budgetary revenue, and they account for up to 20 percent of total funds in some hospitals (Lloyd-Sherlock and Novick 2000). These charges may reduce irrational utilization but may also create access difficulties for low-income groups. Ironically, recovering costs from insured patients—the more obvious channel for increasing revenue—is rarely done. Most public hospitals obtain little more than one percent of their total budgets from billing insurance funds.

Since 1991, the collection and disbursement of social insurance contributions has been centralized through the Ministry of Finance. It was hoped that centralization would make the management of these resources more transparent, increase the regulatory authority of the state, and reduce evasion. Social insurance levies for most funds currently stand at 3 percent of workers' salaries, with a 3 to 6 percent matching contribution from employers, depending on geographical location. However, a ceiling is placed on contributions for those with monthly salaries exceeding U.S.$3,750. Most social funds also require affiliates to make a small copayment somewhere in the range of U.S.$2 to $5 for most ambulatory care services; this copayment is intended to control costs rather than generate revenue.

Social insurance funds have traditionally catered to specific occupational groups, and, as such, some funds would inevitably consist of affiliates with significantly higher incomes (e.g., bank workers) than others (e.g., the construction workers' fund). The Redistribution Fund was established to develop an element of uniformity and solidarity among the funds and their affiliates. Ten percent of total insurance contributions were devoted to the Redistribution Fund. Unfortunately, the Fund operated according to political criteria rather than to actual need and mainly supported the richest, highest-spending, and most powerful funds. Due in part to this, levels of spending per affiliate varied considerably among the social insurance funds, ranging from U.S.$5 to $80 per month in the mid-1990s.

In the past, most social insurance funds paid providers on a fee-for-service basis. Fees were set by a schedule known as a nomenclador that assigned points and monetary values to each medical procedure. However, the system retained an element of flexibility, and prices were usually negotiated between insurers and large groups of providers. A combination of this payment system and poor regulation was blamed for a severe cost explosion. In response, reforms in 1993 granted social insurance funds greater freedom to negotiate their own contracts with individual service providers; it was hoped this would promote competition among providers and drive down costs. However, a continued absence of effective state regulation is thought to have led to corruption and inequitable provision for affiliates in different funds.

Historically, the PAMI fund for older people has been financed through a range of sources including a 5 percent wage levy divided equally between the employer and employee. In 1994, as part of the government's broader neoliberal program of reducing labor costs, the employer contribution to PAMI was discontinued; this has proved to be a major factor in PAMI's financial collapse. By 1995, the fund had accumulated a deficit of U.S.$1.5 billion.

PAMI contracts with service providers through a combination of fee-for-service and capitation payment systems. The latter became more prevalent during the 1990s, but the financial collapse of PAMI illustrates that, although capitation is widely seen as more effective in controlling costs, these savings can only be readily realized in an environment of accountability and regulation. Both were lacking in 1992, when the basic capitation payment in Buenos Aires was raised by 70 percent on the basis of what were later described as "groundless arguments."

Virtually no financial data exist for the private healthcare sector, and official estimates vary widely as regulation is almost absent. However, in 1993, an estimated 35 percent of private payments were accounted for by private insurance plans and 65 percent consisted of out-of-pocket spending. All forms of private health insurance have experienced an unprecedented boom in recent years, although information about the dimensions of this change is unavailable. The recent imposition of a 22 percent value-added tax (VAT) levy on private health insurance payments may slow this expansion. Expansion may also be restricted by high costs: the cheapest packages currently offered start at around U.S.$200 a month, which is well beyond the means of most Argentines.

Health Resources

No national register of health professionals is available in Argentina, but rough estimates show that the health sector employed around 400,000 people in the mid-1990s. This constitutes approximately 3 percent of the national labor force and is fairly typical for a country at Argentina's level of development. However, the distribution of personnel, detailed in Table 5.5, reveals a number of peculiarities and serious problems.

Clearly Argentina has an overabundance of physicians, who represent almost one-fourth of all health workers. Estimates from the Argentine Medical Association show that the total number of physicians now exceeds 100,000. This represents 1 doctor per 370 inhabitants and, when taking into account Argentina's GDP, is higher than for any other market economy. The great majority of these physicians choose to specialize, and general practitioners are virtually unknown. This oversupply of doctors creates a variety of problems, including inflated salary costs, low utilization rates (particularly for more senior physicians), and an extreme curative bias in service provision. No concerted efforts to rectify this situation have been attempted. Indeed, the establishment of medical faculties in several new private universities coupled with expectations of high earnings in the growing private healthcare industry has fueled a sharp increase in supply in the late 1990s. A current reform program funded by the Inter-American Development Bank has sought to promote the conversion of specialists into generalists, but this will have little overall impact in reducing labor market distortions (IADB 1998).

In contrast, the healthcare system is suffering from a clear shortage of trained nurses. Nurse training has been neglected, and the profession suffers from very low status and salaries. Recent data are not available, but Argentina had roughly 18,000 qualified nurses in 1992, yielding a ratio of approximately one qualified nurse for every five doctors; a ratio of three

				TABLE 5.5
Physicians	88,800	Nurses	18,000	**Estimated**
Dentists	21,900	Nurse assistants	51,000	Health Sector
Pharmacists	10,500	Technicians	90,000	Human
Biochemists	7,500	Administrative staff	95,000	Resources,
Obstetricians	4,000	Social workers	3,000	1992
Physiotherapists	6,000	Sanitary engineers	1,000	
Psychologists	32,000	Nutritionists	4,000	

SOURCE: FINOSPORT (1998).

nurses to every doctor is more typical. As a result, doctors and nursing assistants must perform tasks that are usually carried out by qualified nurses.

In addition to physicians and with the exception of nurses, the supply of other health professionals is relatively generous: Table 5.5 shows an estimated 29,000 pharmacists, 22,000 dentists, 9,500 biochemists, 4,000 midwives, and 30,000 psychologists. These groups are politically well-organized, and their respective associations usually ally themselves with physicians to obstruct labor market reforms. Epidemiologists are the only other professionals who are in very short supply, and this fact perhaps reflects the lack of emphasis on public health in Argentina.

The geographic distribution of doctors and other health professionals is grossly uneven. As in other countries, marked concentrations are found in urban areas and richer provinces, with more than four times as many doctors per inhabitant in Buenos Aires as in the poorer north. No reforms are currently proposed to address these disparities.

Argentina has a well-developed network of hospitals, health centers, and other facilities. Overall, between 1980 and 1995, the number of health-care institutions increased from 9,051 to 16,085 (Table 5.6). The lion's share of this growth occurred within the private sector. Unfortunately, years of underfunding in the public sector have led to growing obsolescence and problems in maintenance and quality. The public sector saw a more modest increase and the number of institutions directly owned by social insurance funds decreased. Over the same period, the proportion of institutions providing only ambulatory care experienced a surge, from 66 to 80 percent; this trend was particularly apparent in the public sector and reflects efforts to increase the role of primary health centers. At 64 percent, private ambulatory institutions are much more likely to be specialized than public ones, which are at 3 percent.

Medical equipment in publicly funded hospitals has been described as poorly maintained and outdated (World Bank 1987; EIU 1998). In response, a World Bank–funded reform program recently devoted U.S.$24.5

million to re-equipping selected public hospitals. The quality of equipment in public hospitals contrasts sharply with that used by private providers, whose equipment levels are on a par with high-income countries.

No significant medical equipment manufacturing industry exists in Argentina, but private-sector providers have been able to import equipment at a relatively low cost because of trade liberalization and the strength of the local currency. Although publicly available information about importation of medical equipment is incomplete and not entirely reliable, the national statistics agency estimates that these imports totaled U.S.$207 million in 1996, which represented a 15 percent increase over the preceding year. Obtaining a breakdown by purchasing agencies is not possible, but the bulk of these imports were likely destined for private providers.

The total number of hospital beds fell by approximately 10,000 between the 1980s and 1995 (Table 5.6); this was driven by sharp declines in public and social insurance institutions, and it contrasts with an overall increase in private-sector beds. The fall in the public sector reflects increased emphasis on primary healthcare and restricted budgets. However, the public sector still controls the largest number of beds, including 62 percent of those in specialized care.

By the mid-1990s, Argentina was spending U.S.$3.7 billion a year on drugs and medicines. This represents U.S.$113 per person and is more than three times greater than per capita drug spending in Mexico and four times that of Brazil. In addition, it accounts for 29 percent of total healthcare spending and 57 percent of direct household health expenditures. Total drug expenditures are estimated to have risen by more than 50 percent during the 1990s, due primarily to increases in price rather than the number of units purchased, as the average unit price rose from U.S.$2.4 in 1989 to U.S.$9.4 in 1994. Despite such high levels of drug consumption and expenditures, the only effective drug for Chagas' disease was withdrawn from the market in the late 1980s because the affected popu-

TABLE 5.6
Total Number of Health Service Facilities and Total Number of Beds, 1980 and 1995

Sector	Total Number of Institutions		Total Number of Beds	
	1980	1995	1980	1995
Total	9,051	16,085	145,690	155,822
Publicly funded	4,648	6,971	91,034	84,094
Obras sociales	364	222	8,045	4,403
Private	4,039	8,873	46,611	67,243

SOURCE: INDEC (1999).

lation, estimated to be as high as 13 percent of Argentines, was unable to afford it.

The state regulatory authority has nominal control over drug price schedules, but it has little influence in practice. Since 1991, the status of the agency and allocated funding have been substantially downgraded (Stillwaggon 1998). Part of this failure to regulate pharmaceuticals reflects the strength of the industry in Argentina. By the late 1980s, approximately 351 pharmaceutical manufacturers were registered in the country. Of these, 50 (mostly foreign-owned) accounted for 90 percent of total production. The consumption of imported drugs has likely increased during the 1990s because of trade liberalization and the overvaluation of the domestic currency.

Service Delivery

Primary health services are largely the responsibility of individual provinces. As a result, the quality and extent of these services vary considerably. Overall, Argentina's health services have been characterized as highly curative. According to the World Bank (1987), "Heavy reliance on curative medicine and little concern for preventive care raise costs unnecessarily." The only clear exception to this has been the southern province of Neuquén, where significant attention has been given to this level of care for three decades.

The lack of emphasis on primary care is reflected and reinforced by the structure of human resources and the recent expansion of private provision, as discussed previously; it is also a key factor in Argentina's high infant mortality rate in relation to its total health spending levels. By the early 1990s, levels of child immunization coverage for conditions such as measles were well below the Latin American average. Recent reforms have sought to bolster primary healthcare and include a World Bank–funded maternal and child health nutrition project in several of the poorest provinces. However, the relatively small scale of these schemes suggests that their overall effect on the orientation of the country's health system will be small.

Utilization data are not available for the health sector as a whole. Information for publicly funded facilities is provided in Table 5.7, which shows a sharp rise in outpatient consultations since 1980 and a more gradual one for inpatients. The increases may result in part from reduced insurance coverage (which pushes people into the public sector). However, very probably a combination of population aging and large increases in per capita GDP have led to an overall increase in utilization rates.

With the exception of a small number of flagship hospitals, quality in the publicly funded sector is very poor. This is apparent in inadequate levels of investment, lack of equipment, low staff morale, and badly maintained facilities (Lo Vuolo and Barbeito 1993; World Bank 1997). Delays for public hospital services are a widespread problem; surveys of waiting times in five cities found that more than four hours was not unusual and that poorer patients were particularly subjected to longer waits (INDEC 1990).

Generally, low levels of user satisfaction have been a major factor behind increased use of the private health sector. However, the quality of care given by private providers is highly variable and largely unregulated. Sharp variations in mortality rates have been recorded for private providers serving elderly PAMI patients (Lloyd-Sherlock 1997). Private providers appear to have performed better in terms of the quality of "hotel services" (e.g., office design and decoration, atmosphere) than in actual healthcare.

As might be expected, many equity problems persist in Argentina's healthcare system (Lloyd-Sherlock 1999). Strong regional disparities exist in healthcare indicators (e.g., infant mortality), as well as considerable inequity in financing within the social insurance and publicly funded sectors, as evidenced by sharp variations in per capita spending. The reforms currently being implemented do not appear to have a significant effect on this situation. According to the World Bank (1997), "The problems of transition to a full demand subsidy, giving the poor the same choice of insurer and provider as richer groups, are formidable. However, this could have great potential impact on the neediest part of the population." Unfortunately, the introduction of competition within Argentina's social insurance sector is not primarily intended as a means to increase coverage levels or address the equity issue. This is in contrast with insurance reforms in a number of other Latin American countries such as Colombia which include a demand subsidy for previously unprotected groups (Barrientos and Lloyd-Sherlock, under review).

The reform process also has not included an effective regulatory framework for the burgeoning private health insurance industry, leaving it free to "cream skim" high-income, low-risk groups (Stocker, Waitzkin, and Iriarte 1999). Efforts have been made to enable public hospitals to recover costs for patients covered by social insurance funds, but this may serve a dual, contradictory purpose that both resolves and exacerbates issues of equity. Presently, unpaid use of public facilities by insured groups represents a significant indirect subsidy of the insurance industry from the population as a whole. When costs are recovered, however, the monies are kept separate from core funding and can usually be spent at the discretion of hospital management. Such an arrangement may create incentives for hospitals to target insured groups rather than those who lack coverage, thereby worsening problems of equity and access for the poor.

Prospects for the Future

Given the general level of wealth in Argentina, which involves strong economic performance, a low level of population growth, and a high degree of health spending, considerable opportunity exists for improving the cur-

	1994	1998
Outpatient	52,300,000	74,100,000
Inpatient	1,800,000	2,000,000

SOURCE: INDEC (1999).

TABLE 5.7
Outpatient
and Inpatient
Consultations
at Publicly
Funded
Health Service
Facilities,
1994 and
1998

rent healthcare system and its effect on population health. A range of ambitious reforms are now being implemented, many with the support of international development agencies. However, the prospects for significant progress are threatened by a number of issues.

Income distribution in Argentina is becoming increasingly uneven, and a growing number of people are excluded from secure employment in the formal economy. Consequently, this group is also excluded from private or social health insurance protection. The health of this population may be more readily ensured and the problem remedied by a rapid expansion of secure employment opportunities or a significant upgrading of the publicly funded health sector. However, neither of these seems likely to be explored in the foreseeable future. As a result, diseases of poverty (such as Chagas' disease) will likely remain a significant problem in poor remote regions.

The difficulties that confront Argentina's health system are likely to persist. At present, promotion and provision of primary healthcare is inadequate. New medical schools are being established in various parts of the country, but little is being done to meet the deficit of qualified nursing staff. In addition, current levels of investment in public hospitals insufficiently compensate for a long history of underfunding. Gradual erosion of the role of union-run social insurance funds is expected, as well as a rapid expansion of the private sector as commercial competition is allowed. On the other hand, the regulation of private financing and provision may be strengthened as a growing clientele becomes increasingly aware of irregular quality levels and potential abuses. However, the power of the private medical lobby to resist such change should not be underestimated.

Finally, Argentina is already an aged society as compared with the rest of Latin America, and the health needs of older people will become a significant challenge over the next few decades. The problems associated with PAMI have yet to be resolved despite a number of high-profile and expensive reform efforts made during the last ten years. In response, the newly elected government of January 2000 has made reform of PAMI a leading policy priority. It will be interesting to compare Argentina's progress with this issue to the reform efforts of President Clinton's administration in the United States in the early 1990s.

REFERENCES

Barrientos, A., and Lloyd-Sherlock, P. 2000. "Reforming Health Insurance in Argentina and Chile." *Health Policy and Planning* 15 (4): 417–23.

———. "Health Insurance Reforms in Latin America: Cream Skimming, Equity and Cost Containment." Under review, in *Social Policy Reform and Market Governance in Latin America*, edited by L. Haag and C. Helgo. London: Macmillan.

Belmartino, S., and Bloch, C. 1998. "Desregulación/Privatización: la Relación Entre Financiación y Provisión de Servicios en la Reforma de la Seguridad Social Médica en Argentina." *Cuadernos Médico Sociales* 73: 61–80.

Economist Intelligence Unit. 1998. "Profile—Changing Political Gears in Argentina's Healthcare System," pp. 26–28. London: EIU Healthcare International.

FINOSPORT. 1998. "Argentina. Health Care Sector Overview." Mimeograph. Buenos Aires: FINOSPORT.

Inter-American Development Bank (IADB). 1994. *Economic and Social Progress Report*. Washington DC: IADB.

———. 1998. "Argentina: Programa de Modernización y Reforma del Sector Salud." Retrieved 13 April 1999 from www.iadb.org/exr/doc98/pro/uar0120.htm.

Instituto Nacional de Estadística y Censos (INDEC). 1990. *La Pobreza Urbana en la Argentina*. Buenos Aires: INDEC.

———. 1995. *Situación y Evolución Social. Sintesis No.3*. Buenos Aires: INDEC.

———. 1998. *Statistical Yearbook of the Argentine Republic 1998*. Buenos Aires: INDEC.

———. 1999. *Argentina. Statistical Synopsis, 1999*. Buenos Aires: INDEC.

Lloyd-Sherlock, P. 1997. "Policy, Distribution and Poverty in Argentina since Redemocratisation." *Latin American Perspectives* 94 (6): 22–55

———. 1997a. "Healthcare Provision for Elderly People in Argentina: The Crisis of PAMI." *Social Policy and Administration* 31 (4).

———. 1999. "Health Insurance Reform and Neo-liberalism in Argentina." In *Achieving Universal Coverage of Health Care*, edited by A. Mills and S. Nitayarumphong, pp. 199–215. Bangkok: Thai Ministry of Public Health.

Lloyd-Sherlock, P., and Novick, D. 2001. "'Voluntary' User Fees in Buenos Aires: Innovation or Imposition?" *International Journal of Health Services* 31 (4): 709–28.

Lo Vuolo, R., and Barbeito, A. 1993. *La Nueva Oscuridad de la Política Social. In Del Estado Populista al Estado Neoconservador*. Buenos Aires: Miño and Dávila.

Pan-American Health Organization (PAHO). 1995. "Country Health Profiles. Argentina." Retrieved 3 July 2000 from www.paho.org/english/argentin.htm.

Stillwaggon, E. 1998. *Stunted Lives, Stagnant Economies. Poverty, Disease and Underdevelopment*. New Brunswick, NJ: Rutgers University Press.

Stocker, K., Waitzkin, H., and Iriarte, C. 1999. "The Exportation of Managed Care to Latin America." *New England Journal of Medicine* 340 (14): 1131–36.

World Bank. 1987. *Argentina. Population, Health and Nutrition Sector Review.* Washington, DC: World Bank.

———. 1997. *Argentina. Facing the Challenge of Health Insurance Reform.* Washington, DC: World Bank.

REPUBLIC OF KOREA

Hanjoong Kim, Euichul Shin, Hye-young Kang,

and Kwang-ho Meng

Background Information

The Republic of Korea, also known as South Korea, is a relatively small country located in the southern half of the Korean peninsula (35 to 40 degrees north latitude and 125 to 130 degrees east longitude). The country, with its area of 99,313 square kilometers, is comparable in size to the U.S. state of Indiana. Its population of 46,429,817 gives it a density of 467.2 people per square kilometer (1998), which is 7.5 times denser than that in Indiana. Seventy percent of the country is hilly or mountainous.

Korea's 5,000-year history includes the rule of several kingdoms, but it has maintained a continuous culture throughout all this time. In the nineteenth century, Korea was thrown open to the outside world when China, Russia, and Japan competed for expansion into the Korean Peninsula. Japan eventually annexed Korea, ruling the peninsula from 1910 until the end of World War II. Under Japanese control, Korea began a modernization process through importation of Western culture.

After its liberation from Japanese control, the nation was divided into two Koreas, South and North. In 1948, South Korea (hereafter simply called Korea) became the Republic of Korea and maintained a democratic government, whereas North Korea became the Democratic People's Republic of Korea, a communist country. The Korean War, from 1950 to 1953, devastated almost everything in both of these new nations.

The Korean economy has grown dramatically since its first five-year economic plan was implemented in 1962. This economic success is often referred to as the "Miracle of the Han River," which compares it with Germany's "Miracle of the Rhine River." Per capita gross national income (Korea no longer uses gross national product) increased from U.S.$100 in 1963 to U.S.$1,011 in 1977 and to U.S.$11,380 in 1996 (Table 6.1). During that time, the Korean labor market underwent a drastic restructuring. The percentage of the labor force employed in agriculture, forestry, and fishing (formerly the economic underpinnings of the nation) has dropped to only 11 percent of the total labor force in 1998 (National Statistical Office 1999). The international community has recognized Korea as a developed country since the late 1980s. In 1991, both North and South Korea joined the United Nations. That year, South Korea also became a member of the Organization of Economic Cooperation and Development. Table 6.1 shows some basic economic indicators for South Korea.

The Korean population has been aging during this period of economic development; statistics from 1999 showed that 6.6 percent of the total population was more than 65 years old. Ongoing migration to cities for better jobs and improved living conditions has contributed to greatly increased urban populations as well. In 1960, urban populations accounted for only 28 percent of Korea's total population; by 1995, that number had increased to 78.5 percent. The literacy rate in Korea is nearly 100 percent, and school enrollment at primary and secondary levels approaches 100 percent. The proportion of university students (415 per 100,000 population) in Korea is the highest in the world (Table 6.2). Additional demographic factors are reported in Table 6.2.

Context: Health Needs

The Korean population's general health status has improved greatly with the economic advances of the past 40 years. The infant mortality rate has decreased from 61 per 1,000 live births in the 1960s to 7.7 per 1,000 live births in 1996. The 1998 mortality rate under age 5 was 1.7 and 1.6 per 1,000 for males and females respectively, and the total fertility rate for that year was 1.5. Life expectancy was 71.0 years for men and 74.9 years for women (see Table 6.2) in 2000.

The current panorama of health problems in Korea is similar to that of other developed countries, with infectious diseases no longer the most common causes of death. The proportion of deaths due to infectious and parasitic disease is only 2.5 percent, ranking eighth among the leading

TABLE 6.1

Economic Indicators, 1996

GDP	$520.0 billion
Per capita gross national income	$11,380
Percent unemployment rate	1.6
Total national health expenditures	16.4 billion*
Percent GDP on health	5.14
Percent health budget in public sector	46.23
Per capita expenditure on health services	353.3**

* 22,855.23 Korean Won.
** 492,300 Korean Won.
SOURCE: National Statistical Office (1999); Korea Institute for Health and Social Affairs (2000).

Population (1998)	46.4 million	
Population density per square kilometer (1998)	467.2	
Percent population 65 and older (1998)	6.6	
Percent urbanized (1995)	78.5	
Infant mortality rate per 1,000 live births (1996)	7.7	
Under-five mortality rate per 1,000 live births (1998)		
Male	1.7	
Female	1.6	
Life expectancy at birth (years), male (2000*)	71.0	
Life expectancy at birth (years), female (2000*)	74.9	
Total fertility rate (1998)	1.5	

TABLE 6.2
General Demographics, 1995–98

* Projected estimation.
SOURCE: Ministry of Health and Welfare (1999).

causes of death. The major causes of death for Koreans are cerebrovascular diseases, malignant neoplasm, heart disease, and other chronic diseases (Table 6.3). However, stomach cancer and chronic liver diseases are more prevalent among Koreans than people of other developed countries. The high proportion of deaths due to chronic diseases is anticipated to become more pronounced as the population ages, changes its diet, smokes more, and exercises less.

In 1998, 35.5 percent of Koreans smoked; the rate was much higher for men (67.6 percent) than for women (6.7 percent). Korean drinking behavior is often interesting to foreigners, because it is considered a social tool for making friends and conducting business. This makes drinking socially acceptable and in some cases is encouraged; this obscures its role in the development of health problems. The 1998 alcohol consumption rate was high among the general population at 68.4 percent (83.4 percent of men and 54.9 percent of women); about one-third (35.1 percent) of male drinkers consume alcohol at least 11 to 20 days per month (Ministry of Health and Welfare 1999).

The government provides infants and children with free, mandatory immunization services that target diphtheria, pertussis, tetanus, poliomyelitis, measles, tuberculosis, and viral hepatitis B. Immunization rates for these diseases are estimated to be more than 95 percent.

The first case of HIV was diagnosed in 1985, and the first AIDS case was confirmed in 1987. In 1998, the number of HIV-infected Koreans was 876, and among them were 131 cases of full-blown AIDS (National Institute of Health 1999). Although the prevalence appears to be moderate, the

TABLE 6.3

Major Causes
of Mortality,
1998

	Number of Deaths	Death Rates per 100,000
Diseases of the circulatory system	57,439	123.7
Neoplasm	51,449	110.8
External causes of mortality	32,011	68.9
Diseases of the digestive system	15,745	33.9
Diseases of the respiratory system	12,439	26.8
Endocrine, nutritional, and metabolic disorders	10,822	23.3
Mental and behavioral disorders	7,288	15.7
Certain infectious and parasitic diseases	6,072	13.1
Diseases of the genitourinary system	2,837	6.1
Diseases of musculoskeletal system and connective tissue	2,452	5.3
Total (all causes)	240,254	517.4

SOURCE: National Statistical Office (1999).

number of HIV/AIDS cases is on the rise. The primary route of infection for Koreans has recently shifted to sexual contacts with Koreans from those with foreigners. These findings suggest that HIV/AIDS may soon become the most serious health problem in Korea.

Organization and Management of the Health System

The Korean healthcare system can be characterized as a privately controlled delivery system in combination with a publicly regulated financing system. The Korean system is a hybrid of the Japanese and U.S. systems. Components of the healthcare infrastructure such as the social insurance program, closed hospital system, and health administration structures follow the Japanese system, whereas the U.S. system is reflected in entrepreneurial characteristics of private sectors and in such functional components as the training of health professionals.

Until the 1970s, Korean society was not prepared to address social and welfare concerns. The government's primary focus was economic development aimed at recovering from the devastation of the Korean War. Government expenditures on healthcare during that period were less than one percent of the total national budget. Most of the money was devoted to implementing public health activities such as family planning, tuberculosis control, and maternal and child healthcare through public health organizations.

Owing to sharp economic growth within a short period of time, the government began in the 1970s to pay attention to social welfare programs, especially for medical care and housing. As a result, the Korean government initiated a mandatory health security program for part of the Korean population in 1977. With gradual expansion of coverage, the entire population became entitled to the health security program in 1989, the progression of which is shown in Figure 6.1.

In Korea, the private sector plays a major role in delivering healthcare services and has grown substantially since the introduction of the health security program. For example, when the health security system was first implemented in 1977, about 46.8 percent of all hospital beds were private. However, just 19 years later in 1996, that figure had increased to 86.8 percent (Table 6.4). According to 1996 records, only 6.5 percent of Korean hospitals were government-operated; the remaining 93 percent were owned or operated by private or not-for-profit organizations.

Three sectors—patients as consumers, physicians as providers, and the government as a payer—contributed to the rapid growth of the private sector. As per capita income increased, consumers began to demand more healthcare services. The aging population, improved education, and the expansion of health security plans have also contributed to this trend.

FIGURE 6.1 Development of the National Health Security Program in Korea

Year	Contents
1977	• Insurance compulsory for firms with more than 500 employees • Government program for low-income individuals (Medical Aid) enacted
1979	• Insurance compulsory for government and private school employees • Insurance compulsory for firms with more than 300 employees
1981	• Insurance compulsory for firms with more than 100 employees • Three demonstration societies for the self-employed established
1982	• Three additional demonstration societies for the self-employed established • Insurance compulsory for firms with more than 16 employees
1988	• Insurance compulsory for self-employed in rural areas • Insurance compulsory for firms with more than 5 employees
1989	• Insurance compulsory for self-employed in urban areas

SOURCE: Shin and Lee (1995).

TABLE 6.4
Hospital
Facilities

	1977	1996
Public	13,582 (53.2%)	21,229 (13.2%) 10,796 (6.7%)
National*	8,504 (33.3%)	10,460 (6.5%)
Local government/ not-for-profit	5,078 (19.9%)	
Private†	11,941 (46.8%)	139,603 (86.8%)
Total	25,523 (100.0%)	160,832 (100.0%)

* Includes national leprosy, mental, and tuberculosis hospitals.
† Includes for-profit corporate, for-profit proprietary, not-for-profit welfare organizations, and private university hospitals.
SOURCE: Yang (1996); Ministry of Health and Welfare (1999).

Physicians, who are major contributors to private hospitals in Korea, were encouraged to invest in health facilities and equipment to meet the increased demand from patients. The government has also used financial incentives to encourage private sectors to invest in healthcare to meet a demand that is growing beyond current capabilities.

Nature of Health Planning, Administration, and Regulation

The Ministry of Health and Welfare (MOHW) is the central governmental office for healthcare, and it has the primary responsibility for making and regulating healthcare policy in Korea. It coordinates private and public health activities for the prevention and treatment of diseases, licenses healthcare professionals and facilities, supervises drug manufacturers, and provides other related services. Additionally, the MOHW has responsibilities in health insurance administration, including the setting of fee schedules and determination of benefit packages. However, because most health resources belong to the private sector and a relatively low priority is placed on government health issues, the Ministry's power to affect health policy is sometimes limited.

At the local level, 16 provincial health departments and 243 health centers are in charge of public health administration for their respective jurisdictions. Besides public health administration, these health centers also provide primary health services for the indigent and those living in rural areas. The regional public hospitals, the national public hospitals, and the veterans administration's system of hospitals also provide healthcare services. However, this market is quite small as compared with the private sector (The Korean Society for Preventive Medicine 1999).

Locus of Responsibility for Curative Services, Preventive Care, and Training

Whereas almost all convalescent care is provided by the private sector, the government takes primary responsibility for prevention. Health centers and their satellites offer free vaccinations for recommended childhood immunizations as well as discounts for adult vaccination. For enrollees of the Industrial Accident Compensation Insurance, the government covers the cost of physical examinations for employees and supports worksite measures to prevent occupational injuries. In addition, the government has recently established health promotion funds and operates a variety of activities targeting behavioral changes.

Financing

National Health Security System

Korea implemented universal health insurance for the entire population in 1989. The National Health Security System is administered in two tiers: Medical Insurance and the Medical Aid program. As of 1998, Medical Insurance was a wage-based contributory insurance program covering 97 percent of the population, whereas Medical Aid was a government-subsidized public assistance program for the poor and the medically indigent. Medical Insurance was further subdivided into three separate programs for (1) industrial workers; (2) government and private-school employees; and (3) the self-employed. Interestingly, these programs cover the parents as well as the children of the insured. Table 6.5 summarizes the distribution of population by health security programs in 1998. Beginning July 1, 2000, these programs were integrated into a single system under the heading of National Health Insurance. Thus far the integration has been in name only, although additional integrative actions are expected in the future.

Major Funding Sources for Personal Health Services

Personal health services in Korea are financed through several funding sources:

1. insurance premiums that each enrollee pays for universal health insurance programs
2. government subsidies including government support for insurance premiums of enrollees in the Medical Insurance program and costs incurred by the Medical Aid program
3. private funds and out-of-pocket payments by individual patients

The third category includes copayments for covered health services and payment for uncovered services. As compared with other countries that have national health insurance, Korea has a relatively high rate of direct

Type	Number of Population (Unit: 10,000), %		Contribution (percent)			Number of Insurance Societies
			Insured	Employer	Government Subsidy	
Medical Insurance	4,472	97.0				
Industrial workers	1,614	35.0	50	50	—	145
Government and private-school employees	503	10.9				1
Government			50	50	—	
Private School			50	30*	20	
Self-employed						
Rural area	340	7.4	54	—	46	92
Urban area	2,015	43.7	66	—	34	135
Medical aid	139	3.0	—	—	100	
Total	4,611	100.0				373

* School board.
SOURCE: Ministry of Health and Welfare (1999a).

TABLE 6.5
Medical Care Assurance, 1998

payment because of the limited coverage and high copayment rate. In 1998, Koreans paid 41.6 percent of total healthcare expenditures out of their own pockets. This is significantly higher than that found in most countries with universal health insurance coverage (Korean Institute for Health and Social Affairs 2000).

Management Structure for Health Insurance Programs

Management bodies known as "insurance societies" are responsible for collecting Medical Insurance premiums, determining benefits, and providing administrative support. The 145 industrial workers' insurance societies each include individual societies for large industries plus a common insurance society that covers a number of smaller companies. The program for government and private-school employees was managed by a single insurance society called the Korean Medical Insurance Corporation (KMIC). The self-employed program included 227 insurance societies organized in line with local political jurisdictions. In all, in 1998, 373 insurance societies served a membership ranging from 30,000 to 200,000 workers.

Each society manages its funds independently. If the society shows a negative balance at the end of the year, enrollees and their employers must pay higher premiums for the following year. Fiscal soundness varies depending on the society's financial capacity and the health status of each society's members. Unlike Medical Insurance programs, the Medical Aid program is administered by local governments, which determine the eligibility of enrollees and reimburses providers.

All insurance societies are required to join the National Federation of Medical Insurance (NFMI). NFMI provides a certain amount of administrative support to individual insurance societies; it also collects fees for provider reimbursement from all the insurance societies except KMIC, which has its own reimbursement system.

Each of the programs (industrial workers, government and private-school employees, and the self-employed) has its mechanism for collecting premiums. For the industrial workers and the government and private-school employees, the insurance premiums are set at a fixed percentage of monthly wages (3.1 to 3.8 percent). For the self-employed, the individual contribution is based on income, property, and family size. Table 6.5 summarizes the proportional contribution of premium that the individual, the employer, and the government paid by health security program in 1998. Although these insurance programs are expected to be integrated into one system in July 2002, developing a uniform premium rate will be a critical issue in equity that still needs to be addressed.

Reimbursement Mechanisms

Both hospital and physician services covered by insurance are reimbursed on a fee-for-service basis, which offers a strong incentive to provide extensive services. All healthcare institutions in Korea are designated by NFMI to provide health services to the insured.

However, the Korean National Health Security program does not provide full coverage for all health services. The government-determined benefit packages exclude many preventive services and certain high-technology services such as magnetic resonance imaging (MRI). Since 1987, limited coverage has been offered for Eastern/oriental medicine services. Prescription medicines are included in the benefit package. However, meals for hospitalized patients are not, because personal needs are considered the family's responsibility.

Providers file their monthly claims with NFMI for services rendered. The Medical Fees Review Committee of NFMI compares each claim with the Standard Unit Cost for All Services and Other Items published by the Ministry of Health and Welfare. NFMI then pays the providers with funds deposited by insurance societies. Providers usually receive reimbursement from NFMI within a month after filing the claims. Figure 6.2 demonstrates the flow of funds from premium collection to provider reimbursement.

FIGURE 6.2

Medical
Claims Review
and
Reimbursement
Procedures

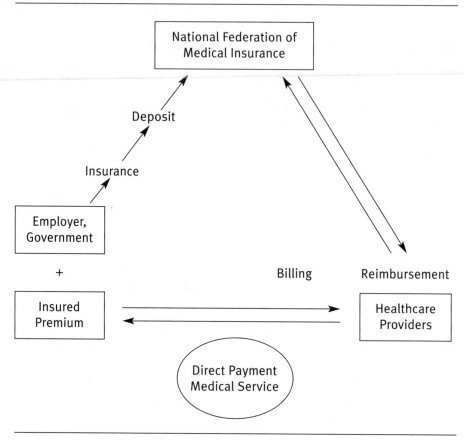

Cost-Containment Efforts

Korea has developed several cost-containment mechanisms including cost sharing, exclusion of certain services from coverage, flexible adjustment of cash benefits, fee scheduling by the government, and utilization review.

The features of cost sharing adopted by the Korean system are different according to each care setting (inpatient or outpatient) and the level of healthcare institutions. For outpatient care provided in clinics or small-sized hospitals, patients pay a flat fee of U.S.$2.50 per visit if they are charged at less than or equal to 10,000 Korean Won. If the charge goes over 10,000 Won, the patient pays 30 percent of the charge. For outpatient care in hospitals and general hospitals, coinsurance rates of 40 percent and 55 percent of the charges are applied, respectively. For inpatient services, patients pay 20 percent of the charges at all types of healthcare institutions. As compared with inpatient care, outpatient care has greater cost sharing as well as differential coinsurance rates for different types of institutions. This is intended to discourage individuals from seeking unnecessary care or from bypassing the primary healthcare level and going directly to specialty, secondary, or tertiary medical facilities.

In setting the fee schedule, the government must balance providers' requests for higher fees with those of consumers and employers for minimizing their payments. NFMI conducts utilization reviews for selected bills to detect inappropriate claims for covered services as well as payment requests for uncovered services.

National Health Expenditure

In 1996, Korea's total national health expenditure was about U.S.$16.4 billion (22,855.23 billion Korean Won), 5.14 percent of the gross domestic product. Per capita health spending for the same year was U.S.$353.3 (492,300 Korean Won), which is relatively small in comparison with other countries that have similar gross national product levels. The public sector share of total healthcare outlays was about 46.2 percent in 1998 (see Table 6.1). Korea has seen a rapid rise in healthcare costs in recent years; this is attributable to the rapid growth of the economy, the expansion of health insurance coverage, and the fee-for-service reimbursement system. Increased investments in health services staff and facilities have also contributed to the increases.

Health Resources

Korea has experienced extensive expansion of healthcare resources in several areas during the past 30 years.

Healthcare Professionals

Healthcare professionals in Korea include physicians, oriental medical doctors, dentists, pharmacists, midwives, nurses, and allied healthcare workers. All professionals are required to be licensed for practice. Table 6.6 shows the number of health professionals, their training levels, and the number of educational institutions for each profession.

Physicians

Korea has two types of physicians: Western and traditional medical doctors. At present, Western physicians are the majority of providers, but a preference for oriental physicians in dealing with certain conditions persists. Physician training begins with six years of medical school education following high school. Medical school graduates become licensed physicians through national examinations. Following these examinations, which permit physicians to become general practitioners, a doctor must complete an additional four to five years of training to become a specialist; this additional training includes one year of internship and three to four years of residency. Medical specialists can train in 26 specialty areas.

As a result of the government's decision to increase the number of medical schools, the number of practicing physicians has increased dra-

TABLE 6.6
Healthcare Professionals, 1998

Provider Type	Number of Professionals	Per 1,000 Population	Number of Educational Institutions	Years of Education
Physicians	65,431	1.41	41	6
Dentists	16,126	0.35	11	6
Oriental medical doctors	9,914	0.21	11	6
Pharmacists	46,998	1.01	20	4
Midwives	8,590	0.18	9	1
Nurses	141,094	3.04	111	3 to 4
Nursing aides	218,718	4.71	113	1
Medical technicians	81,539	1.76	44	3 to 4
Medical records officers	6,811	0.15	30	2
Opticians	18,220	0.39	14	2
Dietitians	73,989	1.59	51	2 to 4
Social workers	21,244	0.46	Unknown	2 or more

SOURCE: Ministry of Health and Welfare (1999).

matically. Numbers of medical doctors and medical school enrollments have almost tripled in the past two decades. Nevertheless, the doctor-to-population ratio continues to be lower than that of most developed countries. The number of physicians per 1,000 population was about 1.4 in 1996, only half the median value for OECD countries of 2.8 (Anderson and Poullier 1999). Meanwhile, some are concerned that the medical education capacity has grown too much and that the country may face a surplus of physicians in the near future if the current level of medical school enrollment is maintained.

Oriental (Traditional) Medical Doctors

Oriental physicians were the primary healthcare providers in Korea before 1885, when Western medicine was introduced and they were replaced with Western physicians. Oriental medical doctors receive their medical training in medical schools separate from the Western medical schools. Since the founding of the first oriental medical school in 1948, oriental medicine has become a specialty in Korea. As shown in Table 6.5, 9,914 oriental medicine physicians were licensed in Korea in 1998, considerably fewer than the number of physicians trained in Western medicine (65,431). The proportion of use of oriental medical care to the total care provided is only 4 to 5 percent of all medical visits.

Pharmacists

Pharmacists complete a four-year baccalaureate degree program. Most pharmacists own their own pharmacies or are employed at community pharmacies (Korean Pharmaceutical Association 1998). Besides dispensing medicines, community pharmacists may prescribe without a doctor's prescription. For the public, community pharmacists are often their first-contact healthcare providers. This was even more true before national health security was introduced because many people could not afford to visit physicians or hospitals.

Nurses and Nursing Aides

Nurses in Korea attend either a four-year university or a three-year junior college. Of the 141,094 licensed nurses (Table 6.5), the majority (about 70 percent) practice in clinical settings such as hospitals and clinics. The next largest proportion works in public health.

Korean nursing aides are a crucial component in nursing care; nursing aide training requires one year beyond high school. Almost 90 percent of nursing staff working in local clinics are nursing aides (Kim et al. 1999). As a result of the steady expansion of the nursing programs, Korea no longer has a nursing shortage. Rather a problem of oversupply is expected in the near future.

Allied Healthcare Professionals

Allied healthcare personnel include medical technicians (clinical pathology technicians, radiological technicians, physical therapists, occupational therapists, dental technicians, dental hygienists), medical records officers, opticians, dieticians, and social workers. Educational programs for these personnel range from two-year college programs to four-year university programs. Because supply is outstripping demand, these groups face strong competition in the labor market.

Health Services Facilities

Medical care institutions are classified as general hospitals; hospitals, dental hospitals, and oriental medical hospitals; and medical clinics, dental clinics, oriental medical clinics, midwifery clinics, and dispensaries. Table 6.7 shows the number of facilities and beds by type of medical care institution.

TABLE 6.7

Number of Medical Care Facilities and Beds by Type, 1998

	Number of Facilities	Number of Beds
General hospital	255	101,137
Hospital	517	52,355
Dental hospital	31	80
Oriental hospital	107	5,952
Specialized hospital		
Tuberculosis	2	818
Leprosy	1	2,600
Mental	42	16,913
Clinic	17,041	55,663
Oriental clinic	6,590	225
Dental clinic	9,653	1
Dispensary	216	510
Midwifery clinic	133	133
Public health centers		
Health centers	243	—
Health satellites	1,266	—
Primary healthcare posts	1,941	—
Total	38,037	220,427

SOURCE: Ministry of Health and Welfare (1999).

Hospitals, General Hospitals (Western)

Hospitals are required to maintain more than 30 inpatient beds. General hospitals are required to have 100 or more inpatient beds and, at a minimum, specialized departments in internal medicine, general surgery, pediatrics, obstetrics, anesthesiology, clinical pathology, psychiatry, and dentistry. Although hospitals and general hospitals are primarily responsible for providing inpatient care, they may also provide outpatient care. About 71.2 percent of inpatient care is provided in hospital or general hospital settings; the remaining care takes place in clinics.

Korean hospitals are quite well equipped. According to a 1990 Korean Ministry of Health and Social Affairs survey, 154 of the 159 general hospitals had at least one computed tomography scanner; 36 had extracorporeal shock wave lithotripsy (ESWL); 32 had linear accelerators; 58 had one or more lasers; 82 had gamma cameras; and 22 had MRI machines. Physicians working at hospitals and general hospitals are salaried employees of the hospitals. Physicians at local clinics do not have privileges to see their patients at hospitals or general hospitals.

Clinics

The approximately 20,000 private local clinics distributed across Korea play a major role in providing outpatient care. Public health centers and health satellites also provide outpatient care, particularly primary care that is comparable to that provided by local clinics. Altogether, local clinics and public health centers provide 77.3 percent of all outpatient care.

Oriental Medical Facilities

In 1998, 107 hospitals and 6,590 clinics specialized in oriental (traditional) medicine, the majority of which were single-practitioner practices. Acupuncture and herbal medicines are the predominant services offered. Because of cultural preferences for tonic medicines, Koreans have a substantial demand for herbal medicines in spite of the fact that these medicines are somewhat more expensive because they are not covered by the national insurance.

Western and oriental medicines have distinctly separate healthcare delivery systems, which results in little collaboration in treating patients. For example, Western general hospitals may not have oriental medicine departments.

Public Health Facilities

Three kinds of government-owned facilities serve as community healthcare resources at each level of administrative district: 243 health centers at the county level, 1,266 health satellites, and 1,941 primary healthcare posts at local levels (Ministry of Health and Welfare 1999). Government facilities also support public health programs not offered by private providers, such as disease prevention activities.

Medical Commodities

Necessary medical equipment is rarely unavailable to Koreans. Korea has been importing newly developed, high-cost medical equipment at a rapid pace with little governmental regulation. Korea has more MRI machines and computed tomography (CT) scanners per 1,000,000 population than do most European countries (Table 6.8). The rapid proliferation of medical technologies has led to sharply increasing healthcare costs and wasteful duplication of technology; this is one of the major problems for the Korean healthcare system.

Several factors may contribute to the rapid adoption and diffusion of high-cost medical technologies. First, most high-technology medical equipment is not covered by the national health insurance, so healthcare

TABLE 6.8
Availability of
Selected
Medical
Technologies
by Country
(per million
population)

	Germany (1987)	France (1990)	U.S. (1988)	Japan (1990)	Korea (1993)	Korea (2000)
CT (whole body)	—	7.2	17.7	40.3	11.8	13.6
MRI	0.9	1.2	11.7 (1992)	13.5 (1993)	1.7	5.0
ESWL	0.3	0.6	0.9	2.3	1.2	3.1

SOURCE: Yang (1996); Korea Institute for Health and Social Affairs (2000).

providers are willing to purchase and use more of these types of equipment to generate greater profits. Second, a strong cultural tendency exists for people—providers included—to perceive high-technology equipment as prestigious and as providing better medical services; this type of equipment is seen as a competitive tool for attracting patients. Third, the government regulation requiring a certificate of need for medical equipment was abolished in 1995, which means that virtually no mechanism is in place to limit the adoption and acquisition of high-technology equipment.

Drugs

Another feature of healthcare resource use in Korea is the high usage levels of pharmaceutical products. Korea shares with Japan the highest pharmaceutical healthcare expenditure ratio in the world (31 percent) (Yoo 1999).

As with high-technology equipment, physicians are compelled to use more drugs as a way of maximizing profits; this may be in part because they can sell medications directly to patients at clinics or at hospitals. A reported 38 percent of physician revenues in private clinics comes from medicines dispensed in the clinics (Ministry of Health and Welfare 1999a). Additionally, pharmacists sell drugs, including antibiotics and steroids, to customers without a physician's prescription, and Koreans commonly self-medicate.

From the patient's perspective, having health problems managed from diagnosis to treatment, including the ability to obtain medicine, at one place is convenient. However, this practice increases the risk of misuse and overutilization of pharmaceutical products. Currently, the Korean government is trying to enact a new law prohibiting physicians from dispensing medicine and pharmacists from prescribing medicine; enactment of this law is expected to reduce the risk of drug misuse.

Service Delivery

The general features of the Korean healthcare delivery system are the absence of the level-of-care concept, the predominance of expensive specialty care over primary care, and the disparity between urban and rural areas.

Nature and Distribution of Primary, Secondary, and Tertiary Care

The concept of primary care physicians (PCPs) as gatekeepers hardly exists in Korea. Patients choose their providers and the level of care they believe they need. If PCPs are defined as including general practitioners, family medicine physicians, internists, and pediatricians, Korea had approximately 14,726 PCPs in 1998, which provided a ratio of 32 per 100,000 population (Kim 1999).

Primary outpatient services and simple cases are generally expected to be handled at local clinics and outpatient departments of small-sized hospitals; however, such cases are instead often treated at general or university hospitals. For example, Korean patients with a cold commonly go directly to a specialist or an outpatient department of a general, tertiary hospital. This happens because the range of services provided by each institution is not clearly defined. In reality, Korean general and university hospitals treat all levels of care, from primary to tertiary. Because a large proportion (about 40 percent) of their revenues comes from outpatient care, these institutions have strong incentives to see outpatients.

Most hospital admissions occur as a result of ambulatory care situations. Referred admissions are the exception rather than the rule in Korea. General and university hospitals are overcrowded and have bed shortages; this phenomenon stems from the Korean people's preference for large hospitals coupled with inadequate regulatory mechanisms.

Several regulatory provisions were created in 1989 to correct uncontrolled use of inappropriate healthcare services and to improve the efficiency of healthcare delivery. The new government policy does not cover care when patients go directly to tertiary institutions without a referral from a primary care physician. At the same time, the coinsurance rate for ambulatory visits to hospitals was raised to 50 percent. Unfortunately, these regulations had little effect on patient behavior, in part because most people were accustomed to paying the full price for health services and were not sensitive to coinsurance rates.

Availability, Access, Equity, and Quality

Although the availability of healthcare has not reached the level of that in major industrialized countries, healthcare staffing, facilities, and equipment have increased substantially since the late 1970s. Overall, the current availability of healthcare in Korea appears to be relatively good.

Because of Korea's universal healthcare system, few financial obstacles exist to accessing basic medical services for most people. Also, because Korea is a small country with a well-developed road system, people can easily reach healthcare settings. For these reasons, most rural residents are able to access city general hospitals within a few hours.

Although Korea has adopted national health insurance coverage, high coinsurance rates as a mechanism to contain healthcare costs have created equity problems across income groups. Low-income groups use substantially fewer services than do high-income groups; this phenomenon is more marked in the case of expensive new medical technologies that are often not covered by health insurance. Studies show that the utilization rate for MRI for people with monthly insurance premiums of less than 10,000 Korean Won was only one forty-fifth of that for those with a monthly premium of more than 40,000 Korean Won (Kim and Moon 1992).

Currently many of the Korean hospitals conduct quality assurance in-house. Also three external institutions monitor quality control. The Korean Hospital Association has been conducting quality control of hospitals since 1981 in an effort to provide criteria for hospital accreditation. The second program is the Evaluation of Services in Health Care Institutions, initiated in 1995 by the government. Finally, the quality of hospital services in terms of consumer satisfaction is assessed by lay organizations. The major criticism of all of these systems is that they lack appropriate mechanisms for feedback to correct inadequacies. In addition, the credibility and reliability of the quality control tools used by these systems are not satisfactory.

Urban versus Rural Contrast

In Korea, equity in the apportioning of healthcare resources between urban and rural areas has been improved, although a concentration of healthcare facilities is still in urban areas. As shown in Table 6.9, less than 10 percent of hospital beds and physicians are located in rural areas. However, as a result of the massive population shift toward urban areas during the past two decades, the proportion of rural residents has dropped to 20 percent; this has, in effect, made the distribution of healthcare resources in rural areas more equitable. Improved roads help rural residents access urban hospitals. The location of many of the public health centers, health satellites, and primary care clinics in rural areas has also increased the accessibility of healthcare for rural Koreans. This improvement is reflected in recent data showing that the utilization rates of healthcare services are similar for rural and urban residents.

Governmental efforts to improve the availability of physicians in rural areas have focused on increased physician supply through expansion of medical schools. However, physician shortages in rural areas have not been resolved by this increase because newly qualified physicians generally prefer to work in urban areas. To counteract this trend, the government has public physicians, who practice medicine in underserved areas as a substitute for their three-year mandatory military duty. However, this is not a long-term solution because these physicians generally leave the area after they have completed their tours of duty.

	Urban Areas (percent)	Rural Areas (percent)
Population (1995)	78.5	21.5
Number of hospital beds	91.1	8.9
Number of physicians	90.7	9.3

TABLE 6.9
Regional Distribution of Healthcare Resources, 1997

SOURCE: Ministry of Health and Welfare (1999a).

Prospects for the Future

Because of universal health insurance coverage and the increased availability of healthcare resources, general accessibility to healthcare services has improved in Korea. Now the government is focusing its attention on the balance between cost and quality of services. Major expected changes and issues in the near future are described in this section.

Unification of Medical Insurance Programs

On July 1, 2000, the three medical insurance programs (industrial workers, government and private-school employees, and the self-employed) were unified into a single system called the National Health Insurance System. The rationale behind this merger was to ease the burden of the government subsidy for the self-employed programs. The insurance societies for the salaried workers (industrial workers and government and private-school employees) are financially stable because their insurance pool is composed of relatively wealthy and healthy workers. On the other hand, the insurance societies for the self-employed program, particularly in poor rural areas, often struggle because workers have low wages and are proportionately older. Another motivation for the merger was cost savings resulting from eliminating the inefficiencies inherent in a fragmented decentralized administration. On average, administrative costs in relation to total insurance societies' expenditures was 15.6 percent, which is very high as compared with Canada (1.5 percent), the United Kingdom (2.6 percent), and the United States (10 percent) (Yang 1996). Figure 6.3 presents the organizational diagram of insurance societies before and after the unification.

Re-evaluation of Pharmaceutical Provision

The roles of the three groups of healthcare professionals (Western physicians, oriental medical doctors, and pharmacists) overlap with respect to prescribing and dispensing medicine in Korea. This overlap results in intense competition among the three groups as a survival strategy. A

FIGURE 6.3

Organizational
Reform of
Health
Insurers in
Korea

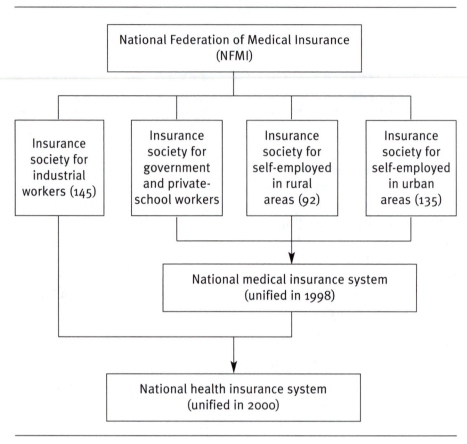

heated dispute has erupted between pharmacists and oriental medical doctors over the right to dispense oriental medicines. In 1994, the government modified pharmacy legislation and created a new profession to resolve the conflict between the two professions; this new group of pharmacists specializes in oriental medicine. However, the conflict between the two professions persists.

The same issue is contested between Western physicians and pharmacists. To resolve the tension, representatives for the government, physicians, pharmacists, and several lay organizations instituted a "separation of dispensing from prescribing" provision which prohibits pharmacists from prescribing medications and at the same time prohibits physicians from dispensing medicines from their offices. Effective July 2000, the provision contributes to the prevention of drug-related accidents and reduces the risk of misuse and overutilization of drug treatments. Also, it is expected to save healthcare costs by discouraging unnecessary drug treatments. However, this provision is strongly contested by the stakeholders, especially physicians and pharmacists, who are concerned that the new provision will greatly decrease their earnings.

New Reimbursement System

To correct the undesirable practice pattern described above and counter-act rising healthcare costs caused by the fee-for-service payment system, the Korean government has considered introducing an alternative payment method under the national health insurance. Since 1995, a case payment system has been used for selected services as a demonstration program; this system has applied the diagnosis-related group payment system adopted from the United States. Some people argue that the efficiency of care can be achieved under the new payment system only by sacrificing quality of services and restricting the physician's professional judgment and freedom. Nevertheless, considering an alternative payment system is imperative to meet Korea's need to control rising healthcare expenditures.

Finally, the Korean government recently focused its attention on disease prevention and health promotion. The 1999 Health Promotion Act employs models to modify health behaviors such as smoking and alcohol consumption.

REFERENCES

Anderson, G. F., and Poullier, J. P. 1999. "Health Spending Access and Outcomes: Trends in Industrialized Countries." *Health Affairs* 18 (3): 178–92.

Kim, B. Y. 1999. "Primary Care Physicians and Residency Training Programs in Korea." *Korean Journal of Health Policy and Administration* 9 (2): 139–56.

Kim, J. S., Choi, E. Y., Park, H. A., and Lee, W. B. 1999. "The Supply and Demand Projection of Nurses in Korea." *Korean Journal of Health Policy and Administration* 9 (3): 33–52.

Kim, L., and Moon, O. R. 1992. "A Study on the Socio-economic Characteristics of Magnetic Resonance Image (MRI) Uses in Korea." *Korean Journal of Health Policy and Administration* 2 (2): 194–220.

Korean Institute for Health and Social Affairs. 2000. "Korea's National Health Expenditure Account." Seoul: Korean Institute for Health and Social Affairs.

Korean Pharmaceutical Association. 1998. *Statistics of Korean Pharmaceutical Association Membership.* Seoul: Korean Pharmaceutical Association.

The Korean Society for Preventive Medicine. 1999. *Preventive Medicine and Public Health.* Seoul: Gae Chook Moon Wha Inc.

Ministry of Health and Social Affairs. 1991. "National Health Expenditure Patterns." Seoul: Ministry of Health and Social Affairs.

Ministry of Health and Welfare. 1999. *Yearbook of Health and Welfare Statistics.* Seoul: Ministry of Health and Welfare.

———. 1999a. *Major Programs for Health and Welfare, 1998–1999.* Seoul: Ministry of Health and Welfare.

National Institute of Health. 1999. *Communicable Diseases Monthly Report* 10 (3): 25–36.

National Statistical Office. 1999. *Korea Statistical Yearbook.* Seoul: National Statistical Office.

Shin, Y., and Lee, K. 1995. "The Health Insurance System in Korea and Its Implications." *World Hospitals* 31 (3): 3–9.

Yang, B. M. 1996. "The Role of Health Insurance in the Growth of the Private Health Sector in Korea." *International Journal of Health Planning and Management* 11 (3): 231–52.

Yoo, C. S. 1999. "The Welfare Effect of Mandatory Prescription in Korea." *Korean Journal of Health Policy and Administration* 9 (4): 65–86.

GERMANY

Gerhard Brenner and Dale Rublee

Background Information

When Otto von Bismarck imposed compulsory health insurance in Germany some 115 years ago and mandated its support through separate, primarily occupation-based funds known as "sickness funds," under the joint control of employers and employees, he created what would eventually become the most widely emulated medical delivery system in the world. Indeed, Germany was the first nation to adopt a national healthcare program. This system has greatly influenced Eastern European countries, which are currently importing selected features of the German system into their own health systems. Long admired by policy experts, the German system has undoubtedly contributed to good industrial relations in the health sector of the economy through a decentralized structure that has served to integrate numerous groups into administration and policymaking.

Today, health policy is increasingly shaped by the requirements of macroeconomics as a whole, and few wealthy countries have passed through a period of economic change equal to the change faced by Germany. This difficult phase can be attributed to a variety of factors that include the following:

- fiscal adjustment and major structural change arising from the integration of the new eastern states (Länder)
- the transformation of Central and Eastern Europe
- a rapidly evolving world economy
- the completion of the European single market

These external changes have placed great pressure on German institutions—particularly its venerable healthcare system—that require increased flexibility and adaptation to these new circumstances.

General Demographics and Education

On the European scale, Germany is a large country in terms of area (more than 350,000 square kilometers) and population. With 82 million people, Germany outnumbers all of its European neighbors. It has the most foreign-born residents, and it is one of Europe's most densely populated countries at 229 people per square kilometer. Germany had a population growth rate of 0.3 percent between the years 1995 and 1996 (Table 7.1).

TABLE 7.1
Selected
Demographics
and Education
Data

Total area (square kilometers)	357,000
Population	
Population in millions	82
Foreign-born population in millions	7.4
Population per square kilometer	229
Population growth rate (percent), 1995 to 1996	0.3
Life expectancy at birth	
Female	79.9
Male	73.6
Infant mortality (percent of live births)	0.50
Total fertility rate	1.26
Education	
Percent of population with at least upper-secondary education	83.7
Expenditure on educational institutions, percent of GDP (1994)	5.8

SOURCE: OECD (2000); Statistisches Bundesamt (1998).

Other demographic data indicate that the most conspicuous fact about Germany is how inconspicuous it is among the wealthy countries. In general, Germany remains more or less hidden in a middle group, with figures close to the average. Every third person is under the age of 15 years or over the age of 65 years. Children under six years old comprise about 6 percent of the population. Life expectancy at birth is nearly 80 years for women and about 74 years for men. At age 60, women retain the life expectancy advantage with 23 years versus 19 years for men. Continuing a long downward trend, the infant mortality rate stood at 0.5 percent of all live births in 1996. The fertility rate (the average number of children for a woman between the ages of 15 and 44 years) was 1.26.

Literacy in Germany is nearly 100 percent. Almost all youth enroll in some secondary schooling as well. Reflecting the high value placed on educational achievement in the country, more than 80 percent of the working-age population have the equivalent of at least a high school education. Nearly 6 percent of the nation's gross domestic product is spent on educational institutions.

Employment and Economic Dimensions

As suggested in the introduction to this chapter, current health policy is framed against a background of ongoing structural change. In response, policy experts are seeking to reduce the size of the health sector and make it more efficient. This is not simply a matter of improving budget procedures and caps across all sectors of the system but also of examining the effectiveness of the regulatory structure and identifying those organizational features of insurance and healthcare delivery that distort incentives at all levels of the German federal system. In this respect, German health policy problems are not unique, as all health systems must constantly address the problems of meeting demands with limited funds.

The rationale for the basic restructuring of healthcare is found in the current labor market. As shown in Table 7.2, the total labor force in 1996 consisted of 39 million workers, 9 percent of whom were unemployed. Long-term unemployed people (perhaps a more meaningful economic indicator in the context of health than overall unemployment) constituted almost half of the total unemployed labor force in 1996. Germany's high level of unemployment creates severe revenue problems because health insurance is financed largely through wage-based premiums, and weak employment, especially in the eastern Länder (states), has been the country's main policy problem throughout the 1990s.

Nevertheless, as also shown in Table 7.2, Germany is a relatively affluent country. At more than U.S.$2 trillion, the gross domestic product is immense. Total health spending in 1996 amounted to 10.5 percent of the nation's gross domestic product, which was the highest level in the European Union that year, with 8.2 percent spent on publicly funded healthcare. The nation's estimate of total healthcare spending depends crucially, of course, on the concept of healthcare used. In this case, as is traditional, the concept is restricted to in-kind healthcare benefits (direct payments to all healthcare providers and suppliers). In this context, a very interesting perspective on total healthcare spending in Germany was recently provided by the Federal Bureau of Statistics, which has expanded the concept of healthcare to include all health-related cash benefits (like sickness benefits paid by employers), all healthcare capital and construction costs, and all private and out-of-pocket health costs. This inclusive definition of healthcare led to an estimated total health spending as a share of gross domestic product in 1996 of 14.9 percent. In fact, because most of Germany's healthcare is funded through the public social security system, nearly 80 percent of total health spending came from public sources. Despite these figures, what effect Germany's level of health spending has had on the health of the population is difficult to judge because many other factors influence health.

Context: Health Needs

Table 7.3 shows the leading categories of mortality in Germany in 1996 calculated in number of deaths per 100,000 people. The data clearly show that diseases of the circulatory system are the leading cause of death.

TABLE 7.2
Selected
Employment
and Economic
Indicators
(1996)

Total labor force (millions)	39
Unemployment rate	
Percent of total labor force	9
Long term (12 months or more), percent of total	47.8
Gross domestic product	
Total in billions of U.S.$ at current exchange rates	2,354
Per person in U.S.$ using P.P.P. $	21,200
Consumer prices December 1997 (Index 1990 = 100)	123.4
Health spending	
Share of total GDP, percent	10.5
Share of GDP in public, percent	8.2

SOURCE: OECD (2000); Statistisches Bundesamt (1998).

Neoplasms are also a major source of mortality at 267.5 deaths per 100,000. Occupying a middle group are diseases of the respiratory and digestive systems, along with endocrine and metabolic diseases.

As is found elsewhere in the world, the major health issues of concern in Germany are chronic diseases of an aging population. Table 7.3 also shows the mean age at which death occurs in Germany according to disease groups and the estimated share of such deaths for those less than 65 years old. The major causes, diseases of the circulatory system and neoplasms, have average ages of death that are quite high.

However, some younger people also have diseases, and, to a certain extent, deaths among the nonelderly are "avoidable." Decreasing the deaths attributable to such causes requires a focus on these avoidable deaths. Indeed, there is room for improvement in German mortality rates for these diseases. For instance, about 12 percent of all deaths from circulatory diseases are in people who are less than 65 years old. Likewise, more than 30 percent of all neoplasms are in people 65 years old or younger. More than 40 percent of all deaths from infectious and parasitic diseases and mental and behavioral disorders are in the nonelderly.

Organization and Management of the Health System

The federal nature of the constitution in Germany has created a complex administrative structure that includes special provisions for employers and employees. The focal point of the social insurance system is the sickness funds, which are administered by employers and employees in accordance

	Deaths per 100,000	Mean Age of Death	Deaths in Those Younger than 65 Years (percent)
Diseases of the circulatory system	520	79	11.8
Neoplasms	267.5	70.8	30.9
Diseases of the respiratory system	65.8	78	13
Diseases of the digestive system	51.2	68.9	39.3
Endocrine and metabolic diseases	33	77.3	12.9
Diseases of the nervous system	19.5	—	—
Mental and behavioral disorders	14.4	66.1	40.5
Diseases of the genitourinary system	11.7	77.5	14.2
Infectious and parasitic diseases	10	63.3	45.9
Diseases of the musculoskeletal system	2.7	—	—
Diseases of the blood and immune system	2	—	—

TABLE 7.3
Causes of Mortality (1996)

SOURCE: OECD (2000a); Kassenaerztlich Bundesvereinigung (2000).

with the arrangement of equally divided financing among them. As in many European countries, Germany's system is part of a larger set of social structures designed to ensure a minimum level of economic protection and social welfare for all residents. The social welfare system consists of social health insurance, pension funds, unemployment insurance, long-term-care insurance, and worker's compensation. The system is funded through monthly payroll deductions shared by employees and employers.

The present federal system was originally based on the principles of subsidization and self-administration, which granted considerable fiscal and administrative independence to the sickness funds, the hospital association, the medical profession, state governments, and other suppliers of services. However, the macroeconomic objective to keep health spending under close control has, in reality, resulted in a system that has grown away from local autonomy and pluralism. The government increasingly defines health finance matters through laws and regulations, although details of the content continue to be delegated to healthcare providers.

The health of the population is primarily the responsibility of the Länder, but mandatory health insurance and hospital financing are controlled by federal laws. Hospital care is administered jointly among individual hospitals, sickness funds, and Länder governments; authority for hospital planning and capital investment rests with the Länder. Although the sickness funds have responsibility for covering operating costs, they have little influence over hospital management, planning, and service utilization.

The ambulatory sector of the healthcare system is administered by associations of physicians and sickness funds. More than 750 sickness funds, which are traditionally organized by occupation or region, provide comprehensive healthcare to 90 percent of the population. All ambulatory care physicians who treat social health insurance patients are required by law to belong to the Länder (or regional) medical association, a public organization self-administered by physicians. The main purpose of the medical association is to contract with the sickness funds to guarantee, in terms of quality and quantity, the provision of ambulatory care to the population. The medical associations review and can sanction member physicians whose practice patterns or billings exceed the norm. The medical associations, hospitals, and sickness funds have representation at the national level.

Financing

Germany's healthcare system operates under a pay-as-you-go financing system. It is not a fully funded system, and it does not accumulate age reserves to compensate for increasing expenditures as the population ages. Contribution rate stability, which links the healthcare budget to the business cycle, is the cornerstone of German health policy. Under this principle, healthcare contributions should not rise faster than the total sum of wages. That is, the goal is to maintain a stable relationship between the growth of health expenditures and the growth in the wages of workers. Coupling sickness funds' expenditures with payroll tax payments accomplishes this objective. As for ambulatory care, the political mandate that increases in health expenditures not be greater than the increase in contributions by workers is fulfilled by extensive use of budgets. In turn, healthcare providers and suppliers' outlays are fixed through budgets.

Germany's financing and delivery structure is shown in Figure 7.1. For the most part, sickness funds are financed by a tax equal to a flat percentage of wages, up to a limit (DEM6,300 per month in 1998), which is adjusted annually. In contrast with more conventional insurance systems, the contribution does not increase when a spouse or dependents are covered. In addition, the size of the contribution depends entirely on the worker's income. Each sickness fund sets its own contribution rate at a level necessary to cover the fund's projected expenditures each year. Rates vary significantly across funds; the range in 1995 was from 9 percent to 15.5 percent in the west, although only a handful of rates are less than 10 percent or more than 14 percent (a risk adjustment system is now in place that will narrow differences in rates among sickness funds). The average contribution rate was 13.2 percent in 1995. This means that an average worker with gross monthly earnings of U.S.$2,000 makes a contribution of U.S.$129 (6.6 percent); the other half (6.6 percent) is paid by the employer.

Table 7.4 shows health insurance coverage by source of payment. About 88 percent of the population (72 million people) obtain coverage from the public sickness funds; about 8 percent and 4 percent obtain coverage through private insurance and central public sources, respectively.

Retired people belong to the social insurance system if, for most of their wage-earning life, they belonged to a sickness fund or were married to someone in this fund. Contributions made on behalf of retirees are equal to the national average contribution; however, this contribution does not cover the full cost of care for retirees because the health expenses of older people are significantly above the average. Reductions in death rates over the last few decades have resulted in greater longevity, which has placed financial stress on the health insurance system. Outlays for retired people are balanced among all funds through a government-sponsored fund to relieve the burden on those sickness funds (and their working members) with a high proportion of retirees.

For employed (earning at least DEM6,300 per month) privately insured people, the premium is also shared with the employer, but only to a maximum equal to the amount the employer would have paid if the person were socially insured. People frequently choose private insurance coverage because the premium cost is less than they would have to contribute to the sickness fund. For example, because private insurance premiums are calculated on a health risk basis rather than income-based criteria, a young, unmarried employee with a relatively high salary may have significantly lower premiums under private coverage than he or she would be required to pay into the sickness fund, thereby reducing both the employee's and the employer's payments.

Hospital Care

Hospital operating costs and capital costs are paid through separate mechanisms, and funding comes from different sources. Hospital capital is supplied by area government funds out of general taxation. Hospital operating budgets are negotiated at the regional level, hospital by hospital, with sickness funds. The sickness funds are obligated to meet hospitals' historic operating costs, and, in turn, hospitals are obligated to provide necessary and economical services. Payments to hospitals are based on a prospective budget negotiated between each hospital and the sickness funds; the Länder then approves all hospital budgets. Budgets are determined through a detailed review of operating costs (about 70,000 items) including drug costs, physicians' salaries, and expected occupancy in conjunction with reviews of comparably efficient hospitals. In addition, recommendations of the hospital association and the guidelines of Concerted Action, an expert advisory board, are also taken into account.

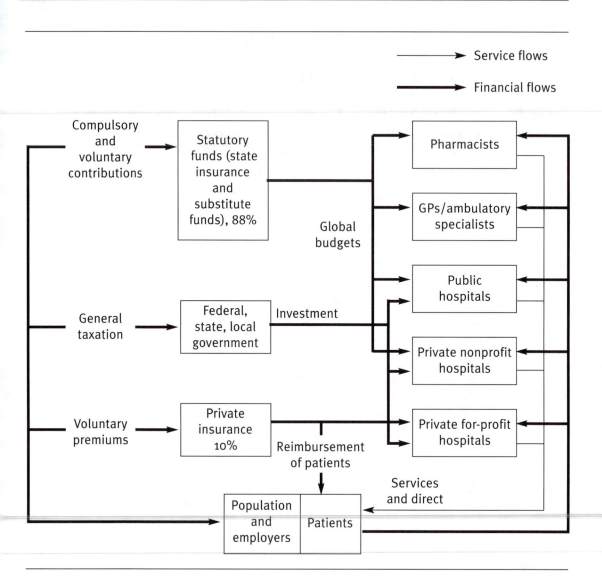

Service flows

Financial flows

FIGURE 7.1
German Service and Financing Flows

Germany's hospital sector has moved from a daily rate system of financing operating costs, which encouraged long hospital stays and high costs, to a mixture of retrospective and prospective remuneration based on costs and prices per case, diagnosis, procedure, or day. The prospective system is based on specific reimbursements and case payment. For additional services or amenities, patients are charged directly. Hospitals claim reimbursement from the sickness funds on the basis of one or a combination of the following reimbursement methods:

- Fallpauschalen payment (per case): Reimbursement is made for the complete treatment of a case relating to a specific diagnosis (including pre- and postoperative care). The reimbursement rate per case is binding for all hospitals within a particular Länder. Should a patient need to stay in the hospital for more than a specific number of days, additional daily payments can be made available. About 60

TABLE 7.4 Insurance Coverage (1996)		
Public mandated insurance		
Number insured (millions)	71.9	
Percentage of total population	87.7	
Private voluntary insurance		
Number insured (millions)	6.9	
Percentage of total population	8.4	
Central publicly funded		
Number of insured (millions)	3	
Percentage of total population	3.7	

SOURCE: Statistisches Bundesamt (1998).

Fallpauschalen treatments are identified, and these include preoperative and postoperative care.

- Sonderentgelte payment (per procedure): Reimbursement is provided for surgeries only. Surgical costs included are specialists' fees, anesthesia, use of the operating room and equipment, and other costs directly relating to the operation. In addition to a procedure payment, the hospital claims a reduced departmental per diem to cover the hospital stay. About 140 different Sonderentgelte procedures have been defined.
- Departmental per diem: With this method, a daily reimbursement rate is paid for all procedures not covered by case and procedure payment. This rate differs from department to department.
- Basic per diem: This provides a reimbursement method for all remaining nonmedical expenses.

Each hospital must project how many of these federal Fallpauschalen and Sonderentgelte will be carried out in a year, as the numbers a hospital can claim are limited. The total sum of money involved with these cases is first deducted from the departmental budget, leaving a remainder. The remainder should cover the treatment of all remaining inpatient days estimated for a year in that department, resulting in an average per diem, which is different for each department. Hospital-based physicians are paid salaries from the hospital budgets. No hospital organizations exist that are comparable to the physicians' organizations described above.

Ambulatory Care

In terms of payment and financing, Germany manages office-based and hospital-based physicians differently. Physicians in independent practice do not usually have hospital privileges; in contrast, hospital physicians do not usually care for ambulatory patients, are salaried, and are normally not allowed to bill patients.

In Germany, all physicians must be members of a regional chamber of physicians to obtain a license to practice medicine; similar organizations also exist for dentists and pharmacists. All office-based physicians can accept privately insured patients, but physicians must be authorized to treat sickness-fund members. Most office-based physicians accept regulation (including standardized fees) and oversight from the sickness funds and the regional associations to be allowed to treat sickness-fund members. In addition to the regional association of sickness-fund physicians, these physicians must also join a chamber of physicians. By law, these associations assume responsibility for providing medical care in each region to all sickness-fund members. They also negotiate fees with the sickness funds, distribute payment to physicians for services, and monitor service use.

The total statutory health insurance system budget for services provided by members of regional associations of sickness-fund physicians is based on a standard allowance for each sickness-fund member in the region. A sickness-fund physician's income is derived from the number of services rendered annually and the level of reimbursement for each service. Reimbursement is determined by the Uniform Evaluation Standard fee schedule, which defines charges for about 2,000 items and determines their relative point value to one another. Along with the physician's own payment, each fee item includes the overhead costs of supporting a practice, costs for single-use items like gloves and syringes, and costs incurred when equipment is used during procedures. In addition, each physician has a separate budget for medical products in his or her specialty such as disinfectants, wound dressings, suture material, and several types of disposable catheters. The Uniform Evaluation Standard fee schedule has three functions:

1. It is the basis upon which a "conversion factor" (a multiplier that converts a number of points allocated to an individual fee item into an amount of money to be paid to the physician) is used to determine the amount to be paid by the sickness funds to physicians for services rendered to patients (historically, this is its most important function).
2. It distributes a budget to physicians.
3. It defines a budget for the total remuneration for all services for all costs of running a medical care practice, including staff salaries, office rental, data processing, and other factors.

In addition to these budgets for services provided by the physician are budgets for prescription drugs and auxiliary items such as physical therapy or eyeglasses.

Cost Sharing

Germans have one of the most comprehensive health insurance benefit programs in the world. According to the health insurance law, sickness-fund benefits include ambulatory, hospital, and preventive care and screening programs; physiotherapeutic, maternity, and preventive care; drugs prescribed by physicians; family planning; rehabilitation; eyeglasses; medical appliances; and dental care, including prostheses. However, as shown in Table 7.5, these benefits are subject to certain cost-sharing requirements.

Health Resources

Germany is generously supplied with both hospitals and physicians (Table 7.6). In fact, the supply of hospital beds and specialty physicians is probably greater than that which can be efficiently deployed. There were 2,325 hospitals in 1996, which resulted in 7.5 beds per 1,000 people. The average length of stay is slightly greater than 12 days. In addition, Germans use the hospital relatively often. There were more than 185 admissions per 1,000 people in 1996 and more than 2,000 hospital days per 1,000 people.

One of the distinguishing features of Germany is its high rate of physician employment and its low rate of health paraprofessional employ-

TABLE 7.5

Cost Sharing in the Statutory Sickness Fund System (1 July 1997)

Benefits/Services	Cost Sharing
1. Drugs	DEM9, DEM11, or DEM13 per drug, depending on the package size
2. Physiotherapy	15 coinsurance
3. Bandages, inserts, compression therapy	20 coinsurance
4. Prostheses, eyeglasses, and hearing aids	No copayment for eyeglasses, hearing aids, and prostheses up to the reference price (100 copayment for eyeglasses frames)
5. Hospital care	DEM17 west/DEM14 east per day for a maximum of 14 days per calendar year
6. Inpatient preventive cures	DEM25 west/DEM20 east per day
7. Maternity rest cures	DEM17 west/DEM14 east per day
8. Rehabilitation that follows medical treatment	DEM17 west/DEM14 east per day for a maximum of 14 days per calendar year (including the copayment rates for in-hospital treatment)
9. Dentures	55% coinsurance
10. Transportation costs	DEM25 copayment per ride

SOURCE: Schneider et al. (1998).

ment. Germany had nearly 280,000 practicing physicians in 1996, which resulted in 3.4 physicians per 1,000 people. Ambulatory care is also used a great deal; in 1996, each insured person made approximately 12 physician visits. Some experts point to a shortage of nurses in the German system, as nurses numbrered only about 4.8 per 1,000 population in 1996. Likewise, a low supply of midwives was found in the same year.

The oversupply of physicians has been one of Germany's most intractable problems. In ambulatory care, physicians have had free access to the system and the right to practice in locations of their choosing. In principle, the license to treat patients who subscribe to the sickness funds is not limited. Access to the medical profession by opening a medical practice is guaranteed by the German constitution. However, as of 1989, measures were implemented to limit the number of ambulatory care physicians. In cooperation with the regional associations of sickness funds, the regional medical associations can close specific geographical areas where a greater than 10 percent excess supply of physicians exists. In each specialty, a maximum physician-to-population ratio is calculated to serve as a baseline on which to determine oversupply in the specialty. Presently, about 60 percent of geographical areas in Germany are closed. In these areas, new physi-

TABLE 7.6
Health Resources and Use (1996)

Inpatient care	
Hospitals (1995)	2,325
Beds per 1,000 population (1995)	7.5
Average length of stay in days (1995)	12.1
Admissions per 1,000 population	185.7
Hospital days per 1,000 population	2,117
Physicians	
Total (thousands)	279
Physicians per 1,000 population	3.4
Ambulatory physician contacts per insured (sickness funds)	12
Nurses	
Total (thousands)	450
Nurses per 1,000 population	4.8
Midwives	
Total (thousands)	74
Midwives per 1,000 population	.09

SOURCE: OECD (2000); Statistisches Bundesamt (1998).

cians wishing to bill the funds must make formal application to assume responsibility for a retiring physician's practice.

Service Delivery

When a patient visits the office of an ambulatory physician, he or she gives the receptionist a health insurance card containing a memory chip. This card stores all relevant administrative data, including the name, address, insurance identification number, and authorization information for services to be paid by the patient's sickness fund. Germany places a high priority on access to healthcare, and, for the most part, the system affords ready access to all medical, hospital, and dental care.

Germans have a free choice of office-based physicians (both general practitioners and specialists) for most medical care. These office-based physicians are well-equipped with medical technology, and virtually all diagnostic and many therapeutic procedures can be performed in an ambulatory setting. In addition, finding a physician specialist in Germany is not difficult because about 60 percent of office-based physicians fit into this category. However, in contrast with ambulatory care, access to a hospital typically requires referral by an office-based physician, and sickness funds normally mandate that these referrals be to the closest suitable hospital.

An important issue in Germany is the separation between ambulatory and hospital care. Ambulatory physicians generally do not treat patients in the hospital, and few physicians employed by the hospital are allowed to see patients after they leave the hospital. (The system tends to duplicate certain specialized healthcare because most medical specialists in office-based practice do not visit patients in hospitals and most hospital-based physicians do not have an office practice.) Three notable exceptions to the division between ambulatory and hospital sectors in healthcare delivery are the following. First, some office-based clinicians (Belegärzte) are allowed to contract with a local hospital to use the hospital's facilities for both inpatient and outpatient treatment of their own patients who are both publicly and privately insured. Second, about 11,000 senior hospital subspecialists (ermächtigte Krankenhausärzte) can obtain permission to provide outpatient services in their hospitals and then pay the hospitals a percentage of their earnings. Third, university medical centers have outpatient departments (polyclinics) that provide ambulatory treatment for the training of medical students and junior physicians.

Prospects for the Future

A great deal was achieved during the last decade, but to translate short-term cost savings into longer term gains, the sickness and private funds must be allowed greater freedom to deal directly with health providers and suppliers. A public debate on improving quality and efficiency is underway; this may result in greater variety and perhaps more competitive choice. The current coalition government of Social Democrats and Greens has pledged to stimulate integration among different provider sectors. They also want to promote cooperation and quality management and reduce overcapacity in the system. The existing German healthcare system will no doubt continue to change. Other major developments that should be realized soon (or are currently being explored) include the following:

- discussion of volume and extension of publicly financed medical services
- implementation of some elements of competition between sickness funds and providers
- incorporation of guidelines for specific diagnostic and therapeutic procedures in hospitals and physicians' offices
- incorporation of benchmarking systems for selected diseases
- improvements in "network" cooperation between physicians' offices and hospitals in a region to reduce hospital referral rates
- definition of measures for cost-effective drug therapy and the organization of 24-hour access to ambulatory services
- change in the monopolistic contracting structure between sickness funds and physician associations to allow contracting between individual providers and sickness funds
- implementation of electronic communication platforms with centralized medical records
- abolishment of the strict separation between inpatient and outpatient treatment by allowing hospitals to organize ambulatory care
- movement away from a fee-for-service system to a case-related or disease-related remuneration system
- development of a "positive list" with recommended and reimbursable selected drugs
- stabilization of wage contributions to sickness funds through the use of global and regional budgets for drugs and hospital services

In Germany, the 1990s were characterized by major efforts to curb the growth of healthcare costs. Providers and suppliers faced increasing burdens as a result of the country's economic restructuring, and the challenges posed by the world economy and the subsequent reduction in healthcare expenditure growth have left their mark, especially on the hospital sector of the healthcare economy.

REFERENCES

Kassenaerztlich Bundesvereinigung. 2000. Grunddaten zur VertragsaerztlichenVersorgung in der Bundesrepublik. Deutschland: Koeln.

Organization of Economic Cooperation and Development (OECD). 2000. *OECD in Figures, 2000 Edition*. Paris: OECD.

OECD. 2000a. *Health Data 2000: A Comparative Analysis of 30 Countries*. Paris: OECD.

Schneider, M., Beckmann, M., Biene-Dietrich, P., Gabanyi, M., Hofmann, U., Koese, A., Mill, D., and Spaeth, B. 1998. *Gesundheitssysteme im internationalen*. Vergleich, Übersichten, Augsburg: BASYS.

Statistisches Bundesamt. 1998. "Gesundheitsbericht fuer Deutschland." Wiesbaden: Statistisches Bundesamt.

ITALY

Laura Marti Dokson Gaydos and Roberto Zanola

Background Information

Italy has been a democratic republic since June 2, 1946, when the monarchy was abolished by popular referendum, and it has a written constitution dating back to 1948. The Italian state is highly centralized, which is evident by the fact that the prefect of each of the 103 provinces is appointed by and answerable to the central government. In addition to the provinces, the constitution provides for 20 regions with limited governing powers. Five regions (Sardinia, Sicily, Trention-Alto Adige, Valle d'Aosta, and Friuli Venezia Giulia) function with special autonomy statutes. More regional autonomy is expected to be introduced as a consequence of a new fiscal federalism law passed in 2000. Under the law, new governing powers will be assigned to regions, and both the quota of national taxes transferred directly to them and the collection of new local taxes will increase correspondingly.

Italy comprises 301,225 square kilometers (116,303 square miles) of mostly mountainous terrain and is about the size of the U.S. states of Georgia and Florida combined, making it relatively large by European standards. Occupying this area is a population of 57.6 million people, of whom the large majority are ethnically Italian, although small ethnic enclaves of German-, French-, Slovene-, and Albanian-Italians are scattered throughout the nation.

Italy is a founding member of the European Union (EU) and shares many of the characteristics of most Western European nations, including a highly developed society with strong health indicators, such as an average life expectancy of 75 years for men and 81.3 for women (WHO 2000). Further demographic information is provided in Table 8.1.

Economy

The Italian economy has changed dramatically since the end of World War II, developing from an agriculture-based economy into a ranking industrial power with approximately the same total and per capita output as France and the United Kingdom. However, despite productivity levels that are higher than the EU average throughout much of the 1990s, real per capita gross domestic product has grown only one percent per year from 1993 through 1998, which is significantly slower than the European average.

TABLE 8.1
General
Demographics

Population in millions	56.9
Infant mortality per 1,000 live births	8
Under-5 mortality per 1,000 live births	6
Life expectancy at birth	74
Fertility rate	0.31
Percent urbanized	67

SOURCE: UNDP (1999).

This capitalist economy is still divided into a developed industrial north dominated by private companies and a lesser-developed agricultural south overspecialized in low-value-added activities. This division between north and south is demonstrated by a high variability in employment rates, with seasonal workers in the south accounting for approximately 30 percent of the overall workforce in industry and services.

Italy has relatively few natural resources. Although it maintains 150,000 square kilometers for farming, the nation is a net food importer. Italy has no substantial deposits of iron, coal, or oil. Natural gas reserves, which are mainly offshore in the Adriatic, have grown in recent years and constitute the nation's most important natural resource. As a result, Italy's economic strength is in the processing and manufacturing of goods, primarily in small and mid-sized family-owned firms. Major industries include precision machinery, motor vehicles, chemicals, pharmaceuticals, electronic goods, and fashion. Italy underwent a substantial privatization program between 1994 and 1999, one of the largest heretofore seen among Organization for Economic Cooperation and Development (OECD) nations. Further economic indicators are provided in Table 8.2.

Education

At present, five years of primary school and three years of secondary education are mandatory, with nearly 100 percent of eligible children attending primary school. This system will change in 2001, expanding to seven years of primary school and two years of secondary school. University requirements will also be reformed to introduce a first-level degree granted after three years of study, followed by a second-level degree after two additional years. The percentage of public expenditure on public education was 9.5 in 1995, one of the lowest rates in the European Union.

The number of individuals attending higher secondary education and university has been increasing steadily throughout the past two decades. However, because of a lack of comparable data, whether this represents a

GNP per capita (U.S.$)	20,170	**TABLE 8.2**
Real GDP per capita	19.363	Economic/
Human Development Index score	0.921	Social
Percent of GNP given to health	8.45	Indicators
Percent of health budget in public sector	70	

SOURCE: UNICEF (2000); UNDP (1999); Mossialos and LeGrand (1998).

real increase or only reflects larger birth cohorts is unclear. The percentages of men and women in higher education are identical.

As is found in many Western European nations, approximately 74 percent of students in upper secondary education are in vocational programs (Eurostat 1995), which indicates a willingness to train the majority of citizens in nonacademic fields. Table 8.3 shows further details about educational levels in Italy.

Context: Health Needs

Health Status

Overall health status in Italy is quite high, with indicators generally near the European average. As expected in a highly developed nation, access to basic necessities and health-enhancing factors is openly available. Specific indicators are shown in Table 8.4.

However, a comparison of the population's health status with 18 EU reference nations shows that, despite improvements in both absolute and relative terms during the 1980s and 1990s, Italy's position remained at or below average for several key indicators (WHO Europe 1998). The infant mortality rate remained one of the highest in the EU, despite the second largest reduction among nations surveyed (from 8.2 per 1,000 live births in 1990 to 5.3 per 1,000 live births in 1998); standardized death rates (SDRs) for all cancers in people up to 64 years old and for lung can-

Adult literacy rate	98%	**TABLE 8.3**
Primary school enrollment	99%	Education
Secondary school enrollment	81.4%	Indicators

SOURCE: ISTAT (1999).

Access to health services	99%
Access to safe water	99%
Access to sanitation	99%
Immunization levels	95%

TABLE 8.4
Access to
Health-
Enhancing
Factors

SOURCE: UNDP (1999).

cer specifically remain substantially higher than EU averages. Italy's position among the EU reference countries for deaths due to external causes (e.g., accidents, violence, poisoning) slipped, although it remained lower than that of a number of countries. The SDR for all external causes is lower than the EU average; the specific SDR for traffic accidents is above average, whereas the SDR for suicide is the second lowest in the EU (WHO Europe 1998).

In 2000, WHO assessed how health systems in WHO member states achieve primary health goals including risk sharing; financial protection; fairness in financial contribution; and respect for people's dignity, autonomy, and confidentiality of information. The overall attainment indicator calculated for each country ranked Italy second, although a 1998 EU study indicates that only 16.3 percent of adults were satisfied with the Italian National Health System (INHS); 59.4 percent reported being unsatisfied.

Leading Causes of Mortality

Noncommunicable diseases including cardiovascular diseases, cancers, chronic obstructive pulmonary disorders, and mental health disorders represent the greatest burden of mortality and morbidity within the EU as a whole and also within Italy. Cancers are the most frequent cause of death for people less than 65 years old, followed by cardiovascular disease (CVD). However, CVD is the leading cause of death across all age groups, accounting for 43.7 percent of all deaths. A more detailed analysis of age-specific mortality patterns shows that the causes of up to 80 percent of all deaths in each age group can be classified in three main categories: accidental or other injuries are the primary causes until age 35, then cancers, then CVD (WHO Europe 1998). According to the nine Italian cancer registries, cancer incidence varies widely across the regions; the highest rates occur in the north/central-eastern areas for both men and women and the lowest rates in the southern areas (Ministry of Health 1994).

The most striking feature of Italian age- and sex-specific death rates is the difference between male and female mortality in the population between the ages of 15 and 64 years: the male death rate is more than three times higher than the female rate for people between 15 and 34 years of age, and it is more than twice as high in people between the ages of 35 and 64 years. The analysis of age-specific mortality patterns shows that some potential for reducing mortality lies in the prevention of cancers at all ages, accidents in the younger population, and CVD in older people. Notably, however, a marked decrease has occurred in all three primary causes of mortality since 1970; the decreases correspond with similar statistics for all EU nations (WHO Europe 1998).

External Causes of Death and Injury

This category covers all deaths not due to illness and primarily refers to accidents, accidental poisoning, violent acts (homicide), and suicide. The trend throughout the EU and in Italy has been a consistent reduction the these types of deaths. However, in Italy, deaths due to automobile accidents are more frequent than the EU average, especially for males. By contrast, the risk of being injured in such an accident is somewhat lower than the EU average, with 6,226 automobile deaths and 270,962 injuries in 1997. During the last ten years, male homicide rates were among the highest in the EU; Italy had the second highest homicide rate in Europe during the early 1990s (ISTAT 1995).

AIDS

The numbers of AIDS cases are rising in all of the northern and western European countries, and Italy is no exception. Taking into account reporting delays, Italy had an incidence rate of 9.6 cases per 100,000 people in 1994, the third highest rate in the EU. The majority of cases are estimated to have been contracted through the sharing of infected syringes.

Disability

The prevalence of long-term illness and disability is an important measure of a population's health-related quality of life. A comparative study of EU countries using national disability pension records found that 10.3 percent of the Italian population suffered from disabilities that resulted in a handicap in social or socioeconomic terms; the average is 11.5 percent for the EU (Eurostat 1995a). The distribution of disabilities varies as a function of geographical and sociodemographic criteria. According to a 1995 ISTAT survey, disabilities are most frequent in the southern part of Italy (7.4 percent); the rates are somewhat lower in the center (6.5 percent), the northeast (5.3 percent), and the northwest (5.1 percent). (The ISTAT survey estimates a much lower disability rate than the Eurostat findings above.)

Arthritis is the most frequent chronic degenerative disease, with a prevalence of 14 percent in the population that is more than 60 years old, followed by hypertension, bronchitis/emphysema and respiratory insufficiency, mental health problems, and diabetes. Table 8.5 shows causes of morbidity and mortality in Italy.

TABLE 8.5

Mortality and
Morbidity
Measures

Leading Causes of Mortality (percent of death per 100,000 population)

	1991	1992	1993	1994	1995
Infectious diseases	0.3	0.4	0.4	0.4	0.5
Cancer	27.2	27.7	27.9	28.1	27.7
Mental disorders and diseases of the five senses	2.8	3.0	3.0	3.2	3.4
Cardiovascular diseases	43.6	43.4	43.8	43.6	43.7
Respiratory diseases	6.1	6.0	5.8	6.1	6.1
Digestive tract diseases	5.1	5.0	5.1	5.1	4.8
Other diseases	7.1	7.1	6.8	6.8	7.3
Other not-well-defined diseases	2.2	2.1	2.0	1.7	1.5
Accidental or other injuries	5.5	5.4	5.1	5.0	5.0

Leading Causes of Morbidity, 1993–97

	1993	1994	1995	1996	1997	Northern-central	Southern	Italy Overall
Diabetes	3.4	3.4	3.4	3.4	3.4	3.1	4.3	3.5
Hypertension	10.0	9.7	10.2	10.3	10.1	10.7	9.7	10.3
Bronchitis	7.4	6.9	6.9	6.9	6.3	5.8	6.5	6.0
Arthritis/ arthrosis	20.5	19.7	20.3	20.6	19.3	17.7	17.9	17.8
Osteoporosis	4.6	4.6	4.8	5.2	5.2	5.2	4.8	5.0
Cardiovascular diseases	3.7	4.0	3.8	3.8	3.7	3.8	3.3	3.7
Allergy	6.8	6.3	6.8	7.2	7.1	7.4	5.2	6.6
Mental disorders	5.1	5.2	4.9	4.9	4.4	3.7	4.1	3.8
Duodenal and gastric ulcer	3.8	4.0	3.9	3.9	3.5	3.1	2.9	3.0

SOURCE: CENSIS (1999); ISTAT (1995).

Aging

Although Italy had one of the highest fertility rates in the 1960s, it currently has the lowest of all OECD countries. Furthermore, Italy has one of the highest life expectancies as compared with other OECD countries. These circumstances have resulted in a large and growing elderly population with specific geriatric health needs that must be addressed.

Policymakers have been conscious of this issue since 1992, when the government introduced a plan for the protection of the health of the elderly. More recently, the 1999–2000 National Health Plan focused attention on finding the best balance between needs and costs of chronic care, with options varying from home help to hospitalized intensive care.

Organization and Management of the Health System

The Three INHS Reforms

The INHS, which is a compulsory social insurance plan, was first reformed in 1978 to provide comprehensive health insurance coverage and uniform health benefits for all citizens and legal residents. The transition to a universal system was motivated by the fundamental belief that health services should be made available to everyone on the basis of need, with no differentiation or discrimination among citizens and no barriers at the point of use (Mossialos and Le Grand 1999).

One goal of the health system reform was to involve the different tiers of government in managing health services. In particular, three different organization levels were identified:

1. The Ministry of Health is responsible for planning, budgeting, and general administration. The Ministry has the responsibility of monitoring, supporting, and assessing the fulfillment of health objectives, and it serves as a guide for the uniform implementation of prevention and care services throughout the nation to ensure equitable access to the INHS.
2. Twenty Regional Health Authorities are responsible for delivering services and ensuring the provision of healthcare to all citizens in their jurisdictions.
3. Local health units are responsible for the daily management of health services and for coordination between hospitals. The 659 local health units are also in charge of the delivery of primary care services, including contacts with general practitioners, occupational health services, health education, disease prevention, pharmacies, family advice, child health, and information services (Mossialos and Le Grand 1999).

Although public healthcare expenditures only grew from 5.2 percent of gross domestic product in 1978 to 6.5 percent in 1992, the need to reduce and rationalize public expenditure has driven the central government to reform healthcare provision once more. In 1992, a second reform was introduced, and its effects were evident by 1995. The key outcomes of the reform included the following:

- separation of the purchasing and providing functions through the creation of 228 Aziende Sanitarie Locali (ASLs) (the purchasers) and Aziende Ospedale (AOs) (the providers)
- implementation of regional budget limitations within which ASLs must function, although they retain full autonomy in organization, administration, financing, accounting, and management
- formation of the Council of Health Professionals, a new health authority that represents physicians and other health professionals; the general manager of each ASL must consult the Council for major health decisions, but it has no legally binding power
- replacement of a payment-per-bed-day system of hospital reimbursement with a prospective payment system based on diagnosis-related groups (Bevan, France, and Taroni 1992)
- replacement of the payroll tax with the regionally imposed Imposta Regionale Attività Produttive, thereby granting regional governments more autonomy

The huge deficit, the still-unsatisfactory and unequal quality of healthcare services, and the limited application of the new system of healthcare delivery necessitated the introduction of a third INHS reform aimed at improving healthcare quality and efficiency through the implementation of new rules (Lorenzini and Petretto 2000). Some of these new rules, in particular, are as follows:

- Regions may now decide the quantity and mix of health services to be provided and are constrained only by a federally mandated minimum level of coverage.
- Public physicians and medical institutions are now subject to a system of "quality certification." In short, the system supports two types of providers: accredited producers, which include both public and private hospitals that sell their services to regions, and nonaccredited producers, which are designated private hospitals that serve only private clients.
- A new form of financing, INHS Integrative Funds, has been implemented to pay for previously uncovered costs of specialty services from accredited facilities.
- Physicians in public hospitals are now required to choose between private, freelance practice and an exclusive relationship with the INHS.

Financing

The health budget is determined centrally, and it is partially financed by employer and employee contributions, with the government paying the balance directly. Funds are allocated to regions according to a formula that considers the type of expenditure and population structure of the region, with adjustments for regional supply and demand factors. The formula has been revised several times since its initial implementation in 1979.

Ambulatory and outpatient hospital services are paid for on the basis of a diagnosis-related-group-type system. Hospital services are usually free at the point of usage, but patients are responsible for a portion of the cost of such nonhospital services as dental care, pharmaceuticals, and diagnostic examinations. Notably, essential drugs are free, and so are most drugs for indigent patients. Fee scales for nonessential drugs are based on average prices in Germany, Spain, France, and the United Kingdom and also on a reference price system (Mossialos and Le Grand 1999).

The INHS is financed through the National Health Fund, which is determined annually as part of the government budget and distributed to the regions for allocation to local health units. As of 1995, the majority of funding (64.6 percent) for the INHS came from general taxation; another 31.2 percent came directly from user copayments, including direct payments to providers. Less than 3 percent of financing came from voluntary health insurance or other private means (Mossialos and Le Grand 1999).

Collection of financial resources for the INHS remains a national responsibility, and each region receives funding on the basis of the resident population. The national level of government also defines a set of basic services to be provided throughout the country. Officials at the regional level plan healthcare activities and organize services in relation to the needs of the population. Each region is accountable to the national tier for providing the designated basic services. Regions are also financially accountable and are responsible for covering any deficit incurred during the medical treatment of their population. Each region allocates to all the agencies within its territory a part of the National Health Fund budget that has transferred from the Ministry of Health using two criteria: historical need and patient mobility across regions.

The Private Sector

In addition to the INHS, the private sector accounts for 20 percent of total health expenditures. People wishing to use private facilities must obtain private insurance in addition to their obligatory INHS contributions. Private service providers may also contract with the public sector to provide services within public institutions; citizens may then use these contracted private services as they would other public services. The private sector provides services not available under the INHS for those who can afford to pay, and it may also relieve pressure on the public sector when waiting lists become too long. Nationwide, approximately 16 percent of the population has private insurance, and, correspondingly, about 16 percent of hospital beds are private. However, the prevalence of private hospitals varies greatly among regions (Bevan, France, and Taroni 1992).

Health Resources

The Italian health system suffers an imbalance in available providers, with too many general practitioners and a relative scarcity of community nurses, social workers, and hospital nurses, especially in public hospitals. In 1997, about 480,000 people were employed in local health agencies throughout Italy; of these, approximately 65 percent were physicians, dentists, or nurses. An additional 302,000 people were employed in hospitals or similar institutions, and there was an average physician-to-nurse ratio of 2.63. Tables 8.6 and 8.7 offer further details on human resources and facilities in the INHS.

Medical training requires three years of post-high-school study for nurses, five years for a degree in dentistry, and six for a degree in medicine. Physician specialization requires an average of four years after the medical degree has been obtained, with the exception of general practice, for which only one year is required. However, anticipated changes in the university system are likely to mean that both physician and dental degrees will soon require five years of additional study.

Although data suggest that the total numbers of beds and doctors per capita are reasonably distributed across the country, areas in the southern part of Italy may be less well endowed.

Service Delivery

In Italy, healthcare services are provided through a combination of public and private hospitals and specialists, general practitioners (GPs), and pharmacies.

Primary Healthcare

Primary healthcare includes diagnosis, treatment, and first-level rehabilitation together with prevention, health promotion, and education activities. Primary healthcare is generally provided by GPs, including GP pediatricians, on-call services, pharmacies, and home caregivers. Some services generally considered primary care in other nations fall under specialist services under the INHS, including clinics and laboratories, family planning clinics, addiction and rehabilitation services, departments for mental health, and physical rehabilitation treatment centers.

All patients are registered with a GP who acts as a gatekeeper to specialist services. GPs contract with ASLs and are paid on a capitation basis. By law, GPs are restricted to patient lists of 1,500 to 1,800 people. Patients

Physicians	97,659
Dentists	171
Teaching and organization staff	1,773
Medical-technical staff	31,071
Control staff	8,457
Rehabilitation staff	16,680
Druggists	2,246
Veterinarians	5,471
Biologists	4,195
Chemists	1,102
Physicists	346
Psychologists	5,743
Nurses	252,163
Professional staff	1,498
Technical staff	152,022
Administrative staff	69,356
Atypical qualification	941

SOURCE: Ministry of Health (1997).

TABLE 8.6
Human Resources and Facilities in the Public Sector, 1997

are registered with individual physicians rather than offices or practices, and GPs typically work alone, although some physicians share offices and resources. Important geographical variations occur in the size of GPs' lists and the availability of their services, especially where pediatricians are concerned, with smaller physician-to-population ratios in the south.

GPs have a statutory duty to provide preventive services; however, in actuality, very few preventive activities are performed. GPs tend to limit themselves to providing very basic medical care, prescribing drugs, ordering diagnostic tests, and hospitalizing patients (WHO European Region 1998). Children who are less than 12 years old are cared for by GP pediatricians, who are GPs with a postgraduate degree in child health. GP services are free at the point of use. However, patients often bypass GPs and go directly to hospital emergency departments in an effort to avoid long waiting lists and charges for pharmaceuticals. A Guardia Medica, consisting of approximately 18,000 physicians, provides after-hours care and services for nonregistered patients at the local health (Unita Sanitaria Locale [USL]) level. Doctors working in the Guardia Medica are not allowed to take extra contracts; physicians in the Guardia Medica are typically young doctors trying to gain experience (McCarthy 1992).

TABLE 8.7
Hospital
Human
Resources,
1997

Physicians per 1,000 population	2.0
Nurses	4.8
Graduate and technical staff	13.5
Social assistance and religious staff	28.2
Other technical staff	12.2

SOURCE: ISTAT (1999).

Public Health Nurses

Public health nurses have the specific duties of safeguarding the health of individuals through public health preventive activities and health education. These nurses try to establish relationships with people in their daily lives and work using such methods as interviews, home visits, and epidemiological investigations. Immunization centers, infectious disease prevention, and school health are a few areas in which public health nurses may focus their resources.

Additionally, about 3,000 occupational health nurses (registered general nurses with in-service training by physicians) administer first aid, provide health education, compile elementary statistics and epidemiology, and conduct common tests (WHO 1995).

Secondary and Hospital Care

The INHS guarantees hospital admission for ailments that cannot be treated in the home or on an outpatient basis as well as treatment in necessary outpatient hospital programs. Hospitals provide inpatient care for one or several specialties, with some laboratory facilities and possibly outpatient care. Hospitals may be public or private. Private facilities may choose whether to contract directly with the INHS; in this case, they must be accredited. Public hospitals are directly managed by the ASLs and financed by a global budget.

The Ministry of Health expects a general hospital to include at least four basic services: general medicine, surgery, pediatrics, and gynecology and obstetrics. Mental health is managed through integrated psychiatric and general healthcare services in hospitals; day hospitals and some mental hygiene centers are also available. Outpatient care is also provided in polyclinics by salaried or contracted specialists and in clinics where specialists see patients for personal (usually ambulatory) consultations.

Care in institutions contracted by the ASLs is free with a GP referral. Patient choice is respected, and as a result, important cross-border flows occur among regions, although most regions maintain at least one general hospital. Private specialists can see patients either privately or through contracts with the INHS.

Community Pharmacies

Pharmacies have the monopoly on drug sales, but they are subject to numerous regulations. Pharmacies may be privately owned and maintain a contract with a USL or belong to a hospital or a local government in which the pharmacists are salaried employees.

Prospects for the Future

In spite of the many improvements in the INHS since the 1992 transformation, the Italian National Health Service still requires many changes, and there is room for improvement.

One of the most important concerns is the need to comply with the financial constraints of the national economic recovery plan, which mandates that all programs must improve their efficiency. Fiscal federalism reform, which was passed on March 15, 2000, was designed to strengthen regional responsibility. However, many scholars complain that the reforms do not prevent future regional revenue shortfalls and therefore will need to be compensated by the central government. In fact, although health services are delegated to the regional governments, the central government maintains the determination of "essential services" to be supplied by regions. Hence, an issue for the future is to introduce full fiscal responsibility on the expenditure side by allowing each region to plan health expenditures and services to be provided; this move, however, would be an abandonment of the central government's goal of providing equal essential health services throughout the country (Reviglio 2000).

A second issue for the future is a consequence of the aging of the population. In 1961, 9.5 percent of the Italian population was more than 65 years old; in 1996, 16.8 percent of the population was in this age group, and the upward trend is expected to continue. In fact, a significant increase in the over-65 population is expected to occur during the next 20 years, with the most rapidly growing segment of the population being people over the age of 80 years.

The growth in the elderly population requires that the INHS prepare to provide services for the elderly at a greater level, including long-term-care services, which are currently severely lacking. The 1998–2000 Italian National Health Plan (INHP) recognized the importance of balancing needs and costs. The development of a broader range of social and medical services for the elderly needs to be encouraged for as long as possible, but the availability of these services must be understood to be limited by economic constraints. This may be resolved by requiring the elderly to pay for some of these services, financial circumstances allowing (OECD 2000).

In addition to economic constraints and an aging population, some additional priorities for the INHS at the beginning of the twenty-first century are outlined in the 1998–2000 INHP. These include strengthening the health service user's decision-making autonomy, promoting the appropriate use of healthcare services, overcoming health inequities, fostering healthy lifestyles and attitudes, combating major diseases, helping patients to actively cope with chronic illness, finalizing the social-health integration process, promoting research, and investing in human resources and quality control.

The complete implementation of the 1998–2000 INHP will require a stable majority in the Parliament. If the outcome of the spring 2001 elections is as predicted, many of the 1998–2000 INHP priorities are expected to be implemented.

REFERENCES

Basch, P. F. 1999. *Textbook of International Health*. Oxford: Oxford University Press.

Bevan, G., France, G., and Taroni, F. 1992. "Dolce Vita: Health Care in Italy." *Health Services* 102 (5291): 20–23.

CENSIS. 1999. *Rapporto Annuale sulla Situazione Sociale del Paese*. Retrieved 06 February 2001 from www.censis.it.

Eurostat. 1995. *Eurostat Yearbook '95*. Luxembourg: Office for Official Publications of the European Communities.

———. 1995a. *Disabled Persons. Statistical Data*. 2nd ed. Luxembourg: Office for Official Publications of the European Communities.

ISTAT. 1995. *The Disabled. Anni 1987–91*. Rome: National Institute of Statistics.

———. 1999. *Compendio Statistico Italiano*. Retrieved 03 March 2001 from www.assofibre.federchimica.it/compend.htm.

———. 2001 *Stili di Vita e Condizioni di Salute—Anno 2000*. Rome: Collana Informazioni.

Levaggi, R., and Zanola, R. 2000. "The Flypaper Effects. Evidence from Italy." University of Eastern Piedmont, Working Paper Series, no. 11.

Lorenzini, S., and Petretto, A. 2000. "Il Finanziamento Pubblico della Sanità in una Prospettiva di Federalismo Fiscale." In *I Servizi Sanitari in Italia*, edited by G. Fiorentni. Bologna: Il Mulino.

McCarthy, M. 1992. *Evolution and Implementation of the Italian Health Service Reform of 1978*. London: Chadwick Press.

Ministry of Health. 1997. *Personale delle U.S.L. e degli Istituti di Cura Pubblici*. Rome: Ministry of Health.

Ministry of Health Italy. 1994. "Italy's Report to the WHO Regional Office for Europe on the 1994 Health for All Monitoring Exercise." Unpublished report.

Mossialos, E., and Le Grand, J. 1999. *Health Care and Cost Containment in the EU*. Burlington: Ashgate Publishing.

Muraro, G. 2000. "Sanità e federalismo fiscale." *Politiche Sanitarie* 1 (1): 17–24.

Organization for Economic Cooperation and Development. *OECD Health Data 1997.* CD-ROM. Washington, DC: OECD.

Reviglio, F. 2000. "Health Care and Its Financing in Italy: Issues and Reform Options." International Monetary Fund Working Paper, no. 166. Retrieved 24 March 2001 from www.imf.org.

UNICEF. 2000. "The State of the World's Children 2000." Retrieved 05 June 2000 from www.unicef.org.

U.S. Department of State, Bureau of European Affairs. 1999. "Background Notes: Italy." Retrieved 11 June 2000 from www.state.gov.

World Health Organization. 2000. "Health in Italy in the 21st Century." Retrieved 20 July 2000 from www.who.it.

———. 2000. "The World Health Report 2000." Retrieved July 2000 from www.who.org.

World Health Organization Regional Office for Europe. 1998. "Highlights on Health in Italy." Retrieved 14 July 2000 from www.euro.who.int.

Zanola, R. 1998. "Il Trasferimento del Fondo Sanitario Nazionale alle Regioni: Un'Analisi Critica." *Economia Pubblica* 28 (6): 91–113.

FRANCE

Julia Field Costich

Background Information

The World Health Organization recently ranked the French healthcare system first in the world for overall performance (WHO 2000). Universal coverage, a fee-for-service system in which the majority of costs are reimbursed, free access for low-income and disabled people, and free choice of physician would seem to describe a medical utopia. Not surprisingly, the French people are more positive about their healthcare system than most other Europeans, with two-thirds responding to a 1997 survey that they are "fairly satisfied" or "very satisfied" as compared with 40 percent of Britons and less than 20 percent of Italians (Mossialos 1997).

However, an undercurrent of concern persists in French analyses of their healthcare system: expenditures, although modest by U.S. standards, far exceed norms for developed countries; out-of-pocket costs are high for those who are required to pay them; quality is variable and poorly monitored; and striking disparities in health status persist across regions and socioeconomic groups. Furthermore, rapid growth in the ratio of dependent elders to working adults will require major expansions in long-term care and home health services, two areas in which the system is already deficient.

At times, the French healthcare system has given the impression of lurching from one scandal or crisis to the next. In 1991, revelations about the failure of high officials to take adequate precautions against HIV transmission in the blood supply led to resignations, arrests, and convictions over the ensuing six years (Breo 1991; Dorozynski 1999). Recurring fears of exposure to bovine spongiform encephalopathy (mad cow disease) since 1996 have suppressed the traditional French affinity for beef and attracted much media attention despite an extremely low incidence of food-based human transmission. Vehement opposition to genetically modified foods—characterized by opponents as "Frankenfoods"—inspired wry comments by American observers about European hostility to scientific advances (Paarlberg 2000).

Despite these shortcomings, the fundamental principle of solidarity across the population makes the French healthcare system exemplary in its attention to the needs of vulnerable populations and those with chronic conditions.

Government

France is a parliamentary republic whose president is elected by direct universal suffrage for a term of seven years. The lower house of the bicameral parliament, called the National Assembly, is elected by direct suffrage, and the Senate is elected by indirect vote. The country is divided into 22 regions and 100 departments, but the health-related activities of lower levels of government are limited to traditional preventive public health functions.

History

The wars and revolutions that have punctuated French history have left their mark on the contemporary French healthcare system. French healthcare policy has been shaped by the same political forces that have given birth to the French republic: the coexistence of pro- and anti-government sentiments, dramatic governmental action following major upheavals, and the emphasis on social solidarity as justification for redistributive social welfare initiatives have all played a role in the design of French health policy.

The legacy of the 1789 French Revolution and subsequent swings toward and away from monarchy have demonstrated a persistent tension between classic liberalism, with its suspicious attitude toward governmental intervention, and the impulse toward a highly centralized structure that characterizes French government in general. The devastation wrought by World Wars I and II precipitated a national emergency and forced change in the healthcare system. Thus, the configuration of contemporary French healthcare originates in actions taken in 1945. The need for social solidarity (again to some extent the legacy of both overt, revolutionary class warfare and the national shame of the Vichy government during World War II) has also shaped the contemporary French healthcare system.

France has made important contributions to public health and medicine, including those of eight Nobel Prize winners in the twentieth century. The most celebrated French contribution to medical science is undoubtedly Louis Pasteur's work in food safety, which culminated in the 1880s. Pasteur's achievements helped public health practice move from the containment approach to disease control and toward more positive, targeted interventions. More recently, France's Luc Montagnier shares credit with U.S. scientists for identifying the human immunodeficiency virus.

Socioeconomic Indicators

France is one of the world's wealthiest countries, with a 1997 gross domestic product of U.S.$23,843 per capita (U.S.$22,465 per capita using the constant purchasing power parity model) (UN 2000). About two-thirds of employed French people work in the service sector, and most of the balance work in industry; only 2.6 percent of the total labor force are farmers or farmworkers. The unemployment rate in the first quarter of 2001 was 8.8 percent (Anonymous 2001), reflecting a persistent French problem, particularly among young women and North African immigrants (WHO/ROE 1997). Unemployed French people are provided with a safety net of comprehensive benefits including family allowances and healthcare coverage. French workers have a guaranteed minimum wage (*salaire minimum interprofessionel de croissance*) of approximately U.S.$5.60 per hour, which is about U.S.$950 per month. A well-known feature of French working life is the statutory entitlement to five weeks of paid vacation per year.

Despite France's reputation for frequent strikes, only 8 percent of the working population belong to unions, the lowest proportion of any European Union country. However, physician associations (*syndicats*) continue to wield great influence in the healthcare system. Additional economic indicators are provided in Table 9.1.

Population Trends

The French population of 59.2 million is growing only because of immigration and increased longevity; at 1.73, the French fertility rate is well below replacement levels. The over-65 population is projected to increase from the 2000 figure of 15.9 percent to some 20.1 percent of the total population by 2020 (Anderson and Hussey 1999). French health authorities are formulating plans to deal with the effects of this rapid growth in tandem with the low fertility rate.

The French territorial "hexagon," as it is commonly called, covers 551,000 square kilometers of diverse terrain, from the marshes of the southwestern Camargue to the Alps in the east. Population is increasingly concentrated in large and mid-size cities, and many small villages survive only by attracting tourism and vacation homebuyers.

TABLE 9.1
Selected Employment and Economic Indicators, France, 2000

Total labor force, thousands	23,529
Unemployment rate	
Percent of total labor force	9.9
Percent under 25 years old	17.9
GDP	
Total in billions U.S.$ at 1999 exchange rates	1,435,629
Per person in P.P.P.$	22,465
Health spending	
Share total in GDP (percent)	7.2
Share public in GDP (percent)	9.4

SOURCE: INSEE (2001); OECD Databank (2001).

The French are a well-educated people: 75 percent of 25 to 29 year olds and 60 percent of the total adult population have completed secondary school. France spends 7.2 percent of its gross domestic product on education (U.S.$5,104 per student). Additional demographic data are available in Table 9.2.

Context: Health Needs

Major Health Problems

The World Health Organization assesses health status and systems in 18 European reference countries: the 15 European Union countries plus Iceland, Norway, and Switzerland. In this context, although notable progress

TABLE 9.2
Selected Demographic and Education Data, France, 1998

Total metropolitan area (square kilometers)		544
Population		
Population in millions		58.5
Population per square kilometer		108
Population growth rate, 1990–99 (percent)		3.14
Age structure of population (percent of total population)		
Under 20		25.7
20 to 59		53.9
60 and over		20.4
Life expectancy (years)	Female	Male
At birth	82.2	74.6
At age 40	43.5	36.7
At age 60	25.2	20.0
Infant mortality per 1,000 live births		5.5
Total fertility rate		1.73
Education		
Population with at least upper-secondary education	63% male,	56% female
Public and private expenditure on educational institutions (percent of GDP)		7.2

SOURCE: OECD Databook (2001); INSEE (2001).

has been made in several areas, France still has high rates of cancer (particularly lung cancer in men) and suicide (particularly in men), and significant health disparities along socioeconomic and geographic gradients remain. Life expectancy for French women is the highest in Europe and second only to Japan worldwide. For men, life expectancy is at the European average. Disability-free years gained over the past two decades have exceeded the number of life-years gained; that is, the health-related quality of life has improved even beyond increased average longevity.

For the French population as a whole, the leading causes of death are cardiovascular diseases (CVD), cancers, and external causes of death (accident, suicide, and other injuries), as shown in Table 9.3. CVD is heavily concentrated in the over-65 population; for French men under 65, external causes rank first. Male death rates significantly exceed female rates at all ages and are nearly triple the female rates in the 15- to 34-year-old age group; again, this is overwhelmingly attributable to causes other than disease.

	Deaths per 100,000	Years of Productive Life Lost per 100,000		
		Male	Female	All
Diseases of circulatory system	181.6	807.5	270.6	535.2
Neoplasms	191.9	1,702.4	914.8	1,302.1
Diseases of respiratory system	43.6	177.7	78.4	127.3
Diseases of digestive system	33.4	335.8	153.3	243.5
Endocrine and metabolic diseases	20.5	346.5	123.4	234.5
Diseases of nervous system	15.2	159.5	104.5	132.0
Mental and behavioral disorders	14.3	160.7	42.9	101.6
Diseases of genitourinary system	7.4	23.8	13.7	18.7
Infectious and parasitic diseases	8.4	72.4	37.5	54.9
Diseases of musculoskeletal system	2.7	8.8	9.3	9.0
Diseases of blood and immune system	3.0	19.1	11.9	15.5
External causes (injury, poisoning)	60.8	1,196.6	1,781.7	606.8
Motor vehicle accident	12.5	586.0	198.4	393.8
Suicide	17.8	580.9	194.7	387.9
Homicide	1.0	41.5	25.8	33.7

TABLE 9.3
Causes of Mortality, France

SOURCE: OECD Health Data (2000).

The proportion of France's population that is more than 15 years old and smokes cigarettes is the second highest in Europe at 35 percent (EC 2000). Among young people between the ages of 15 and 24 years, a majority (54.5 percent) smokes cigarettes, including 58.3 percent of young women. Excess cardiovascular and lung cancer mortality related to the high rate of smoking in France has given rise to sporadic public health initiatives, none of which approach the zeal of the U.S. public health community for tobacco use prevention and cessation. The traditional French reluctance to limit lifestyle choice appears to influence the government's relative inaction in this area.

Data about mental health are much less accessible than those describing physical health. French suicide rates are among the highest in Europe, ranking third for men and fifth for women. In a 1994 survey, 11.2 percent of respondents reported having taken psychotropic medication for at least six months (Service des statistiques 1994); it is impossible to determine whether this figure is attributable to a high level of psychological distress or excessive prescription drug use.

French HIV/AIDS prevalence is second only to that of Spain among European nations (UN/WHO 2000). A recent report estimates that 130,000 residents of France were living with HIV/AIDS at the end of 1999 (adult rate: 0.43 percent) and that 39,000 had died of AIDS since the epidemic began; the current death rate is approximately 2,000 per year. HIV-infected people are disproportionately male (72 percent), reside in the Paris area or the southeast, and are usually infected through same-sex activity or injection drug use. The French dedication to medical privacy (*le secret professionel*) has meant that HIV testing has remained anonymous and voluntary. Clinicians who provide prenatal care are required to offer HIV testing to all pregnant women; seroprevalence among pregnant women who gave birth is estimated at 2.1 to 2.8 per thousand.

Child and adolescent healthcare in France is generally excellent by both EU and U.S. standards, with an infant mortality rate of 5.5 per 1,000 live births and immunization rates against diphtheria, pertussis, tetanus, and poliomyelitis of 95 percent. Immunization against measles, mumps, and rubella has increased to 80 percent for six year olds, with measles immunizations taking hold after an alarming 1989 peak incidence of 823 measles cases per 100,000.

French women's health is better overall than that of French men as evidenced by the striking mean longevity for women (82 years) and their avoidance of excess premature mortality. The extreme male-female disparities in causes of death and years of productive life lost include rates among males of diseases of the circulatory and respiratory systems, endocrine and metabolic diseases, mental and behavioral disorders, motor vehicle accidents, falls, and suicides that are more than double those for women.

French teen birth rates are relatively low at 8.7 per 1,000. This figure reflects widespread access to contraception and a high abortion rate;

the High Commission for Public Health reports that two-thirds of conceptions in women under the age of 18 resulted in abortion (HCSP 1999).

Organization and Management of the Health System

Any analysis of the French healthcare system must first acknowledge its context in the broader national system of social security. The principle of social solidarity, which is a legacy of both the French Revolution and postwar response to the divisive Vichy era, governs a wide array of benefits including unemployment, subsidies for families with children, maternity benefits, disability and retirement income support, compensation for workplace injuries, and survivor benefits (see generally Dupeyroux 1998; Prétot and Dupeyroux 2000). Although most French have access to all these benefits, the classification of funding sources by occupational category means that some groups (notably the self-employed and those who are not part of the workforce such as full-time homemakers without working spouses) have less comprehensive protection. Because healthcare is integrated with a comprehensive social welfare system, patients and families can avoid the coordination problems associated with the United States' separation of funding for healthcare from that of social services and education.

The French healthcare system is made up of a complex array of agencies, representative bodies, and regulatory regimes. The national government has primary control and responsibility for regulating the activities of healthcare organizations and plays an important—albeit limited—role in the direct provision of care.

The national government is responsible for regulating the following:

- financing, coverage, reimbursement, and access for the entire French social protection system, which includes healthcare
- the quality and quantity of health professions education
- the quality of health services
- public hospitals' financing, personnel, and facility development

The Ministry of Health is part of the Ministry of Employment and Solidarity (Ministère de l'Emploi et de la Solidarité), whose very name is an expression of the founding principle of the French social protection system: solidarity among and between generations and social classes.

Important national agencies and organizations include the High Commission on Public Health (Haut Comité de la Santé Publique); the public health policymaking entity; the Health Monitoring Institute (Institut de Veille Sanitaire); the French Health Products Safety Agency (Agence Française de Sécurité Sanitaire des Produits de Santé), which is roughly equivalent to the drug and medical device function of the Food and Drug Administration; and the French Blood Institution (Etablissement Française du Sang), the successor to the agency established after the scandals involving HIV-tainted blood, which is responsible for the quality of blood supply.

Healthcare is regularly delivered in the public schools under the direction of the Ministry of Education. Each school in Paris has its own infirmary that is staffed by a nurse and visited regularly by a corps of pediatricians who work only in the schools (Chayes 2000). These practitioners do not replace private physicians, although they do write some prescriptions and make referrals. All Parisian school children get a health notebook at birth, which travels with them whether they see a private pediatrician or one of the nursery or school doctors. School children receive annual hearing, vision, and speech tests, and they are given full health examinations when they enter kindergarten, middle school, and high school.

Regional and departmental health authorities coordinate local health services planning (particularly medical equipment acquisition), health promotion, and preventive services. Regional "health observatories" perform surveillance and data collection functions to identify changes in local and regional needs.

Until 2000, medical assistance for low-income residents of France was also administered at the regional level. This system was centralized in 1999 to simplify administration and make supplementary coverage more uniformly available. The new universal health insurance (known as Couverture Médicale Universelle) is automatically available to the nearly 3 million recipients of the guaranteed minimum income, which is provided to those who are disabled, unemployed, or otherwise unable to support themselves. Other low-income families are also eligible. Couverture Médicale Universelle frees its beneficiaries of the usual high coinsurance requirements and the need to pay up front and request reimbursement.

Supplementary coverage is available at no cost to those with monthly incomes under about U.S.$500 for single persons or U.S.$1,050 for a family of four. Government estimates put the total number of potential supplemental coverage beneficiaries at about 6 million, which is about 10 percent of the French population.

Division of Control Between Government and the Private Sector

The dual governing principles of national solidarity and freedom of choice are reflected in shared control between the public and private sectors. French national health insurance is a collection of Sickness Insurance Funds (SIFs) that are based primarily on occupational class and secondarily on place of residence and that are augmented by nonprofit insurers or mutual supplementary carriers and some general tax-based funding (Anderson 1998). The organizations responsible for health benefits also have separate branches to deal with old age and family benefits; the health benefit branch includes what U.S. observers would classify as worker compensation and disability benefits.

Administration of the national funds is controlled by the Central Agency for Social Security Organizations (l'Agence Centrale des Organismes de Sécurité Sociale); regional and local administrative entities are also in place. The funds' administrative councils include representatives of employers and employees, who are designated by their various official organizations.

The largest of these occupation-based systems covers 80 percent of the population and includes industrial and commercial employees, government workers, and voluntary enrollees (e.g., the self-employed). A smaller SIF covers farmers and agricultural employees and their families, which make up about 9 percent of the population; another covers skilled craftspersons, small businesses, and professionals, which make up about 6 percent of the population. Specific SIFs are also available for certain government employees, physicians, students, active military personnel, miners, clergy, and other occupational groups. The benefit levels are not quite the same across SIFs: the plans for miners and railroad workers, for example, resemble U.S. HMOs in that those covered do not share cost if they use contracted providers (Chatagner 2000). Additional insurance coverage information is provided in Table 9.4.

Because the income and expenses of the various health insurance funds vary, a complex demographic adjustment system is used to cross-subsidize funds that are in deficit. Variation in contribution rates across the funds has been reduced by the introduction of a statutory standard contribution, but observers of the French healthcare system report that considerable variation persists (Imai, Jacobzone, and Lenain 2000).

Some 84 percent of the French population has supplementary coverage through a mutual insurance fund, which covers cost-sharing amounts and other out-of-pocket expenses (de Kervasdoué 2000). Mutual insurance fund coverage is purchased primarily through the employer. Another 7 percent purchase supplementary coverage through private carriers. Of the remaining 13 percent of the population, most are exempt from cost sharing because of their low income, disability, or unemployment.

TABLE 9.4 Insurance Coverage, Public Mandated Insurance

Percent of total population covered	99.5
Population with supplementary coverage by percent of total expenditure	84
Government-funded other than social security	4
Government-administered social security	72
Supplementary coverage	12
Out-of-pocket costs	13

SOURCE: OECD Health Data (2000).

Universal coverage does not guarantee universal access to necessary services. France has the same problems with healthcare resource distribution as other industrialized countries, modulated to some extent by the availability of more than 2,000 clinics with salaried doctors who provide health education, screening, prevention, and free checkups. One access issue arises because more than one-fourth of French physicians are not required to adhere to the national fee schedule. Some urban areas have few general practitioners who observe the fee schedule, and the extra charges can be a serious financial burden for low-income patients whose supplementary coverage does not extend beyond fee-schedule rates (WHO 1997). Even so, private general practitioners provide the majority of preventive and outpatient care. The very small group of people ineligible for any government program (e.g., undocumented immigrants) receives care through charitable associations and clinics run by *Médecins sans Frontières* and similar organizations.

Public Health

Despite its historical contributions to global public health, the formal public health sector in France is quite limited, amounting to 2.5 percent of total health expenditures (Imai, Jacobzone, and Lenain 2000). A national public health policy–coordinating body, the High Commission for Public Health, was only established in 1990, and its functions are very limited. Public health surveillance is carried out under the auspices of the Health Surveillance Institute (Institut de Veille Sanitaire), which is somewhat comparable to the U.S. Centers for Disease Control and Prevention. The need for a national health policy with disease-specific objectives and greater emphasis on prevention is the subject of many discussions, but as of yet no formal proposals have been made to remedy this situation.

Financing

For the working French population, healthcare funding takes the form of a payroll tax shared between employer and employee and a second fee for supplementary coverage that reimburses out-of-pocket expenses such as coinsurance (ticket modérateur). The French system offers free choice of providers, and less than 10 percent of French physicians take on care coordination functions for any of their patients; coinsurance would thus be an important curb on utilization if it were not reimbursed by supplementary coverage.

Until recently, all but the lowest-income French had to pay for outpatient services out-of-pocket and then apply to their insurance funds for reimbursement. This system imposed at least a modest restraint on unnecessary use because the insured person lost the use of the fee amounts for several weeks while awaiting reimbursement. An increasing number of services now offer third-party billing (tiers payant), which eliminates even this slight deterrent.

Coverage is complete for major surgery and other high-cost interventions, and it declines to about 75 percent for outpatient physician visits and to as little as 35 percent for "lifestyle" drugs such as minoxidil for hair loss. Physician reimbursement also varies according to the "sector" in which they choose to practice. Sector I physicians are reimbursed according to a fee schedule and agree not to bill for additional amounts, in exchange for which they receive government benefits such as free health insurance. Those in Sector II and others who are allowed to charge extra fees lose access to government benefits but can charge significantly higher fees. Participation in Sector II has been very tightly regulated since 1990, and its relative share of physicians has declined from 31 percent in 1990 to 27 percent in 1997 (34 percent of specialists). The excess fees of Sector II physicians are treated differently by the various supplementary insurance plans, which leads to some inequity of access (Imai, Jacobzone, and Lenain 2000).

French physicians earn far less than their U.S. counterparts, with some generalists making just over U.S.$30,000 annually and the most highly paid specialists making no more than U.S.$120,000; the mean physician income across all ages and specialties is about U.S.$60,000 per year (Chayes 2000). An outpatient physician visit of 15 minutes costs the patient U.S.$20 in Sector I, and the fee is fully reimbursable; routine dental care costs an equally affordable U.S.$15 (de Kervasdoué 2000). Hospital care in France is billed to the patient's insurance fund (tiers payant) after payment of a lump sum coinsurance (forfait hospitalier).

France ranks fourth among the nations of the European Union in the proportion of its gross domestic product, 9.6 percent, that is spent on healthcare. The average working household spends 20 percent of gross income on health, including the purchase of supplementary coverage. In response to deficits in governmental healthcare funding in the 1980s and early 1990s, copayments were increased and physician reimbursements lowered. The fee-for-service system responded predictably with increased volume of services, which allowed general practitioners to maintain their real income (Imai, Jacobzone, and Lenain 2000). The increase in coinsurance was likewise ineffective because of the ubiquitous availability of supplementary coverage.

Mandatory clinical practice guidelines (références médicales opposables) were introduced in 1994, and 454 had been promulgated by 1998 (Lancry and Sandier 1999). They were developed under the auspices of an independent organization, Agence National pour le Développement de l'Evaluation Médicale, and involved the collaboration of a wide range of medical organizations (Durand-Zaleski, Colin, and Blum-Boisgard 1997). Doctors who do not abide by the guidelines may have to pay fines that vary with the number of violations and their potential adverse consequences.

The 1996 Juppé Plan reformed French healthcare financing at a level so broad as to require constitutional amendments. The most important cost-containment measure was the Parliamentary adoption of an annual national health spending objective known as ONDAM that included spending targets for private physician fees, prescriptions, public hospitals, private clinics, and the so-called medical-social sector. This administrative category also includes government-funded services for the frail elderly, children's mental health, and people with disabilities. In addition to the economic measures, the Juppé Plan created regional hospital authorities (Agences Régionales Hospitalières) to allocate hospitals' global budgets and coordinate regional health and social services.

Healthcare expenditure increases slowed in the late 1990s in France, either because of these reforms or for more complex economic reasons. Still, the ONDAM plan was exceeded by 11 billion francs (about U.S.$1.5 billion), about 2.5 percent, in both 1999 and 2000 (Cour des Comptes 2000). Juppé Plan provisions are intended to trigger additional cost-containment mechanisms when this level of cost overrun occurs; however, no additional measures have been implemented, apparently because of their lack of political support (Quest Economics Database 2001). This is not surprising: a generous system of coverage with fee-for-service payment and reimbursement of coinsurance gives patients and physicians a joint interest in maximizing insurers' reimbursement.

Health Spending by Category

Figure 9.1 presents French healthcare expenditures by category. The most striking feature is drug expenditures, which are 19 percent of the total as compared with 13 percent for physician services. Overspending for prescription drugs is widely recognized as the source of much of France's excess health expenditure. Ninety percent of physician office visits result in a prescription as compared with 28 percent in the Netherlands (Pellet and Kervasdoué 2000). France has a large pharmaceutical industry, so government refusal to cover a prescription drug has domestic economic consequences that policymakers take into consideration. Many drugs that would not be acceptable formulary entries for U.S. health plans, such as homeopathic remedies, are routinely reimbursed in France. Excess consumption may also be stimulated by heavily regulated prices that tend to be somewhat lower in France than in other European countries (Hartmann, Rochaix-Ranson, and de Kervasdoué 2000).

Health Resources

France has an abundance of health resources; some critics of the French healthcare system claim that excess capacity, particularly with regard to physician specialists and hospital beds, is one of its greatest problems (Duriez

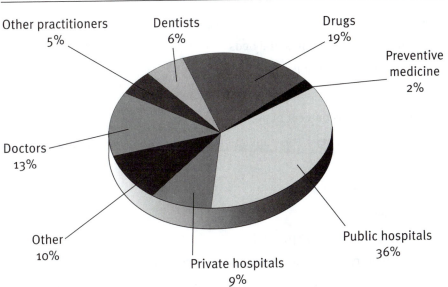

FIGURE 9.1
French
Healthcare
Consumption,
1998

SOURCE: National Health Accounts, Ministere de l'emploi et de la solidarite (2001).

and Sandier 1995). Health services account for 9 percent of all employment in France. According to the World Health Organization, for every 1,000 members of the French population, there are 2.9 physicians, nearly six nurses, one pharmacist (a total of some 24,000 pharmacies), 0.2 midwives, and 0.68 dentists (WHO 1999). See Table 9.5 for additional information on healthcare human resources.

Hospital capacity is difficult to compare among countries because classification of hospital beds as acute care, long term, or specialty varies widely. Figure 9.2 represents French hospitals across two dimensions: type of patient and facility legal status. The latter comprises three basic categories: public hospitals, private hospitals that participate in the national healthcare system, and nonparticipating private hospitals. Twenty-nine regional facilities serve as teaching hospitals and have the greatest technological resources (WHO 1997).

Service Delivery

Ambulatory care is provided primarily by private-practice doctors who are paid on a fee-for-service basis, which is the way physicians practicing in private clinics are also paid. Lower-income people receive checkups, screening examinations, health education, and preventive services at some 2,000 health centers whose priority clientele include the unemployed, retirees, and their dependents. Maternal-child health and school health services are well-developed in France. Nurses provide primary care in municipal health

TABLE 9.5

Health Resources and Use

Inpatient care	
Short-stay general hospital beds	260,276
Beds per 1,000 population	4.45
Average length of stay, all diagnoses (days)	10.8
Admissions as percent of population	2.5
Hospital days per 1,000 population	2,500
Physicians	
Total (1998)	175,431
Female	60,661
Physicians per 1,000 population	2.9
Ambulatory physician contacts per capita (1996)	6.5
Medical student admission quota (2000)	3,850
Nurses	
Total	347,918
Nurses per 1,000 population	5.9
Pharmacists	61,692
Dentists	39,471
Annual dental visits per capita (1996)	1.1

SOURCE: OECD Databank (2001).

centers and in association with other practitioners, and some 5,000 occupational health nurses provide on-site preventive and primary care.

Public hospital outpatient departments and even specialist physicians often provide primary care because the large majority of patients are free to choose any service or practitioner under contract with the social insurance funds. Public hospitals also have a legal duty to provide emergency treatment. France has a high rate of hospitalization: the number of hospital admissions is equal to 22.5 percent of the population, although some of the admissions undoubtedly involve the same patient. The figure of 2,500 hospital days per 1,000 population should not be compared to days-per-thousand figures in the United States, because the French figure includes specialty hospitals and long-term-care facilities. Nevertheless, the French use hospital facilities to a greater extent than Americans do, although their hospital capacity and length of stay are not extraordinary by European standards (European Commission 2000).

	Public Facilities	Participating Private Hospitals	Nonparticipating Private Hospitals	Total
Inpatient Facilities				
Short-term care				
Medicine	97,535	9,805	16,213	123,553
Surgery	51,091	8,505	51,268	110,564
Obstetrics/ gynecology	15,551	1,280	9,328	26,159
Total short-term	164,177	19,290	76,809	260,276
Mental health	50,018	11,229	11,549	72,796
Substance abuse	1,129	163	807	2,099
Rehabilitation and subacute care	39,072	19,949	33,183	92,204
Long-term care	74,115	3,080	3,505	80,700
Total inpatient	328,511	53,711	125,853	508,075
Outpatient Surgery and Partial Hospital				
Partial hospitals other than psychiatric or substance abuse	5,580	1,899	3,124	10,603
Partial hospitals/ mental health/ substance abuse	21,219	3,726	1,673	26,618
Outpatient surgery	869	158	5,508	6,535
Total	27,668	5,783	10,305	43,756

FIGURE 9.2
Hospital Capacity by Sector, January 1997

SOURCE: Adapted from Hartman, Rochaix-Ranson, and de Kervasdoué (2000).

Health Disparities

Despite the wealth of health resources and services in France, socioeconomic and geographic disparities persist (Garros and Rodrigues 2000). Unskilled laborers and the unemployed have higher rates of self-reported disease across nearly all categories, yet they do not visit physicians (particularly specialists) at rates proportionate to their burden of disease. The ultimate disparity appears in the comparison of life expectancy for 35-year-old men: managers and professionals can expect an additional 46 years, whereas unskilled workers can only expect another 37 years.

Cancer death rates vary by socioeconomic strata in the population between the ages of 25 and 64 years, with a higher death rate overall among working-class men and a higher cervical cancer mortality rate among women (Mesrine 1997). Death rates from most external causes (notably traffic accidents) have improved since 1970 but remain the second highest in the European Union, and improvement has been far greater in the upper socioeconomic categories. An unskilled laborer has a 29 percent chance of dying between the ages of 35 and 65, whereas an executive's chances of such a premature death are only 13 percent.

Similar disparities across regions are also well-documented: the male life expectancy in the northeastern Pas de Calais is more than five years lower than that of the males in some of the southern and southeastern regions (Mesrine 1997). Although the northern departments have higher death rates from most causes, they do not have a comparable number of health services and resources. The south of France and the Paris region have significantly higher physician-population ratios than the less-healthy north. Whether this lack of resources contributes to the excess northern mortality is debatable. The rates of cigarette smoking and alcoholism are much more closely matched to premature death rates by department than are the ratios of physicians and hospital beds to the departmental population.

The north-south mortality disparity has given rise to several hypotheses: the so-called "French paradox" (greater life expectancy than lifestyle alone predicts) may be a stronger influence in the south, where the general diet may be healthier, the air quality better, and general attention to physical health more pronounced in a region where the climate is more conducive to outdoor activities (Taboulet 1999; HCSP 2000). Some parts of the south have seen rises in traffic fatalities contrary to national trends, but cancer and CVD mortality rates are considerably lower in these areas.

French men are notably less healthy than French women, as is shown in Table 9.3. Although some of the excess mortality may be attributable to higher rates of alcohol and cigarette consumption among men, this trend has changed: French women between the ages of 15 and 24 have a higher rate of cigarette smoking than men in this age group and comparable alcohol consumption rates. Men are known to seek healthcare less frequently than women in all developed countries, but the excess mortality of French men appears more likely to be a function of lifestyle and fundamental male-female physiological variables than inadequate healthcare use.

Prospects for the Future

The most ambitious recent effort to address problems in the French health-care system was the 1996 Juppé Plan. In addition to limiting health expenditures and increasing revenue, it was intended to improve the quality of healthcare by making structural changes in the French healthcare system. In ambulatory care, the Juppé Plan established the use of medical guidelines and required physicians to use patient-specific medical records (carnets de santé). Various measurement tools were implemented to make more systematic comparisons of hospital activity.

Building on these broad initiatives, the largest of the healthcare funds, the National Sickness Insurance Fund for Wage-Earning Workers (Caisse Nationale d'Assurance Maladie des Travailleurs Salariés [CNMATS]), recently presented an elaborate plan for reforming the French healthcare system (Pellet and de Kervasdoué 2000). Although it has not been implemented, some of its provisions shed light on chronic problems in the French healthcare system.

The objectives of the CNMATS plan include a higher level of patient responsibility, greater attention to quality, and availability of performance-related data, selective contracting, diagnosis-related-group-style hospital payments, and prescription drug reimbursement by therapeutic class. The proposal to require written surgery documentation and coded entries for services and prescriptions suggests that the level of mandatory documentation in the French healthcare system is far lower than in the United States. Physician recertification would be required every seven years, and those who failed to achieve recertification would not be eligible for health insurance reimbursements. An element of selective contracting would be introduced to alleviate the physician surplus in some areas. The CNMATS plan also establishes a portable medical record that the patient presents for physician annotation at each visit, a feature that has been implemented on a limited trial basis. In the absence of these and similar cost-containment measures, the French healthcare system will not likely achieve better control of its rapidly escalating expenditures.

Challenges in improving health status were addressed by the newly appointed health minister, Bernard Kouchner, in a presentation to the March 2001 National Health Conference (Kouchner 2001). He outlined five priorities:

1. chronic illness, with a primary focus on cancer
2. infectious disease, particularly HIV
3. emerging and orphan diseases, a concern highlighted by the mad cow crises
4. addictive disorders
5. special programs for the health of youth, the elderly, women, vulnerable populations, and the incarcerated

Other topics that will receive special consideration include the following:

- patient rights
- compensation for adverse outcomes (l'aléa thérapeutique)
- health system safety measures (la sécurité sanitaire)
- public education regarding health risks
- opening the health system, especially hospitals, to greater public understanding

The general trend toward greater openness and patient empowerment expressed in Kouchner's references to patient rights must be analyzed in the context of the traditional paternalistic nature of the physician-patient relationship in France (Béraud 2000). As is the case in the United States, the better-informed French patient wants a voice in treatment decision making, access to patient records, and adequate physician attention to specific questions and concerns. Whether these trends will give rise to a higher level of cost-consciousness on the part of the French public or simply generate demand for even higher levels of service and drug utilization remains to be seen.

Acknowledgments

The staff of the University of Kentucky Libraries demonstrated remarkable creativity in procuring the necessary data for this chapter.

REFERENCES

Anderson, G. F. 1998. *Multinational Comparison of Health Care*. New York: Commonwealth Fund. Retrieved 01 April 2001 from www.cmwf.org/programs/international/ihp_1998_multicompsurvey.pdf.

Anderson G. F., and Hussey, P. 1999. "Health and Population Aging: A Multinational Comparison." New York: Commonwealth Fund. Retrieved 01 April 2001 from http://www.cmwf.org.

Anonymous. 2001. "Economic Indicators: Output, Demand and Jobs." *The Economist* (U.S. edition) April 7: 120.

Béraud, C. 2000. "La reconnaissance des Droits des Malades va Bouleverser la Relation Médecin-Malade." In *Le Carnet de Santé de la France en 2000*, pp. 213–17, edited by Jean de KervasdouéParis: Editions la Découverte.

Breo, D. L. 1991. "Blood, Money, and Hemophiliacs—The Fatal Story of France's AIDSgate." *Journal of the American Medical Association* 266 (24): 3471–73.

Chatagner, F. (ed.). 2000. *La protection sociale: des réformes inachevées*. Paris: Le Monde.

Chayes, S. 2000. "All Things Considered, August 27, 2000." Transcript on file with author.

Cour des Comptes. 2000. *La sécurité sociale*. Paris: Editions des journaux officiels.

De Kervasdoué, J. 2000. *Le carnet de santé de la France en 2000*. Paris: Editions la Découverte.

Dorozynski, A. 1999. "Former French Ministers on Trial over Blood." *British Medical Journal* 318: 419.

Dupeyroux, J.-J. 1998. *Droit de la sécurité sociale*, 13th ed. Paris: Editions Dalloz.

Durand-Zaleski, I., Colin, C., and Blum-Boisgard, C. 1997. "An Attempt to Save Money by Using Mandatory Practice Guidelines in France." *British Medical Journal* 315: 943–47.

Duriez, M., and Sandier, S. 1995. *The French Health Care System: Organization and Functioning*. Paris: Editions du Service de l'Information et de la Communication.

European Commission. 2000. *Eurostat Yearbook: A Statistical Eye on Europe*. Luxembourg: Office of Official Publications for the European Community.

Garros, B., and Rodrigues, J.-M. 2000. "Regards sur la santé des Français Aujourd'hui." In *Le carnet de santé de la France en 2000*, pp. 13–58, edited by Jean de Kervasdoué. Paris: Editions la Découverte.

Hartman, L., Rochaix-Ranson, L., and de Kervasdoue, J. 2000. "Le systeme de santé Francais: un etat des lieux." In *Le carnet de santé de la France en 2000*. Paris: Editions la Découverte.

Hartmann, L., Rochaix-Ranson, L., and de Kervasdoué, J. 2000. "La Régulation économique du système de santé." In *Le carnet de santé de la France en 2000*, pp. 85–121, edited by Jean de Kervasdoué. Paris: Editions la Découverte.

Haut Comité de la Santé Publique (HCSP). 1999. *La santé en France 1994–1998*. Paris: La Documentation française.

———. 2000. *Allocation Régionale des Ressources et Réduction des Inégalités de Santé*. Retrieved 09 April 2001 from www.HCSP.ensp.fr.

Imai, Y., Jacobzone, S., and Lenain, P. "The Changing Health System in France." OECD Economics Department Working Papers No. 269. Retrieved 17 April 2001 from www.oecd.org/eco/eco.

Institut National de la Statistique et de Etudes (INSEE) Database. Retrieved May 2001 from www.insee.fr/fr/fcc/acceuil.fcc.asp.

Kouchner, B. 2001. "Address to National Health Conference." Retrieved 09 April 2001 from www.sante.gouv.fr/htm/ minister/cns01/33_010327.htm.

Lancry, P., and Sandier, S. 1999. "Rationing Health Care in France." *Health Policy* 50: 23–38.

Mesrine, A. 1998. "Les différences de mortalité par milieu social." In *Indicateurs socio-sanitaires*, pp. 228–35, edited by Pierre Gottely and Jean Mercier. Paris: La Documentation française.

Mossialos, E. 1997. "Citizens' Views on Health Systems in the 15 Member States of the European Union." *Health Economics* 6: 109–16.

National Health Accounts, Ministere de L'emploi et de la solidarité. Retrieved May 2001 from www.sante.gouv.fr/drees/cptsante/resume98.pdf.

OECD Databank. Retrieved May 2001 from www.oecd.org.

OECD Health Data 2000. Luxembourg: OECD.

Paarlberg, R. 2000. "The Global Food Fight." *Foreign Affairs* 79 (3): 24.

Pellet, R., and de Kervasdoué, J. 2000. "L'Etat et la maîtrise des dépenses de santé." In *Le carnet de santé de la France en 2000*, edited by Jean de Kervasdoué. Paris: Editions la Découverte.

Prétot, X., and Dupeyroux, J.-J. 2000. *Droit de la sécurité sociale* (memento), 9th ed. Paris: Editions Dalloz.

Ramsey, M. 1994. "Public Health in France." *Clio Medica* 26: 45–118.

Service des Statistiques, Des Études et des Systèmes D'information. 1994. *Les Français et leur santé*. Paris: Ministère des Affaires Sociales, de la Santé et de la Ville.

Quest Economics Database. 2001. *Société Générale France: Monthly Economic Report*.

Taboulet, F. 1999. "Déterminants de la santé et inégalités." *Soins* 634: 53–55.

United Nations. 2000. "Population Data." Retrieved 06 April 2001 from www.undp.org/popin.

United Nations/World Health Organization. 2000. "AIDS Epidemiological Fact Sheet, France." Retrieved May 2001 from www.un.org.

World Health Organization. 1999. "WHO Estimates of Health Personnel." Retrieved 21 April 2001 from www-nt.who.int/whosis/statistics.

———. 2000. "Health Performance in All Member States, WHO Indexes, Estimates for 1997." In *World Health Report*, Annex Table 10. Retrieved 06 April 2001 from http://filestore.who.int/~who/ hr/2000/en/pdf/ AnnexTable10.pdf.

World Health Organization Regional Office for Europe (WHO/ROE). 1997. "Highlights on Health in France." Retrieved 31 March 2001 from http://www.who.dk/country/country.htm.

10

SPAIN

Ana Rico and Tom Lazenby

Background Information

The Spanish National Health System (Sistema Nacional de Salud) is characterized by the principles of universal and free access to healthcare services, public financing through general taxation, integrated health service networks, and primary healthcare with an emphasis on health prevention and promotion. Healthcare services in Spain are partly decentralized and partly managed by central state authorities. Services are provided primarily by the public sector, with the private sector playing a relatively minor role. In the 1990s, dissatisfaction with healthcare services and rising healthcare costs acted as catalysts for political efforts to reform the organization and management of the system. Despite significant progress, the complexity of providing integrated healthcare to a changing population continues to present challenges for the Spanish National Health System.

Government

The Spanish government is a parliamentary monarchy with a constitution dating back to December 29, 1978. Legislative power rests in a bicameral parliament elected by universal suffrage. The parliament includes the Senate (Camara Alta) and the Congress of Deputies (Camara Baja). The Congress of Deputies and the Cabinet elect a prime minister, who holds executive power. At the regional level, 17 autonomous communities each have their own parliaments. These communities consist of provinces and municipalities (WHO 1997).

Economy

On a per capita basis, Spain's gross domestic product is only three-fourths that of the largest Western European economies. In addition, the country is plagued by the highest unemployment rate in the European Union. As shown in Table 10.1, almost 20 percent of the population was unemployed in 1998.

On the other hand, the Spanish economy has experienced only modest inflation, at 2 percent annually (CIA 1999). Per capita spending for healthcare is 40 percent below the average of OECD Western countries; however, this figure can be misleading because of the differences in income among these countries (Lopez-Casanovas 1998). Healthcare spending as a percentage of GDP has remained fairly constant at 7.5 percent since 1994 following an agreement among central and regional governments to adjust the year-by-year increase in financing at the rate of growth in GDP (Rico and Sabes 2000).

Demographics and Education

Spain's landmass covers 505,955 square kilometers, and its current population is 39,200,000 (Table 10.2). The elderly population (those 65 years old or older) continues to grow and currently accounts for almost 19 percent of the entire population (INE 2001). Life expectancy in Spain is among the highest in the world at 77.9 years. Females can expect to live longer than males, with life expectancies at 81.8 years and 74.2 years, respectively. The infant mortality rate is 5.5 per 1,000 live births (INE 2001). Spain's fertility rate has declined and currently is the lowest in Europe; this is in contrast with 1970 statistics that reported Spanish fertility as the second highest in Europe. After 20 years of steady decline, the fertility rate has reached a plateau over the last few years (INE 2001).

Education statistics in Spain compare favorably with other EU nations. The school enrollment ratio for the 6- to 23-year-old age group is one of the highest among the nations of the European Union (WHO 1997). The literacy rate in 1997 was 97.2 percent, with male literacy slightly higher than female literacy (UN 1999). During the 1997–98 academic year, more than 3.5 million students were enrolled in primary school, almost 2.5 million students attended secondary and professional schools, and more than 1.5 million were enrolled in university-level education (INE 2001).

TABLE 10.1
Selected Economic Data, Spain, 1998 (U.S.$)

Labor force, 1999	16.2 million
Unemployment rate	20%
Inflation	2%
GNP per capita, 1997	U.S.$14,490
GDP per capita	P.P.P. $16,500
Human Development Index score, 1997	.894
GNP given to health, 1997	7.4%
Health expenditure per capita	P.P.P. $1,183
ODA inflow/outflow as percent of GNP 1997	23

NOTE: ODA = official development assistance.
SOURCE: CIA (1999); UNDP (1999); Trias et al. (1998); WHO Regional Office for Europe (2000).

Demographics		**TABLE 10.2**
Population	40,202,160	Selected
Urban population, 1997	76.9%	Demographic
Life expectancy (years)	77.9	Data, Spain,
Male	74.2	2000
Female	81.8	
Fertility rate	1.20	
Birth rate	9.58	
Death rate	9.40	
Infant mortality per 1,000 live births	5.5	
Under-five mortality per 1,000 live births, 1997	5	
Education		
Public expenditure on education as a percentage of total expenditure, 1993–96	12.8	
Literacy rate, 1997	97.2%	
Male	98.4%	
Female	96.2%	
Primary school enrollment, 1997	99.9%	
Secondary school enrollment, 1997	91.9%	

SOURCE: U.S. Census (1999); UNDP (1999); INE (2001).

Health System History

The foundation of the Spanish National Health System was established in 1942 with the Seguro Obligatorio de Enfermedad (Compulsory Sickness Insurance) program. This program began as an insurance policy for industrial workers. In 1963, Spain established a modern social security system, and coverage expanded from 25 percent of the population in 1944 to 45 percent in 1963 (Rico and Sabes 2000). When Francisco Franco died in 1975, nearly 40 years of fascist dictatorship ended, paving the way for a new democratic government that expanded social security coverage and changed the framework for health services in Spain. In 1978, public health became a constitutional right for all Spaniards (Roemer 1991). Autonomous regions were created, and these progressively assumed healthcare powers; in addition, the Institute for the Social Security's Health Services, INSALUD, was founded (Saturno 1998). The contemporary Spanish National Health

System was established by the Ley General de Sanidad (Health Care Act) in 1986. This act merged all of Spain's public health institutions into one entity (INSALUD 2000).

Context: Health Needs

The leading causes of death in Spain are similar to those of other industrialized nations, with chronic diseases accounting for the largest number of deaths (Table 10.3). Diseases of the circulatory system and tumors are the leading causes of death, with the former accounting for 131,362 deaths and the latter accounting for 90,930 deaths in 1997. Other major causes of mortality include diseases of the respiratory and digestive systems, traumas/poisonings, traffic accidents, and AIDS (INE 2001). As the seventh leading cause of death, AIDS represents a growing health problem for Spaniards. Spain has the highest AIDS incidence in the European Union, and the disease is the primary cause of death in the younger population. AIDS is most prevalent among the more disadvantaged socioeconomic classes (Borrell and Pasarin 1999).

Access to healthcare services is quite high in Spain and has recently improved following a steady decline in hospital waiting lists during the late 1990s. However, health prevention and promotion services as well as community care still suffer from serious pitfalls. The Spanish National Health Service provides health coverage to almost 100 percent of the population (INSALUD 2000), although the affluent self-employed and illegal immigrants are excluded. The near universal coverage is the result of a national effort to expand the welfare state. Access to safe water and sanitation is also near 100 percent (WHO 2000). Immunization rates for four major inoculations (polio, diphtheria, tetanus, and rubella) were approximately 94 percent in 1997 (INE 2001).

TABLE 10.3
Deaths by
Major Causes,
Spain, 1997

Circulatory system diseases	131,362
Tumors	90,930
Respiratory system diseases	34,491
Digestive system diseases	18,476
Trauma/poisonings	16,493
Traffic accidents	5,790
AIDS	2,844

SOURCE: INE (2001).

Organization and Management of the Health System

The 17 autonomous communities (CCAAs) were created and their basic laws approved between 1978 and 1983. The timing of the decentralization process, as well as the powers and policy responsibilities transferred, varied among regions. In the health sector, devolution began in 1978 for public health and in 1981 for healthcare. By 1995, seven of the CCAAs (Andalucia, Basque Country, Canary Islands, Catalonia, Galicia, Navarra, and Valencia) had full responsibility for governing health services within their respective regions. These seven autonomous regions provide services to 62 percent of the population (Reverte-Cejudo and Sanchez-Bayle 1999). The remaining ten regions, along with the cities of Cueta and Melilla, receive healthcare services from the Instituto Nacional de la Salud (National Institute of Health or INSALUD). These regions have not yet assumed autonomous control in the healthcare field.

The National Health System consists of hospitals, a network of primary care centers, specialized outpatient clinics, and contracts with other public and private clinics (Trias et al. 1998). Eighty-five percent of service organizations in the system are public, and 15 percent are private (Lopez-Casanovas 1999). The government deals with pharmaceutical regulation, financing of the system, and coordination of health policy at the state level. With the exception of public health functions, which are carried out by local health authorities, the regional authorities handle most other health activities (EHTO 1996).

Almost 10 percent of the population (mostly civil servants and their dependants) is covered under special public insurance arrangements that consist of several mutual funds created in the early 1970s. The biggest of these funds is the Mutua de los Funcionarios de la Administración Central de Estado (MUFACE). MUFACE is a financial intermediary that allows participants to choose either public or private plans. Eighty-five percent of enrollees choose private insurance, whereas 15 percent choose public (Pellise 1994). Insurance carriers are paid on a capitated basis, calculated as the average cost per person in the public insurance system (Puig-Junoy 1999). MUFACE has raised questions of equity because enrollees are permitted to choose insurance carriers while the rest of the population is given no choice.

Financing

Public Financing

Healthcare in Spain is provided through both the public and private sectors. Total health expenditures in 1997, both public and private, were 4.6 billion pesetas, which was 7.4 percent of the GDP. Public spending accounts for 76 percent of total expenditures. As of 1999, the public health system was completely financed by general taxation; before 1999, social insurance contributions were the main source of funding. The shift to tax-based financing was made through a gradual process that began in 1989. The only cost sharing in the public sector is for pharmaceuticals (patient copayment is 40 percent); pensioners and chronic patients are exempted from copayment. Most dental care is provided in private practices because the public system covers only tooth extraction (Rico and Sabes 2000).

The Spanish parliament approves the global health budget on an annual basis. Funds are then allocated to the seven autonomous regions and INSALUD. The seven autonomous regions can only increase their health budgets by increasing their own tax bases because financial transfers from the center are earmarked; however, the issue is currently under judicial examination as a result of recent disputes among the central government and the autonomous regions.

Beginning in the early 1990s, hospitals were budgeted according to a system of Unidades Poneradas de Asistencia (UPAs) or standardized patient days. Each hospital projected UPAs for the coming year and submitted a proposal to the Ministry of Health. The Ministry of Health based the budget on the hospital's actual UPAs for the current year and a negotiated average of the proposed UPAs multiplied by a standard rate per UPA (Feldman and Lobo 1997). A new system of diagnosis-related-group-based prospective payment, introduced in the late 1990s, is still in the pilot stage. Hospitals typically have separate budgets for capital expenditures and operating costs. Once these budgets are determined, administrators may not transfer funds between budgets. Any savings the hospital incurs are returned to the INSALUD budget at the end of the year. For additional information on healthcare financial flows, see Figure 10.1.

Physicians working in public hospitals are salaried; this also applies to most professionals working in private (usually not-for-profit) hospitals that contract with the public sector. In contrast, physicians working in private hospitals that do not hold a contract with the public sector are frequently paid on a fee-for-service basis. Doctors are not permitted to see private patients in public hospitals; however, they are allowed to work part-time in the private sector. For this reason, economic incentives have been offered since the late 1980s to persuade physicians to work full-time in the public sector. Recently promoting access to directive positions has been planned for those professionals fully dedicated to the public system.

Private Insurance

In 1995, 5.7 million Spaniards (15 percent of the population) had supplemental private health insurance with 40 different insurance agencies. This includes civil servants opting for a private carrier, with their policies paid for by the state. Between 1990 and 1997, premiums increased by 105.7 percent. Notably, only 15 percent of private expenditures go to premiums; the other 85 percent comprise out-of-pocket copayments (Rico

FIGURE 10.1
Financial
Flows in the
Healthcare
System

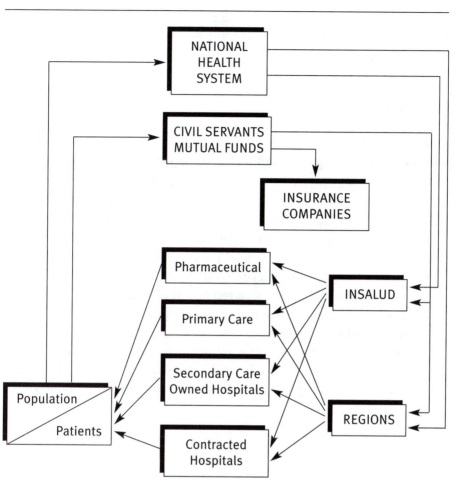

and Sabes 2000). Spain's private expenditure share of total expenditures (25 percent) is slightly below the OECD average. Not surprisingly, private expenditures are usually higher in the wealthier regions. Direct expenditures are highest for dental care (28 percent) and pharmaceuticals (24 percent). Outpatient care is the next highest expenditure at 15 percent (Lopez-Casanovas 1999).

Enrollees in private insurance plans may choose from a network of physicians provided by each insurance company; visits to doctors outside of the network are not reimbursed. A specific historical feature of the insurance sector in Spain is that insurance companies usually own and manage their own network of healthcare centers and contract with private physicians, who provide services directly. Private health insurance in Spain generally has very low copayments; in 1997, the highest copayments were equivalent to U.S.$1.50 (Vera-Hernandez 1999). Spaniards were also allowed to deduct 15 percent of premiums and private health expenditures for tax purposes until 1999. Since that time, only employer-purchased private plans are subject to a tax break. Individuals with private insurance remain eligible to receive healthcare in the public system. Private insurance is often used as a supplement to public insurance. Additional insurance information may be found in Table 10.4.

Health Resources

Health Professionals

Spanish physicians begin medical training with a six-year undergraduate program. In 1996, there were 4,309 students in 26 medical schools (Trias et al. 1998). Although medical schools are separate from hospitals, they have formed special agreements that allow medical students access for training (Lopez-Cassanovas and Saez 1999). Prior to 1995, only an undergraduate medical degree was required for general practitioners desiring private practices; only those physicians wishing to work in public hospitals or wanting to become specialists required postundergraduate training. Now, all physicians must spend three to five years in postgraduate medical training (Gomez and Pujol 1998).

Spain has a surplus of physicians, and this is reflected in high physician unemployment rates. The 111,076 physicians documented in 1998 resulted in a ratio of 3.5 physicians for every 1,000 population (Table 10.5).

TABLE 10.4
Percentages of Healthcare Spending, Spain, 1995

Public	
Inpatient and outpatient care	54.1
Pharmaceuticals	18.8
Primary care	16.5
Research, training, public health, and administration	5.2
Investment	2.7
Other	2
Private	
Insurance	14
Dental	28
Pharmaceuticals	24
Outpatient	15
Inpatient	9
Prostheses	11

SOURCE: Rico and Sabes (2000).

This number is significantly higher than that of France (2.5:1,000) or Germany (2.7:1,000). However, 24,512 physicians were unemployed in 1998 (15 percent of male registered doctors and almost 30 percent of female doctors). In fact, only 83,534 doctors were practicing in 1998, which was a ratio of 2.2 per 1,000 population (Rico and Sabes 2000).

Somewhat paradoxically, high unemployment rates coexist with double employment, as professionals working for the public system also commonly work part-time in the private sector. In addition, measuring the proportion of private physicians who deliver public services is difficult, as they may work for private hospitals that have contracts with the public system. Payments to contracted-out hospitals represent 15 to 20 percent of the total public healthcare expenditure.

Approximately 70 percent of active physicians are directly employed by the National Health System (Gomez and Pujol 1998); this gives a public sector ratio of 1.6 doctors per 1,000 population. One-third of these physicians also work in the primary care sector. In addition, the public sector employs 2.4 qualified nurses, 1.3 auxiliary nurses, 0.1 midwives, and 0.1 physiotherapists per 1,000 population (Rico and Sabes 2000). Additional information about health services personnel is provided in Table 10.5.

Health Facilities

In 1997, Spain had almost 800 hospitals with a total of 166,276 hospital beds (4.2 beds per 1,000 population), which was lower than that found in most OECD countries. The division of beds between public and private hospitals is shown in Table 10.5. Sixty-eight percent of all hospital beds are in the public sector, whereas 32 percent are private beds. Sixty percent of private beds are in for-profit hospitals, and the remaining 40 percent are in not-for-profit hospitals. The hospital occupancy rate is 76.7 percent, and the average length of stay is 11 days. In 1997, Spanish health facilities were equipped with 367 computed tomography scanners, 130 magnetic resonance imaging machines, and 131 units of radiation therapy equipment (OECD 1999).

Pharmaceuticals

The Spanish pharmaceutical market is the fifth largest in Europe and the seventh largest in the world. Drug expenditures account for more than 20 percent of public health spending, which is a higher proportion than in any other industrialized nation. In an effort to slow pharmaceutical spending and raise the quality of public prescription patterns, the Ministry of Health issued in 1993 a list of drugs for which the state will not reimburse (Bastida and Mossialos 1997). As a result, 892 drugs were excluded from public funding (Bosch 1998). In 1998, a second negative list was approved by the Ministry that excluded 831 additional pharmaceutical products considered to have low therapeutic value (Rico and Sabes 2000). In total, the lists have excluded 30 percent of the total pharmaceutical brands registered

TABLE 10.5
Health Resources and Usage, Spain, 1997

Health resources	
Healthcare professionals (per 1,000 population)	
Physicians (registered physicians in 1998)	3.5
Nurses	4.6
Dentists	.4
Hospitals	
Total	799
Per 1,000 population	.02
Hospital beds, 1995	
Total	154,644
Per 1,000 population	3.9
Public beds, 1995	104,432
Private beds, 1995	50,212
For-profit	30,101
Not-for-profit	20,111
Health technology	
Computed tomography scanners	367
Magnetic resonance imaginary equipment	130
Radiation therapy equipment	131
Lithotriptors	72
Resource use	
Bed days per capita, 1996	1.1
Inpatient admissions per 1,000 population, 1996	100
Inpatient occupancy rate, 1994	76.7%
Average length of stay, 1996	11 days
Ambulatory care consultations per capita, 1989	6.2

SOURCE: OECD (1999); WHO Regional Office for Europe (2000); Bosch (1999); Ministerio de Sanidad y Consumo (1997).

in the market. However, the measure has had little success in controlling spending due to shifts in public prescription patterns toward substitute drugs that are often more expensive (Bastida and Mossialos 1997; Crespo, Benedi, and Gómez-Juanes 1999).

One reason for the failure to control growth in pharmaceutical spending is the lack of promotion of generic drugs, although their introduction in the Spanish market was authorized by the 13/1996 and 66/1997 Acts. In 1999, only 0.2 percent of drug sales (in value) were for generic drugs as compared with figures ranging between 10 and 15 percent in countries such as Germany and the United States. Pharmaceutical price setting is under strict governmental control, but pricing policies based on concerted strategies to lower expenditures were not introduced until the late 1990s. Reference prices were finally approved in December 2000, and these required public doctors to prescribe the cheapest drug available in the market. Since that time, patients wishing to receive other pharmaceutical brands were required to pay the difference between the reference price and the price of their preferred brand.

Service Delivery

Patients in the public system register with a general practitioner in their zone of residence. These patients visit their primary care physicians on an outpatient basis in primary health centers. In 1984, a move was initiated toward primary health teams with extended task profiles (including health prevention, promotion, and rehabilitation together with the traditional curative functions) and consisting of general practitioners (GPs), pediatricians, nurses, social workers, and sometimes dentists (WHO 1997). These teams provided care to 85 percent of Spaniards in 2000, with the remainder seen in single clinician practices. The GP acts as a gatekeeper within the healthcare system; patients cannot visit specialists nor be admitted to a public hospital without a referral letter from the GP. In contrast with other EU countries, gatekeeping functions are effective in day-to-day practice in Spain. However, patients frequently skip referral by going directly to the emergency room. As a result, some 50 percent of all hospital admissions are by way of the emergency room (Rico and Sabes 2000).

In comparison with other countries in continental Europe, the Spanish people report a low level of satisfaction with their health system (Mossialos 1997). One reason for this dissatisfaction may be excessive waiting times in the public system. In most public hospitals, wait times are more than a year for surgical problems such as gallstone removal and hernia repair. In the emergency room, patients often wait several hours before they receive attention for acute illness (Trias et al. 1998). INSALUD has focused on internal change to reduce waiting times and, during 1998, average waits for nonemergency surgery decreased to two months, a five-month improvement over the average wait in 1996 (Bosch 1999). Consistent with these changes, Spain is one of four EU countries in which satisfaction with healthcare has increased during the period from 1996 to 1998 (Mossialos, King, and Dixon 2000).

In 1993, Spain established a committee to study the inequalities in the health system. The committee found no inequalities in the use of the national health service (primary care and hospital services). Unskilled workers used the health system as frequently as managers and professionals with university degrees. However, unskilled workers did not visit the dentist as frequently as managers and professionals. This inequality likely exists because dental services are available only in the private system and therefore must be paid for by the individual (Navarro 1997).

The committee did discover class, regional, and gender differences in health status. Health indicators are best for the upper class and worst for the lower class. This might indicate that the working class is under-utilizing health services if utilization is based on need. However, recent research demonstrates that this pattern only applied to the utilization of hospital services in the late 1980s, whereas utilization patterns adjusted by need were the same across social classes during the early to mid-1990s (Urbanos 1999). In addition, health indicators are worse for women than for men.

The committee also found that the average visit time with the GP was 2 minutes in the public system and 20 minutes in private offices. Because MUFACE allows civil servants to participate in the private system, their average visit time is longer than that of the rest of the population. Geographical differences in average visit time have also been reported and can likely be attributed to the variation in private enrollment across regions (Navarro 1997) as well as to the different timing under which the primary healthcare reform was implemented in different Autonomous Communities (Rico and Sabes 2000).

Prospects for the Future

Three of the most daunting challenges awaiting attention from the Spanish healthcare system are information management, managerial autonomy, and the integration of social and community care. Probably the most important deficiency in the Spanish healthcare sector is the weakness in data collection functions, particularly across Autonomous Communities. As a result of the transfers of healthcare powers, these Autonomous Communities have disappeared from statistical data collection sources at the central level; consequently, accessing comprehensive data for the nation has become increasingly difficult. In spite of the significant advances made by all levels of government in this field, the data are of limited use due to the lack of homogeneous codification and common data banks. Critical information such as staffing levels, usage levels and patterns, waiting times, primary care network coverage, and hospital cost profiles are generally not available on a nationwide basis. A related problem is the very low satisfaction levels of the Spanish population regarding the institutional information provided by the public sector on such key issues as user rights, benefits covered, and public health campaigns.

Second, as with most European countries, a pressing need exists to manage health services with greater efficiency through the shifting of risk and responsibility to local budget holders, increasing the autonomy of hospitals and health centers, and involving healthcare professionals (particularly physicians) in clinical management. In addition, available resources must be effectively managed through increased use of ambulatory surgery and the extension of evidence-based medicine into clinical practice. Following the pioneering initiatives undertaken by special Autonomous Communities during the 1990s, the Ministry of Health has laid the groundwork for extending and coordinating some of these innovations, and progress now depends on the extension and consolidation of the reform process.

Third, the extent of social and community care benefits in the Spanish National Health System is problematic. Within this field, only mental health care has been integrated into the public healthcare system and subjected to major reform; in contrast, long-term care for the elderly and disabled is still considerably underdeveloped. Reforms in this area are greatly needed, particularly given the substantial increase in the elderly as a proportion of the total Spanish population. The restrictions in public coverage of dental care and some preventive services should also be reconsidered in the near future.

Since the early 1980s, Spain has undergone significant efforts to expand the welfare state, including broadened access to the National Health System. The country has also sought to improve the health system through a reformed primary care network and reorganization of financing and management structures. These efforts are commendable when one considers the international climate of cost containment, concerns over economic development, and the political transition to a democracy. However, healthcare reform and demographic changes have resulted in a new generation of problems. The Spanish National Health System will be challenged in coming years to effectively address these problems.

REFERENCES

Bastida, J., and Mossialos, E. 1997. "Spanish Drug Policy at the Crossroads." *Lancet* 350 (9079): 679–80.

Borrell, C., and Pasarin, M. 1999. "The Study of Social Inequalities in Spain: Where Are We?" *Journal of Epidemiology and Public Health* 53 (7): 388–89.

Bosch, X. 1998. "Spain Takes Hard Line on Spending on Pharmaceuticals." *Lancet* 351 (9103): 655.

———. 1998a. "Investigating the Reasons for Spain's Falling Birth Rate." *Lancet* 352 (9131): 887.

———. 1999. "Spain Cuts Waiting Times for Surgery." *British Medical Journal* 318 (7181): 419.

———. 1999a. "Spain Leads World in Organ Donation and Transplantation." *Journal of the American Medical Association* 282 (1): 17–18.

———. 1999b. "Too Many Physicians Trained in Spain." *Journal of the American Medical Association* 282 (11): 1025–26.

Crespo, B., Benedi, A., and Gómez-Juanes, V. 1999. "Genéricos, Financiación Selectiva y Nuevos Principios Activos: Análisis en 1999." *Administración Sanitaria* III (2):141–66.

European Health Telematics Observatory. 1996. "Trends in Spain." Retrieved 12 February 2000 from www.ehto.org.

Feldman, R., and Lobo, F. 1997. "Global Budgets and Excess Demand for Hospital Care." *Health Economics* 6: 187–96.

Ferrandiz, J. 1999. "The Impact of Generic Goods in the Pharmaceutical Industry." *Health Economics* 8: 599–612.

Gomez, J., and Pujol, R. 1998. "Changes in Medical Education in Spain." *Academic Medicine* 73 (10): 1076–80.

INSALUD. 2000. "Organización General." Retrieved 19 February 2000 from http://www.msc.es/insalud/introduccion/home.introduccion.htm.

Instituto Nacional de Estadistica (INE). 2001. "Espana en Cifras." Retrieved from http://www.ine.es/espcif/espcifes/espcif00.htm.

Lopez-Casanovas, G. 1999. "Health Care and Cost-Containment in Spain." In *Health Care and Cost-Containment in the European Union*, pp. 401–41, edited by E. Mossialos and J. LeGrand. Burlington: Ashgate Publishing Ltd.

Lopez-Casanovas, G., and Saez, M. 1999. "The Impact of Teaching Status on Average Costs in Spanish Hospitals." *Health Economics* 8: 641–51.

Ministerio de Sanidad y Consumo. 1997. *Catalogo Nacional de Hospitales.* Madrid: Ministerio de Sanidad y Consumo.

———. 1997. *Estadisticas de Coberturas de Vacunacion.* Madrid: Ministerio de Sanidad y Consumo.

Mossialos, E. 1997. "Citizen's Views on Health Care Systems in 15 Member States of the European Union." *Health Economics* 6: 109–16.

Mossialos, E., King, D., and Dixon, A. 2000. "Public Opinion on Health Care Systems in Britain and the European Union." Paper presented to NHS Confederation Annual Conference, June 28–30, 2000, Glasgow, Scotland.

Navarro, V. 1997. "Topics for Our Times: The 'Black Report' of Spain—The Commission of Social Inequalities in Health." *American Journal of Public Health* 87 (3): 334–35.

Organization of Economic Cooperation and Development (OECD). 1992. *The Reform of Health Care: A Comparative Analysis of Seven OECD Countries.* Paris: OECD.

———. 1999. *OECD Health Data 99.* CD-ROM. Paris: OECD.

Pellise, L. 1994. "Reimbursing Insurance Carriers: The Case of 'Muface' in the Spanish Health Care System." *Health Economics* 4: 243–53.

Puig-Junoy, J. 1999. "Managing Risk Selection Incentives in Health Sector Reforms." *International Journal of Health Planning and Management* 14: 287–311.

Reverte-Cejudo, D., and Sanchez-Bayle, M. 1999. "Devolving Health Services to Spain's Autonomous Regions." *British Medical Journal* 318 (7192): 1205.

Rico, A., Sabes, R., and European Observatory on Health Care Systems. 2000. "Health Care Systems in Transition: Spain." Retrieved 19 February 2000 from http://www.observatory.dk,HiTs, Spain.

Roemer, M. 1991. *National Health Systems of the World*. New York: Oxford University Press.

Si Spain. 2000. "Health." Retrieved 22 February 2000 from http://www.docuweb.ca/SiSpain/english/health.

Trias, M., Targarona, E., Moral, A., and Pera, C. 1998. "Surgery in Spain." *Archives of Surgery* 133 (2): 218–22.

United Nations Development Programme (UNDP). 1999. *Human Development Report*. New York: Oxford University Press.

Urbanos, R. 1999. "Es Realmente Redistributivo el Gasto Sanitario Público?" In *Necesidad Sanitaria, Demanda y Utilizacion*. Barcelona: Asociacion de Economia de la Salud.

U.S. Census Bureau. 1999. *International Database*. Washington, DC: U.S. Census Bureau.

U.S. Central Intelligence Agency (CIA). 1999. *The World Factbook*. Washington, DC: CIA.

Vera-Hernandez, A. 1999. "Duplicate Coverage and Demand for Health Care: The Case of Catalonia." *Health Economics* 8: 579–98.

World Health Organization (WHO). 2000. *WHOSIS*. Geneva: WHO.

World Health Organization (WHO) Regional Office for Europe. 1997. *Highlights on Health in Spain*. Copenhagen: WHO.

———. 2000. *HFA Statistical Database*. Copenhagen: WHO.

PORTUGAL

Teresa Durães

Background Information

The nation of Portugal, officially the Portuguese Republic (República Portuguesa), occupies about 16 percent of the Iberian Peninsula, a total area of 92,389 square kilometers. It is bordered on the east and north by Spain and on the west and south by the Atlantic Ocean. The stability of these continental borders, which have remained virtually unchanged since the thirteenth century, have made Portugal one of the oldest nations in the world. To the west and southwest lie the Atlantic islands of the Azores and Madeira, which Portugal governs as autonomous regions. Until the 1970s, Portuguese overseas territories included the Cape Verde Islands, São Tomé and Principe, Portuguese Guinea, Angola, and Mozambique, all in Africa; Macau in Asia; and East Timor in Oceania. Of these, only Macau remained a Portuguese dependency during the late twentieth century (*Merriam-Webster's Collegiate Dictionary* 2000). Portugal has two large cities: the capital, Lisbon (Lisboa), with a resident population of 1,892,891 (2001), and Porto (Oporto), with a resident population of 1,260,679 (2001).

Despite its small size, Portugal boasts a great diversity of geographic features. The River Tagos (Tejo) divides the country into two distinct areas: the North Central region, which is characterized by rivers, valleys, forests, and mountains and where the land rises to an elevation of 1,991 meters at its highest point in the Estrela Mountains, and South Portugal, which is less populated and, apart from the rocky backdrop of the Algarve, much flatter and drier. The climate is temperate throughout mainland Portugal.

Government

Portugal has been a sovereign republic since 1910 and a constitutional democratic republic since 1974, after a revolution ended the dictatorships of Salazar and Caetano. Mainland Portugal is divided into 18 districts, which comprise municipalities and are subdivided into parishes. Each governmental level (autonomous region, district, municipality, and parish) has a representative body elected by universal suffrage.

The primary governing bodies of the state are the president of the republic, the parliament, the government, and the courts. Executive power is vested in the president of the Republic, who is elected every five years by universal suffrage. The president appoints the prime minister on the basis of election results; other members of the Council of Ministers are appointed on the basis of the prime minister's nomination. Legislative power is vested in the unicameral Parliament (the Republic Assembly), whose members are elected by direct universal suffrage under a proportional representation system. As a member of the European Community since 1986 and the North Atlantic Treaty Organization since 1945, Portugal plays a greater role in both European and world affairs than its size would suggest (*Encyclopedia Britannica* 2000).

Demographics

The total population of Portugal in mid-1997 was 9.8 million (WHO 1999), which was a decrease of 1.9 percent from the previous decade. The 2001 population census shows a change in that trend. The resident population has grown to 10,355,824 inhabitants, a 5 percent increase from 1991 to 2001 (INE 2001). The population pyramid shows a decline in the younger age groups. Consequently, the proportion of the population under 15 years old has declined to 18 percent, whereas the proportion of the population 65 years old and older has risen steadily, to 14.9 percent of the population in 1997 (WHO 1999b). The aging trend is much more pronounced in women, who account for 70 percent of the population that is more than 85 years old. For demographic indicators, please see Table 11.1.

The Economy

Although Portugal's economy has benefited from the creation of the European Union, Portugal is still one of the poorest countries in the EU. A program of privatization has been underway since the early 1990s, result-

TABLE 11.1
General Demographics

Population in millions, 2001	10.356		
Infant mortality per 1,000 live births, 1999	5.6		
Under-five mortality per 1,000 live births	6.4		
Life expectancy at birth (years), 1997	75		
Additional life expectancy at 65 years	15.3		
Fertility rate, 1996	1.4		
Percent urbanized, 1993	35		
Dependency ratio (%), 2000	47.4		
Population distribution by age group (%), 2001	0 to 14 years	15 to 64 years	65 years old and older
	16.6	67.9	15.5

SOURCE: OECD (1998); National Statistic Institute (2000, 2001); UNICEF (2000).

ing in a period of economic growth beginning in 1994, with a real gross national product increase of 3.5 percent in 1997 (OECD 1999). Such growth is attributed primarily to improved export capacity and stronger domestic demand. The per capita gross domestic product in 1998 was U.S.$10,574, and the real gross national product per capita (P.P.P.$) was $15,266 (OECD 1999).

The total population unemployment rate in 1997 was 6.9 percent, which was one of the lowest in the EU; the inflation rate was just above 2 percent in that same year (OECD 1999). Agriculture still occupies 12 percent of the civilian workforce, although it accounted for only 6 percent of the GDP in 1994. The industrial sector, which is dominated by the manufacture of textiles and footwear, employs 33 percent of the workforce and accounts for 37 percent of the GDP. Services account for 61 percent of the GDP and employ 56 percent of the civilian workforce. Tourism is one of the most important service areas in Portugal. For further economic indicators, please see Table 11.2.

Education

In Portugal, as in all EU countries, primary education is universal; therefore, the most significant indicator besides the literacy rate for measuring educational achievement is the proportion of the population achieving greater than a lower-secondary education. In both respects, Portugal lags behind other EU countries, with an adult literacy rate of 92 percent, which is also lower than that of other European countries. Only about 25 percent of the adult population attains upper-secondary education (WHO 1997). The situation is improving among younger people, however, as shown by the proportion of the 25- to 29-year-old age group that has completed upper-secondary education (more than 35 percent). A sizable education differential is evident between women and men. In the younger age groups, 15 percent of women (as opposed to only 9 percent of men) achieve a higher degree (WHO 1997). In the 16- to 18-year-old group, 15 percent more girls than boys are enrolled in educational programs (WHO 1997a). Please see Table 11.3 for further indicators.

GNP per capita (U.S.$), 1998	10,574	**TABLE 11.2**
Real GDP per capita (P.P.P.$), 1998	15,266	Economic
Percent of GNP to health, 1996	8.3	and Social
Public health expenditure as percent of total public spending, 1996	10.8	Indicators
Public health expenditure as percent of total health spending, 1995	60.5	
Percent of health budget in public sector (national)	4.9	

SOURCE: OECD (1998, 1999).

TABLE 11.3
Education
Indicators

	Total	Male	Female
Adult literacy rate, % (1995)	92	—	—
Secondary education, higher level, % (1993)			
Total (25 to 59 years old)	—	22	21
55 to 59 years old	—	11	8
25 to 29 years old	—	28	36

SOURCE: UNESCO (2000); WHO (1997).

Context: Health Needs

The health status of the Portuguese population still lags behind EU standards, despite considerable improvements in some areas. Life expectancy at birth has continued to improve over the past two decades and has now reached 75 years. The infant mortality rate, although nearly halved during the preceding ten years, remains among the EU's highest, at 5.6 deaths per 1,000 live births (INE 1999). Maternal mortality has also improved, but Portugal has moved from last only to the next lowest position in the ratings (WHO 1997b). Major causes of death across all age groups are, in order of prevalence, cancers, cardiovascular diseases, and external causes. A standardized death rate chart is presented in Table 11.4.

Portugal's mortality rates for a number of groups are the highest in the EU. Portuguese boys and girls in the 1- to 14- and 15- to 34-year-old age groups have among the highest mortality rates for their age groups in the EU. Portuguese men between 30 and 64 years old and women 65 years old and older have the overall highest mortality rates for their age groups in the EU; Portuguese men over 65 have the second highest.

Deeply rooted dietary patterns stemming from cultural traditions and local agricultural production patterns significantly influence specific premature mortality rates. Changes have occurred in recent years because of internationalized European food markets, which have equalized nutritional differences between northern and southern Europe. As a consequence, Portugal is straying from its typical Mediterranean diet, which is particularly low in saturated fatty acids. The average proportion of energy derived from overall fat intake has been increasing over the past decade and has now reached 34 percent. Nevertheless, Portugal's level of fat consumption remains the lowest in Europe.

Portugal is the fifth largest consumer of alcohol among EU countries. Not surprisingly, Portugal had the highest EU death rate from cirrhosis and other liver diseases in 1993. A positive trend in deaths from liver

Leading Causes of Death	Percent of Deaths
Cerebrovascular disorders	20.86
Ischemic heart disease	8.73
Pneumonia	3.77
Diabetes mellitus	3.03
Cancer of the respiratory tract	2.52
Stomach cancer	2.50
Chronic liver disease	2.50
Motor vehicle accidents	1.92
Colon cancer	1.80
Prostate cancer	1.59
Breast cancer	1.4

TABLE 11.4 Leading Causes of Mortality, 1998

SOURCE: Ministry of Health, Department of Health Studies and Planning (1998).

diseases is developing; the rate has dropped over the past 15 years by 24 percent for women and 22 percent for men.

Cardiovascular disease rates have been falling since 1970, but in 1993 the standardized death rate (SDR) for women from cardiovascular diseases was one of the highest in the EU. Cmparatively small reductions in mortality from ischemic heart disease have been seen, and both sexes had relatively low SDRs in 1993. The geographic pattern for ischemic heart disease reflects a strong north-south gradient for the age group of 0 to 64 years, with values more than two times higher in some southern regions and Lisbon. Geographical differences also are observed for cerebrovascular diseases, with the highest SDRs in the northwest portion of the country.

In 1993, Portugal maintained a strong position with regard to cancer and the second lowest rates of death due to cancer of the bronchus and lung. However, cervical cancer is rising slightly for women, and the incidence of breast cancer is rising faster than the EU average. A geographic variation is indicated for cancer, with relatively low rates in the northeast and the highest rates in Viana do Castelo, Porto, Beja, Lisbon, and Setúbal.

External causes of death and injury include deaths due to accidents. Traffic accidents as a cause of death became more frequent for both men and women until the beginning of the 1980s; the rate started falling thereafter. As a consequence, the risk of dying from a traffic accident has dropped by 16 percent over the last 19 years, but it is still the highest among the EU reference countries.

Psychosocial and mental health conditions and disorders are extremely difficult to measure in any country. Portugal has traditionally had one of the lowest SDRs for suicide. During the last ten years, the decreases in suicide for both men and women were more pronounced in Portugal than in the rest of the EU. In 1993, women had the third lowest and men the fifth lowest SDR for suicide in the European Union.

In 1994, Portugal had an incidence rate of 6.7 cases of AIDS per 100,000 population, which was just below the EU average. According to the European Center for the Epidemiological Monitoring of AIDS, at the beginning of 1995 a total of 2,400 cases had been reported in Portugal, with predictions that 800 to 1,000 new cases per year could be expected thereafter. A 1995 report found that 31 percent of the cases were transmitted by homosexual or bisexual contact and by use of injected drugs, whereas 27 percent were contracted through heterosexual contact. According to estimates from the European Center for the Epidemiological Monitoring of AIDS, there were 15,000 HIV-positive people in Portugal at the end of 1993, 14 percent of them women.

A comparative study conducted in the EU (WHO 1997) estimated that, in 1992, 9.5 percent of the EU population suffered from disabilities that resulted in a personal, social, or economic handicap; this figure was derived from a health survey of those individuals 60 years old or younger on the list of disability pension funds. Portugal, according to the study, had the second lowest proportion of disabled people in the EU, well below the EU average of 11.5 percent. Nevertheless, some bias may have been introduced by the study method, because a relatively high degree of disability is needed for entitlement to a disability pension under the Portuguese system.

Organization and Management of the Health System

Portugal shifted from a social welfare–based system to a tax-financed national health system providing universal coverage, the Serviço Nacional de Saúde (SNS), in the late 1970s. At present, the Portuguese healthcare system comprises three coexisting systems of which the SNS is dominant. These systems include the SNS, special insurance schemes for specific professions, and voluntary private health insurance schemes. The central government, through the Ministry of Health, has primary responsibility for the organization, regulation, and direction of the healthcare system as a whole. Private healthcare providers typically supplement the SNS rather than provide an alternative to it (WHO 1997b). Key institutions include private practitioners; independent charitable institutions (the Misericórdias); private hospitals, clinics, and facilities; and a national network of health centers and hospitals maintained by the Ministry of Health and controlled by the five regional health administrations under the centralized governance of the SNS.

The Ministry of Health is responsible for developing national health policy and for overseeing and evaluating its implementation; it also coordinates health-related activities with other ministries. The Ministry's General Directorate of Health carries out central planning for health on the basis of plans submitted by the five regional health administrations. The boundaries between the main functions in the system—planning, regulation, financing, and management—overlap, because the health system is integrated with the government, which functions as both provider and third-party payer at the same time (Dixon and Reis 1999). Nevertheless, some degree of decentralization is being pursued with the implementation of the 1990 Law on the Fundamental Principles of Health Practice, which allows public facilities to be managed or provided by other companies, public or private. Under the law, private companies may establish a contract with the Ministry of Health that details the annual (public) budget to be managed, against which contracted expected activity and quality benchmarks must be met. This reform aims, among other things, to separate the purchaser and provider roles in the healthcare system. One pilot experiment was implemented in 2000 with good results, and several new hospitals and other health facilities are expected to open using this new management model.

The high degree of regulation in the Portuguese health system reflects the major role of government in funding, planning, and providing care. Control is exerted over pharmaceuticals, technological equipment, and the education, training, and accreditation of health personnel. Although the rules are restrictive, they are not strictly enforced. A Sub-Directory for Quality resides within the general directorate of health, and plans are being made to create a separate institute for quality control for the accreditation of hospitals and other health facilities (Dixon and Reis 1999).

Capital planning and investing are the responsibilities of the General Directorate of Health, and most of the investment in health comes from the Portuguese state budget through the Central Administration's Investment and Development Plan. As a member of the EU, Portugal has participated in some joint funding of hospitals and health centers. The installation of all public and private high-technology equipment must be approved by the Ministry of Health.

Financing

Healthcare is financed through both public and private means (Table 11.5). In 1996, Portugal spent 8.3 percent of the total gross domestic product on healthcare, which was a per capita expenditure of U.S.$1,071 (OECD 1999). The SNS, which provides universal coverage, is almost totally funded by general taxes. Citizens using the SNS pay flat-rate copayments that are widely implemented. Health service users are also charged for auxiliary diagnostic and therapeutic procedures in ambulatory settings, hospital- and health-center-based emergency services and consultations, and other public or specified private health services. Portugal's exemption system is rather complex because it attempts to account for all situations where people might need exemption from users' charges. Thus, exemptions are considered under the following broad categories: children under 12 years of age; low-income people; disability status; pregnant women; medical condition; blood donors; the chronically alcohol- and drug-addicted; and children and young people living in institutions (Ministério do Trabalho e da Solidariedade 1999).

The health subsystems provide coverage to approximately one-quarter of the population and are funded by employer and employee contributions. Sources of private funding include individual out-of-pocket payments directly to health providers, copayments, and voluntary health insurance premiums. Private voluntary health insurance covers only 10 percent of the population, and it is partially tax deductible. Nevertheless, this portion of the population is still obliged to pay health taxes out of their gross income. The 1995 distribution of healthcare funding is detailed in Table 11.5.

On average, the Portuguese have one of the highest out-of-pocket payment rates in Europe; this type of spending accounted for about 45 percent of total health expenditures during the last ten years (Dixon and Reis 1999). More than 50 percent of out-of-pocket expenditures goes toward pharmaceuticals, followed by medical, nursing, and paramedical services at 36.8 percent. In spite of this high personal expenditure, incentive to purchase or use private insurance is low. Most health expenses are fully deductible from personal taxes, and a stand-alone limit on insurance premiums is in place (Dixon and Reis 1999), thereby making out-of-pocket payments favored by the population. Additionally, because private voluntary insurance is not very well developed, the insurance plans available are very restrictive, selective in nature, and lack comprehensiveness, which reinforces a low demand (Dixon and Reis 1999).

TABLE 11.5

Sources of Healthcare Financing as Percentage of Total Expenditures

Source of Financing	1995 Percent Distribution
Public	
Taxes	62.6
Health subsystems	4.8
Private	
Out-of-pocket	44.6
Voluntary insurance	1.4

SOURCE: OECD (1998).

Nevertheless, the use of voluntary health insurance may increase if tax policies change as a result of government efforts to alleviate the public funding burden by diversifying financing sources. Some health economists advise against such measures and argue that the imminent risks of such a policy must be carefully considered. According to Pinto and Pereira (1993), a dangerous political dynamic can be created if a large segment of the population leaves a primary care gatekeeper structure for direct access to specialists: support for the public system could decline and with it funding from the public system.

Since Portugal became a member of the European Community, European lines of funding are also available for health programs. In 1994, a program of investment in healthcare services was developed with EU cofunding, and significant investments have been made. The Portuguese government contributes 25 percent of the funding for each cofinanced project.

Health Resources

All healthcare personnel within the SNS, the major health employer, are salaried civil servants. At 2.9 physicians per 1,000 population in 1992 and 1993, the number of practicing physicians was slightly above the EU average of 2.7 per 1,000 population (WHO 1997b). In 1995, according to the Portuguese Medical Association, Portugal had 29,000 physicians, of which 73 percent were SNS employees (Dixon and Reis 1999). According to 1996 figures (Department of Human Resources 1997), 46 percent of physicians worked in hospital settings and 35 percent were general practitioners specializing in family medicine. In the primary healthcare setting, 74 percent of doctors are general practitioners (GPs) who have dominant roles as gatekeepers to secondary care. The number of active physicians has been increasing during the last decade, and by 1998, 31,087 physicians (National Statistic Institute 1998) were enrolled in the Portuguese Medical Association. Physicians are allowed to practice simultaneously in both the public and private sectors. Although they may choose to work exclusively as public servants, the majority of physicians hold a private practice in addition to their public service in order to augment their income.

Portugal has five schools of medicine, with plans for two new schools. Medical training programs are similar among schools and follow the accepted international academic curricula: two phases of three years each, with a core program covering basic sciences and a clinical program with practical sessions. A curriculum change is underway to shorten the course to five years. After university, all graduates complete internships. The accreditation and certification of physicians is a joint responsibility of the government and the Portuguese Medical Association (Dixon and Reis 1999).

Portugal has a serious ongoing shortage of nurses. In spite of gains made over the last 12 years, Portugal still has a very low nurse ratio at 3.8 per 1,000 population, which is less than half of the EU average (WHO 1997b). One important consequence of the shortage is that primary health-care nursing is underdeveloped. Nurses work mainly in central and district hospitals (which employ 74 percent of the nursing workforce), followed by the primary care setting (20 percent), and the psychiatric setting (3 percent) (Dixon and Reis 1999). Two university education levels for nursing are available in Portugal: a three-year program culminating in a bachelor's degree and a four-year program resulting in a licensed advanced degree. Both grant the title of registered nurse. After becoming a registered nurse, a nurse can pursue specialized degrees in administration, public health, or a specialty track. Nursing aide, nursing auxiliary, and equivalent positions were eliminated in 1978 and 1979. The Portuguese Nurses Association, which has powers similar to those of the Medical Association, was established in 1998.

The number of dentists in Portugal is also very low as compared with the EU average, limiting the services available for dental care at dental clinics and integrated health centers. In spite of these figures, in 1990, 12-year-old children had an average of 3.2 decayed, missing, or filled teeth, which was the EU average (WHO 1997b). Since 1986, three public and one private schools of dentistry have operated in Portugal. An odontology level was created by the government in an attempt to reduce the scarcity of dental services, but this training has been replaced in favor of the primary degree of dental medicine. Before 1986, a stomatologist specialty was available to doctors specializing in dentistry, which required a medical degree plus three years of dental training. The number of pharmacists in Portugal is also low by EU standards; community pharmacists are subject to numerous regulations.

Portugal has a wide geographic variation in the distribution of health professionals. Health personnel tend to work in or near major cities: 60 percent are located in the large metropolitan area of Lisbon, 17.6 percent are in Porto, and 9 percent are in Coimbra, in the center of the country. This leaves the rest of the country with few professionals and a number of districts critically understaffed (WHO 1997b). Additional information concerning health professionals can be found in Table 11.6.

The Ministry of Health in Portugal has not recognized alternative medicine practitioners such as acupuncturists, chiropractors, and homeopaths. Although a trend for healthcare consumers to adopt such alternative medicines has been perceived, Western medicine still prevails as the first choice (Dixon and Reis 1999).

Primary and preventive healthcare is provided by a national network of integrated primary health centers and includes a range of services from health promotion and protection to preventive care and diagnostic and treatment services. A total of 2,424 medical units (Table 11.7) are found

	Total	Per 1,000 Population
Physicians	31,087	3.1
Nurses*	37,747	3.8
Pharmacists	7,505	0.8
Dentists	2,219	0.2

TABLE 11.6
Human
Resources by
Type, 1998

* Portuguese nurses include midwives who have completed a nursing training track before specializing as midwives.
SOURCE: National Statistic Institute (1998).

in the primary care setting, including 382 health centers and 2,042 health posts, with an average of 243.62 units per 1,000 population (WHO 1997b). Facilities vary widely across the country. Some physical structures are well-prepared to provide primary care to a designated population; others were incorporated into residential buildings and do not provide a patient-friendly environment (Dixon and Reis 1999). Centers also vary significantly in terms of services provided; some offer a range of general practice services and basic diagnostic equipment as well as dental care and some specialty care in gynecology and pediatrics. At the other extreme, some rural centers may only have one general practitioner for the entire population in that area.

According to Dixon and Reis, in 1996 Portugal had 211 hospitals, of which 122 were public and 89 private (Table 11.7). Eighty-three percent of all hospital beds are in the public sector (WHO 1997b). Central hospitals are located in the main cities of Lisbon, Porto, and Coimbra. At least one district hospital is located in the main town of each district. The national hospital network includes specialized psychiatric, maternity, oncology, and rehabilitation hospitals (WHO 1997b). Portugal is experiencing a significant shortage of geriatric and nursing home beds. This is an important challenge for the near future, as a rapidly aging population and family life–pattern changes will expand the need for solutions beyond informal family care.

Prescribed drugs are partially paid for by the SNS, with the remaining portion of the cost (0 to 60 percent) paid for by the user (Portuguese Association of Health Economics [APE] 1996). The amount of copayment depends on the therapeutic value of the drug. Pensioners pay a reduced copayment, and the chronically ill are exempted from copayments. Although the SNS has a national formulary of drugs for hospital use, health centers and outpatient services are not obliged to follow the formulary. Therapeutic products are essentially out-of-pocket expenses. According to Dixon and Reis (1999), 90 percent of every household's health expense pays for medical, nursing, or paramedical items. All medical devices are regulated according

TABLE 11.7
Number and
Type of
Health
Services
Facilities and
by Population,
1996

	Number	Per 1,000 Population
Hospitals*	215	21.5
Health centers†	2,424	243.62
Public hospital beds	30,392	3.1
Private hospital beds	8,820	.89

* Table refers only to mainland hospitals; psychiatric and rehabilitation hospitals are not included.
† Total of medical units in primary care setting, including health centers (382) and health posts (2,042).
SOURCE: National Statistic Institute (1998).

to Economic European Committee Directive 93/42 and a national directive of 1995. The regulating institutions are the National Institutes of Health for active medical devices and the Institute of Pharmacy and Drugs (INFARMED) for nonactive medical devices (Dixon and Reis 1999).

Service Delivery

The Portuguese Constitution stipulates that health is a universal right, but healthcare provision is perceived as an elective area for social intervention. The SNS provides a national network of care, from primary to tertiary. Through the SNS, a theoretically comprehensive plan of care is available to every citizen, independent of his or her ability to pay. However, several services (e.g., dental care) are not available within the public network. Consequently, a private sector has been developing to complement the SNS. These services are provided by the private sector with payments partially reimbursed by the SNS and the remainder of the cost paid by the consumer; this has created a growing equity problem (WHO 1997). Patients often pay private practitioners themselves; therefore, more expensive health needs may not be available to poorer individuals.

In Portugal, a mix of private and public providers delivers primary healthcare. Wealthier people seek primary and specialized care privately, with the volume of private care offered increasing over the last 10 to 15 years. The public sector is composed of a network of health centers distributed throughout the country. On average, each health center covers 28,000 citizens and employs 80 health professionals. Health centers vary greatly from region to region both in terms of facilities available and in the number and type of health professionals. Health centers currently have no financial or managerial autonomy, and they are directly dependent on the local regional health administration.

GPs deliver most of the primary care services in the health centers. The range of services includes general medical care, prenatal care, pediatric care, women's health, family planning, first aid, certification of incapacity to work, home visits (very few), and preventive services such as immunizations and breast, cervical, and prostate cancer screenings (Dixon and Reis 1999). Every citizen must register with a GP chosen from among the physicians in the health centers in the household's geographic area. Each GP has, on average, 1,500 patients on his or her list. As a result, long waiting lists for physicians' appointments and for referrals to specialized care characterize primary care provision.

Formally, secondary care is only available through referral by a primary care physician. However, in an attempt to circumvent the long waits, patients frequently go directly to hospital emergency departments to seek a consultation because no financial deterrents exist for the abuse of emergency room care; this has led to one of the largest dysfunctions in the pattern of service utilization. An overconsumption of emergency care for nonemergent situations has led to misuse of expensive resources.

Healthcare resources are inequitably distributed throughout the country, with inland areas lacking health professionals (mainly physicians and nurses), who prefer to work in coastal and metropolitan areas. Patients covered by health subsystems have direct access to the hospital and specialist care allowed by their health plans. Private doctors can also refer patients to SNS hospitals. Diagnostic and therapeutic services in ambulatory care are usually provided by the private sector to the SNS through provider contracts (Dixon and Reis 1999).

Secondary and tertiary care are delivered by hospitals (Table 11.8); most hospital services are provided by the SNS. The number of hospitals in Portugal has been decreasing, as in other developed countries, for the past 30 years. Portugal currently has fewer hospital beds than the EU average. A decrease in SNS hospital beds has been accompanied by a progressive increase in privately owned beds. The utilization rate of hospital beds, however, is comparable to the European average.

Hospitals are classified as central, specialized, district, or district level one according to services offered. Again, hospital resources are concentrated in Lisbon and the coastal areas, with the regions of Alentejo and Algarve the most underserved (WHO 1997b). To reverse this trend, major investments have been made in the interior and rural areas, and today many of the district hospitals inland have better facilities than those in coastal areas.

Elder care provided by the public sector through the SNS is deficient, and public residential care is often of very poor quality (Dixon and Reis 1999). Nursing homes are private and are only affordable to the wealthier population. Several residential homes are run by a private not-for-profit institution, the Misericórdias, which are of better quality and only request a small monetary contribution. However, these institutions are unable to fulfill the demands that exist for these services. A network of day centers, managed and supported by the Ministry of Employment and Social Solidarity (which is responsible for social security affairs), does offer some support

TABLE 11.8
Service Use
and Rates

	Number	Per 1,000 Population
Hospital admissions, 1997	1,184	11.9
Average length of stay (acute beds) in days, 1997	7.3	—
Occupancy rate (%), 1997	75.5	—
		Per capita
Outpatient visits, 1996	32,720	3.3
Consultations		
Primary care visits	24,882,400	252
Hospital visits	6,034,800	61
Emergency room visits		
Primary care	4,586,800	46
Hospital care	5,618,000	57
Patients discharged, 1995		
Primary care	26,400	0.27
Hospitals	848,368	8.6

SOURCE: WHO (1999); DEPS (1995, 1998).

for elder care. In 1998, 41,195 day centers provided a range of services such as meals, meals on wheels, laundry, bathing, or assistance in activities of daily living. Usually, a small means-tested contribution is charged (Dixon and Reis 1999). As with residential care, day center facilities are not able to meet the demand for their services. Home care is now expanding in Portugal, with the development of the Integrated Support Plan for the Elderly, a joint venture between the ministries of Health and Employment and Social Solidarity that is developing infrastructures for the delivery of home care (Dixon and Reis 1999).

Prospects for the Future

The Portuguese health system faces several challenges. The main problems in the system are waiting lists and unmet needs due to the elective cost-control mechanism of budget caps on healthcare expenses that results in the SNS being chronically underbudgeted. The public system as it currently operates provides few incentives for healthcare professionals to provide quality care in a cost-effective manner. Also, the lack of coordination between GPs and hospitals results in inefficiencies and the frequent duplication and misuse of resources. Decentralization is key to current health-care reform efforts, which include initiatives designed to separate purchaser and provider roles, introduce competition incentives, and find new financing mechanisms.

The decree of 1993 started a process of change within the Portuguese SNS, and with it came the decentralization of health management. Five health regions, known as the regional health administrations, now work autonomously from the central government to coordinate care (Dixon and Reis 1999). Health centers and hospitals are also organized into health units, which are accountable for providing all needed care to a specific geographic population. The concept of a health unit was expanded by a 1994 law that created Local Health Systems and by 1999 legislation that further expanded the concept. Under the local health systems, health centers, hospitals, public or private health providers, and nongovernment organizations intervening in health matters can coordinate efforts in exchange for specific management privileges (Ministério da Saúde 1998). The 1993 decree also opened the door for the creation of an alternative health insurance scheme whereby private companies receive a capitation payment from the government for each person opting out of the SNS in exchange for paying a premium. However, the project did not evolve, primarily because of a lack of interest from insurance companies but also because of a change in government and consequent ministerial rearrangements (Dixon and Reis 1999).

The 1993 decree introduced competition into the health market for the first time by allowing public facilities to be managed by other public or private companies. The goal of this reform is to create controlled competition within the market as different companies compete for government contracts. These organizations will manage healthcare facilities to meet population needs within defined budgets but will remain part of the public system at the point of delivery of care. Each regional health administration will monitor facilities operating under private management contracts. Under this reform, the first public hospital to be privately managed, the Hospital Fernando Fonseca, opened in January 1996. This hospital has become financially accountable for the quantity and quality of care provided to the population in its geographic region.

Portugal is striving to clearly separate the roles of purchaser and provider. If management organizations contracting with the Ministry fail to meet budgets, they are still accountable for the provision of all needed and contracted care. The facilities are retained as public property, and health professionals are free to choose between public or private contracts. Patients access health services at Hospital Fernando Fonseca following the rules of the public system, namely GP referral and current copayment requirements. The contract allows for the management company to establish other private contracting with third-party payers or serve private out-of-pocket patients along with public system consumers. The aim is to allow for the most efficient use of installed capacity while meeting public needs and maintaining equity. The system also adds an incentive for management companies to excel in the efficient use of resources. Under negotiation is an extension of the management umbrella of the Hospital Fernando Fonseca to the total health unit, thereby allowing for the integrated management of the continuum of healthcare delivery.

Despite the extensive program of legislative reform of the healthcare system in Portugal, several important challenges must still be addressed. One important challenge remains in the existence of multiple subsystems of coverage that operate in an uncoordinated manner. Lack of coordination allows patients to shop around for care using either their SNS status or the subsystem under which they are covered (Dixon and Reis 1999). As a consequence, cost-control mechanisms are not working as designed, and duplication and fragmentation of care persists. A nationally unified system of identification—the user's card—is now being implemented to effect change in this area.

Portugal, like many other developed countries, is in a period of transition and reform. Change has been implemented incrementally, with the emphasis of 1990s legislation on the role of the state as a health purchaser rather than provider in a mixed economy of provision (Dixon and Reis 1999). The coming decade will focus on the health strategies, goals, and desired outcomes set for the nation in the "National Health Strategy" (Ministry of Health 1996).

REFERENCES

Associação Portuguesa de Economia da Saúde (Portuguese Association of Health Economics [APE]). 1996. *Actas do IV Encontro Nacional da APES.* Lisbon: Associação Portuguesa de Economia da Saúde.

Department of Health Studies and Planning. 1998. *Portugal Saúde 1996, Statistic Division.* Lisbon: Ministry of Health.

————. 1995. *A Saúde em Portugal.* Lisbon: Ministry of Health.

Department of Human Resources. 1997. Annual publication. Lisbon: Ministry of Health.

Dixon, A., and Reis, V. 1999. *Health Care Systems in Transition—Portugal.* Copenhagen: European Observatory on Health Care Systems, World Health Organization.

Encyclopedia Britannica. Retrieved 14 May 2000 from http://www.britannica.com.

Merriam-Webster's Collegiate Dictionary. 2000. Retrieved 14 May 2000 from http://www.m-w.com/cgi-bin/mweb.

Ministry of Health. 1996. *A Saúde em Portugal—Uma Estratégia Para o Virar do Século, 1997–2001, Orientações Para 1997* (Health In Portugal—A Strategy for the Turning of the Century, 1997–2001, Orientations for 1997). Lisbon: General Directorate of Health.

Ministério do Trabalho e da Solidariedade (Ministry of Employment and Social
 Solidarity). 1999. Portugal home page for Social Security data. Pensões e
 Protecção Especial na Invalidez. Retrieved 02 June 2000 from
 http://www.seg-social.pt.

———. 1998. *O Hospital Português* (The Portuguese Hospital). Lisbon: General
 Directorate of Health.

National Statistic Institute. 2001. "População Residente" (Resident Population).
 Retrieved 25 February 2002 from http://www.ine.pt/prodserv/indi-
 cadores/quadros.asp?CodInd=65.

———. 2000. "Principais Indicadores Demográficos" (Main Demographic
 Indicators). Retrieved 04 June 2000 and 25 February 2002 from
 http://www.ine.pt/prodserv/indicadores/quadros.asp?CodInd=17.

———. 1998. "Health Indicators." Retrieved 04 June 2000 and 25 February
 2002 from http://www.ine.pt/prodserv/Indicadores/
 quadros.asp?CodInd=.

———. 1998. "Data on Country's Mainland plus Madeira and Açores Islands."
 Retrieved 04 June 2000 from
 http://www.ine.pt/prodserv/Indicadores/ultindic.asp.

Organization of Economic Cooperation and Development (OECD). 1998.
 Health Data 98. Paris: OECD.

———. 1999. *Main Economic Indicators, National Accounts Division, STD.*
 Paris: OECD.

Pinto, C. G., and Pereira, J. 1993. "Equity in the Finance and Delivery of
 Health Care in Portugal." In *Equity in the Finance and Delivery of
 Health Care. An International Perspective,* edited by E. V. Doorslaer.
 Oxford: Commission of the European Communities, Oxford University
 Press.

Portuguese Ministry of Education. 2000. "Department of Prospective Appraisal
 and Planning." Retrieved 02 June 2000 from http://www.dapp.min-
 edu.pt.

UNICEF. 2000. "Indicators by Country, Portugal." Retrieved 02 June 2000
 from http://www.unicef.org/statis/Country_1Page141.html.

United Nations Development Programme (UNDP). 1996. *Human Development
 Report 1996.* New York: Oxford University Press.

United Nations Educational, Scientific and Cultural Organization. 2000.
 "Statistics Database." Retrieved 02 June 2000 from
 http://www.unesco.org.

World Health Organization (WHO). 1997. *Eurostat 1995c.* Copenhagen: WHO
 Regional Office for Europe.

———. 1997a. *Eurostat 1995d.* Copenhagen: WHO Regional Office for Europe.

———. 1997b. *Highlights on Health in Portugal.* Copenhagen: WHO Regional
 Office for Europe.

———. 1999. *Mid-Year Estimate 1997, Health for All Database.* Copenhagen:
 WHO Regional Office for Europe.

———. 1999a. *Council of Europe 1995.* Copenhagen: WHO Regional Office for
 Europe.

———. 1999b. *Eurostat 1996.* Copenhagen: WHO Regional Office for Europe.

ISRAEL

Arie Shirom and Revital Gross

Background Information

Israel was established as an independent state in May 1948. It succeeded the British administration, which ruled Palestine under a League of Nations mandate from 1920 until 1948. The newly established Jewish State culminated the half-century struggle by the Zionist movement to reestablish an autonomous community of Jews in their Promised Land, which was at that time called Palestine. This Jewish resettlement effort was powered by waves of immigration from Europe and from Arab countries in Asia and Africa to the Promised Land beginning in the nineteenth century and accelerating after World War II and the Holocaust.

Israel is a small country on the European scale: it occupies 22,145 square kilometers, a narrow strip of territory on the eastern shore of the Mediterranean Sea. At the end of 1999, some 6,220,000 people were living in Israel; about 80 percent were Jews who speak Hebrew, and about 20 percent were Muslims, Christians, and Druze who speak Arabic (and therefore would be referred to as Israeli Arabs). It is a densely populated country, with about 281 people per square kilometer. Israel is bordered by Egypt to the west, Jordan to the east, Lebanon to the north, and Syria to the northeast. The climate is Mediterranean, with hot, dry summers, and it tends to be subtropical on the coast but extreme in the Negev Desert, in the south, and near the shores of the Dead Sea.

Israel's system of government is essentially a parliamentary democracy, with supreme legislative authority resting with the Knesset (Israel's parliament). The Knesset's 120 members are elected for four-year terms (subject to self-dissolution via special legislation) based on proportional representation. Executive power lies with the Cabinet, which is led by a directly elected prime minister. The president of Israel is a constitutional head of state elected by the Knesset for a five-year term, fulfilling mostly ceremonial duties and with minimal formal authority. The Cabinet takes office after receiving a vote of confidence in the Knesset, to which it is responsible. Elections for mayors and municipal council members in the country's system of local government are held separately from those for the Knesset.

In 1998, according to estimates of the World Bank, Israel's gross national product was U.S.$95,200 million, or about U.S.$15,940 per capita. Israel's gross domestic product increased, in real terms, by an average of

3.5 percent per year from 1980 to 1990 and by 5.4 percent from 1990 to 1994, largely because of the massive influx of Jews from the former USSR during the early 1990s. During this last wave of Jewish immigration, which occurred from 1990 through 1995, 685,683 immigrants arrived in Israel, mostly from the former USSR, increasing the population by 14 percent. Among the effects of this large-scale immigration was a doubling of the number of physicians (11,280 immigrant physicians joined the 13,000 veteran physicians [Nirel 2000]) and the creation of special health needs. In 1996, a period of economic slowdown began, and real GDP increased by 4.6 percent in 1996, by 2.6 percent in 1997, and by 1.7 percent in 1998. The years 1999 and 2000 were a time of economic recovery spearheaded by the booming exports of the high-technology industry. Table 12.1 details the country's economic indicators.

The age distribution of the population has important implications for its health status because of the different health needs and different patterns of healthcare utilization of the various age groups. The age and sex distributions of the Jewish and Arab population groups differ markedly (based on 1995 data of the Bureau of Labor Statistics). The Arab population has a large proportion of children (40 percent are under the age of 15) and a small proportion of elderly (5.1 percent are over the age of 65). In comparison, the Jewish population is much older, with only 27 percent under the age of 15 and 11.1 percent over the age of 65. The proportion of elderly (65 years old and older) in the population as a whole is 9.5 percent, which is lower than in the countries of the European Community and in the United States. In comparison with these countries, Israel has the highest proportion of children under 15: about 30 percent in 1996. In 1996, 61 percent of the Jewish population was Israeli-born. The total fertility rate was 2.9 in 1996; among Jews it was 2.6, whereas among Muslims it was 4.6. Total fertility rates are higher in Israel than in all of the countries of the European Community. Table 12.2 shows Israel's demographic profile.

Employment patterns in Israel mirror those of the OECD countries, with a growing proportion of women employed outside of the home (about 47 percent in 1999). At postsecondary educational levels, almost no difference is found between the proportion of women and men in the labor force. Unemployment, as in the other industrialized market economies, has been a serious social problem in Israel during the last decade, with unemployment rates exceeding 8 percent for the period from 1997 through

TABLE 12.1
Economic
Indicators

GNP per capita (U.S.$), 1998	15,940
GDP to health, 1999 (%)	8.3
Percent of health budget in public sector (national, regional, local)	48

TABLE 12.2
General Demographics

Population in millions, 1998	6	
Infant mortality per 1,000 live births, 1996	3.6	
Under-five mortality per 1,000 live births, 1996	Male	0 to 1 year: 7.4
		1 to 4 years: 0.4
	Female	0 to 1 year: 6.6
		1 to 4 years: 0.4
Life expectancy at birth in years, 1996	Male	76.3
	Female	79.9
Fertility rate, 1996	2.9	
Percent urbanized	91	

2000. A consistently higher percentage of women are unemployed as compared with men, and a consistently higher percentage of the Arab minority is unemployed as compared with the Jews.

Israel has a high standard of literacy and educational services. Free compulsory education is provided for all children between 5 and 15 years of age. Postprimary education, which is also free, lasts six years. Enrollments at primary and secondary schools exceed 96 percent of children between the ages of 6 and 17. Among women, ethnic differences in educational status are very marked: 39.1 percent of Arab women in 1997 had less than nine years of education as compared with only 15.4 percent of Jewish women. Because the educational status of women is closely associated with their health status and with that of their children, these differences have important implications for the health of different population groups. Table 12.3 illustrates education levels in Israel.

The waves of immigration in the early twentieth century sparked the establishment of networks of community welfare and health organizations. These health organizations, established in the early 1920s, largely followed the central European model of sick funds. The sick fund model of health provision has persisted in Israel to this day, although the 1994 National Health Insurance (NHI) Law made all sick funds regulated subcontractors

TABLE 12.3
Education

Adult literacy rate (%)	Male: 97
	Female: 93
Primary school enrollment, 1999	640,000 pupils
Secondary school enrollment, 1999	535,000 pupils

of the state, thereby providing healthcare services to the country's residents under government regulation.

The descriptive and analytic literature on the Israeli healthcare system is not extensive (for useful sources, see Chinitz and Cohen 1993; Ellencweig 1992; Gross, Rosen, and Shirom 2001; Shuval 1992; Steinberg and Bick 1992). Most of this literature describes features of the healthcare system that were prevalent before the 1994 NHI Law. In this chapter, recent sources are drawn upon to describe different facets of Israel's healthcare system (Central Bureau of Statistics 1999; Hadassah 1999; Kop 1999; State of Israel, Ministry of Health, Israel Center for Disease Control 1999; Pilpel et al. 2000). Other sources will be specifically referred to in the following sections.

Context: Health Needs

This section provides an overall view of some of Israel's major health needs. However, descriptions of these major needs should be balanced from the outset by an appreciation of the quality of Israel's highly developed healthcare systems. The scope of services, technical level, and quality of labor in the various medical professions contribute to health standards that are among the highest in the world. The World Health Organization's report for the year 2000 ranked Israel 28th in health system performance and attainment among 191 countries based on 1997 data on eight different criteria (WHO 2000). The system has been developed through voluntary sick funds, not-for-profit institutions, and the state itself. To a large extent, the nature and achievements of the Israeli health system stem from its foundation in organized social arrangements and the general consensus that society as a whole is responsible for the health of its citizens. For this reason, the state has played an active role in the development and financing of the service network beyond the activities of public bodies and into the private sector.

Israel's healthcare system has distinguished itself in several areas. In 1998, an evidence-based process for adding new technologies, especially newer drugs, to the basic basket of services was instituted. As a result, noninvasive medical technologies have replaced invasive ones over the last two years as indicated by the major reduction (about 30 percent) in the number of open-heart surgeries and the increase (about 27 percent) in the number of therapeutic catheterizations in 1999 as compared with 1998.

The last four decades have seen a continuous decline in the incidence of and mortality from most infectious diseases, particularly vaccine-preventable diseases. The Israeli healthcare system has made significant achievements in the area of immunization. In comparison with the European Community, Israel is ranked second, sixth, and seventh for coverage of immunizations

Percent access to health services		100
Percent access to safe water (urban areas)		100
Percent access to sanitation (urban areas)		100
Immunization levels, 1996		
	Hepatitis B	96%
	Measles-mumps-rubella	94%
	Oral polio virus	92%
	Injected polio virus	93%
	Diphtheria	92%

TABLE 12.4
Access to Health-Enhancing Factors

against polio, diphtheria, and measles, respectively. Table 12.4 details access levels to immunization and other health-enhancing factors.

As in most Western countries, life expectancy in Israel is higher for women than for men, among both Jews and Arabs, with significant differences between ethnic groups. In 1996, the average life expectancy at birth was 76.3 years for men and 79.9 for women. Life expectancy at birth among Jews was 80.3 years for women and 76.6 for men, whereas among Arabs it was 77.7 years for women and 74.9 for men. The shorter life expectancy for Arabs is due primarily to higher rates of infant mortality and of age-adjusted mortality from heart disease and infectious disease. For Israeli men, life expectancy at birth is higher than in most European Community countries; this is probably due in part to the virtual absence of alcohol-related mortality in Israel, which comprises a significant part of male mortality in most European countries.

The favorable gap between female and male life expectancies, enjoyed by women in most Western countries, is considerably smaller for Israeli women. In 1996, this gap was 3.8 years in Israel and 6.4 years in the European Community. This may be attributed to excessive mortality from heart disease and a high incidence of breast cancer as compared with women in the European Community. The stress of immigration, which presents particular psychological difficulties for women, also may contribute to the higher mortality rate.

During the period from 1993 through 1997, the infant mortality rate among Israelis was 7 per 1,000 live births (10.3 in the Arab sector and 5.5 among Jews). In general, infant mortality rates have been declining steadily over the past decade, but the rates have remained twice as high in the Arab population. The disparity in infant mortality rates between the Arab and Jewish populations is primarily attributable to markedly higher rates of mortality associated with congenital abnormalities among Arab newborns because of the high frequency of consanguineous marriage and less frequent use of prenatal screening in this population group. Infant mortality due to external causes (e.g., accidents) is also twice as high in the Arab population as in the Jewish population; this indicates a salient need to increase the safety of the infants' environments in the Arab sector.

Table 12.5 lists morbidity measures for Israel. The leading causes of death are heart disease, malignant neoplasm, cerebrovascular disease (stroke), and external injury, in that order. In 1997, these diseases were responsible for 70 percent of all deaths in Israel. The ten leading causes of death in Israel were similar to those reported for the United States for the same year. A 1996 study of knowledge, attitudes, and health behavior found that the proportion of the population reporting their health as "not good" or "fair" was higher in Israel than in the United States.

Among factors related to health behaviors, several indicators of relatively high levels of certain risk factors in Israel suggest areas in need of improvement. The few studies that have been conducted on the health behaviors of large samples of Israelis largely concluded that about 25 percent of the population is overweight and that the prevalence of overweight adults increases with age. A 1998 national telephone survey of a large sample found that about 33 percent of men and 25 percent of women were habitual smokers. Smoking rates were relatively high among those with lower levels of education and among the Arab population. Additional areas of public health concern are the considerable increase in the proportion of adolescents who reported consuming drugs in several surveys conducted during the 1990s and the rising levels of smoking and eating disorders among adolescent girls.

Organization and Management of the Health System

The Ministry of Finance plays a major role in Israel's health system and in the government as a whole (Gross and Harrison 2001). It allocates the budget to all ministries, and its approval is required for all decisions made by the Ministry of Health that have budgetary consequences, such as overtime arrangements and outpatient fee schedules at government hospitals. The NHI Law assigns a senior role to the Ministry of Finance in policymaking with regard to health finance, including defining the funding level of the sick funds and the yearly updates of that funding.

The Ministry of Health has historically been responsible for the supervising, licensing, and overall planning of services. In addition, it has assisted the sick funds and other bodies by subsidizing operations as well as by directly providing some services not offered or inadequately provided by the sick funds, such as mother and child health centers, psychiatric services, and hospitalization of chronically ill patients. The state has developed a network of state-owned general hospitals; the Ministry of Health is in

TABLE 12.5
Leading
Causes of
Morbidity

Leading Causes of Death, 1998	Rate per 100,000 Population	
	Male	Female
Heart disease	161	150
Cerebrovascular disease	61	71
Malignant neoplasms	148	147
External causes	46	23
All other	213	198

Proportion of deaths due to communicable diseases, noncommunicable diseases, and injuries, 1997

	Percent of deaths	
	Male	Female
Communicable diseases	2	2
Noncommunicable diseases	91	95
Injuries (accidental, intentional, and other external causes)	7	3

effect the owner of approximately half of the acute care hospital beds in the country. These hospitals, together with hospitals developed by the General Sick Fund (now called the General Health Services), provide hospitalization services to members of all the sick funds throughout the country on the basis of mutual agreements between the sick funds and the state.

In most industrialized countries in the western hemisphere, the healthcare system has several distinct traits. It is the single industry that is projected to grow continuously in the next decade to become one of the largest industries; it affects every person in these countries; and it is, perhaps, the industry least affected by modern management techniques and behavioral science knowledge. In the Israeli healthcare system, the last feature is undergoing a change in the wake of the introduction in 1995 of managed competition among the country's four sick funds. These sick funds, under the NHI Law of 1994, provide healthcare to the country's residents. At the end of 1999, 6.3 million people were members of the four sick funds. General Health Services, the largest, accounted for 57.2 percent of the insured population; Maccabi, Leumit, and Meuhedet accounted for 22.4 percent, 10.0 percent, and 10.4 percent, respectively (Bendelac

TABLE 12.6
Medical Care
Insurance
Coverage by
Type (percent)

Private voluntary insurance, 1999	25
Public mandated insurance	100
Sick fund supplemental insurance, 1999	51

2000). Approximately one percent of members switched funds during 1999 (Bendelac 2000). Table 12.6 shows coverage rates by type.

Under the NHI Law, all of the country's residents are insured and have access to a comprehensive basket of services of a generally high standard. Sick funds may charge extra premiums only for supplemental insurance for services not provided in the basic basket. Currently, supplemental health insurance policies are sold by all sick funds and also by several for-profit insurance companies. These supplemental insurance policies cover such items as second opinions, private hospitalization and surgery, and long-term geriatric care.

Most services are available on the basis of need and not ability to pay. Patients are generally not deterred by a price barrier from seeking primary care treatment. However, in 1999, the funds were allowed (by an amendment to the NHI Law) to introduce user charges for visits to specialists and higher copayments for prescribed drugs. A survey conducted to evaluate the effects of these new charges found that 6 percent of the respondents have forgone treatment due to the price barrier and 11 percent did not buy medications prescribed by a doctor because of the copayments (Gross and Brammli-Greenberg 2001).

The NHI Law centralized the regulation and control of the sick funds in the Ministry of Health. However, it did not cover the hospital sector, where government ownership and operation still predominate, particularly in acute care hospitals. The management and control of a sizeable part of the country's hospital sector by the Ministry of Health has had several major consequences. One of these has been the preoccupation of the Ministry with its direct service provision responsibilities to the relative neglect of its ministerial duties in the areas of regulation and control of the country's health resources. Thus, the regulative and control mechanisms of the Ministry of Health in areas such as quality assurance, new health technologies, and re-registration and recertification of professional health labor are still in an embryonic stage of development. Establishing a mechanism to regulate recertification or re-registration of physicians or nurses necessarily involves other stakeholders, such as the professional associations representing these groups. Because the Ministry of Health was mandated by the NHI Law to act with regard to sick fund quality assurance, this case will be used to illustrate the Ministry's failure to develop appropriate regulative functions.

The NHI Law was intended to promote competition among the four sick funds with regard to quality of service. The law requires that all sick funds offer the same basic basket of services and refrain from assessing membership fees. Freedom of movement among the four sick funds was granted to each resident of the country once a year, and the sick funds were enjoined by law to accept any applicant as a member without enrollment barriers. The law mandated quality assurance of the sick funds by the Ministry of Health. However, no mechanisms were established in the Ministry of Health to measure quality or disseminate information about quality improvement to the sick funds or to consumers, although mechanisms were established to monitor and assess the financial performance of the sick funds. Although the Ministry does provide incentives to the sick funds to operate in an economically efficient way, without the dissemination of comparative quality information to the members of the sick funds, the law cannot achieve the goal of providing incentives to improve quality of care.

Financing

Israel is in a period of restrained national spending on health and will remain so for the foreseeable future. During the last two decades, the share of gross domestic product devoted to the health sector has continuously increased, mirroring similar trends in OECD countries (OECD 1993). In the 1980s, health expenditure as a share of GDP rose from about 6 percent to 7.5 percent. From the mid-1980s to the mid-1990s, it rose toward 8.5 percent and remained at this level until 1999. A gentle downward trend appeared during the period of 1996 to 1997 and a gentle upward trend during the period of 1998 to 1999. In 1999, the share of GDP devoted to health expenditure was 8.3 percent, which was equal to the level of health spending in the Netherlands and Portugal in the same year but lower than that of Germany, Canada, and France, each of which spent about 10 percent of GDP on health (Central Bureau of Statistics 2000). However, this figure is somewhat misleading in light of Israel's relatively low GDP. The absolute per capita expenditure was U.S.$1,510 in 1997, adjusted by P.P.P.$ of GDP (Central Bureau of Statistics 2000), which was below the OECD average, thereby giving rise to concern among those who believe that society should place a high priority on healthcare. The growth in per capita expenditure must also be examined in light of the age structure of the Israeli population, which is relatively young as compared with other countries and consequently consumes fewer health services. However, the Israeli population has been aging at a particularly high rate. From 1955 to 1996, the share of those aged 65 years old and older in the Jewish population increased from 4.7 percent to 11.1 percent; this population sector consumes at least three times more health services than the general population.

Israel's experience as the first country to allocate 100 percent of the nation's health insurance monies on the basis of a needs-based capitation formula is of interest. One of the major innovations brought about by the NHI Law was the introduction of a capitation formula for allocating the annual public health budget to the sick funds. According to this formula, the sick fund revenues became a function of the age mix of their members (rather than their financial status). The capitation formula was intended to ensure that those funds accepting elderly members have the resources necessary to cover the higher-than-average healthcare costs of this population segment. It was also intended to provide the sick funds with an incentive to compete for the elderly and poor just as they compete for healthier population segments.

As an illustration of the age-weight allocation system, sick funds receive more than 3.5 times the allocation for each member aged 75 years old or older than they receive for the average member. In addition to allocating money based on age, special rates have been established that reflect the estimated average annual cost of caring for people with five major diseases: thalasemia, Gauche's disease, end-stage renal disease, multiple sclerosis, and AIDS.

In 1997, 41 percent of total health expenditures was spent on hospitals and research, and 39 percent was spent on public clinics and preventive medicine. Yet another 13 percent went to private physicians and dental health services, and an additional 6 percent was spent on medications and medical equipment purchased by households. The main source of income for acute care or general hospitals has been the sale of services to the sick funds, primarily on the basis of government-set per-diem rates. For some (mostly operative) procedures, hospitals are paid on the basis of a diagnosis-related-group-like prospective fee-for-service schedule. Additional sources of income have been the sale of out-of-basket services through affiliated public bodies and donations. Hospital outpatient clinics have a special price list. Since 1996, the government has used a capping system to control the rising costs of hospitalization.

National health expenditures were funded in 1998 and 1999 by three major sources. The health tax collected from the country's residents (3.1 percent of taxable income up to the minimum wage and 4.8 percent of income above that level) constituted about 25 percent of total expenditures. The second was the state budget, which contributed about 48 percent of the total. The third, which made up about 27 percent of total expenditures, was paid by households on such items as copayments or user charges paid to the sick funds, dental services (which are not part of the basic basket of health services under the NHI Law), private physicians, and drugs. Thus, the government covered less than three-quarters of national health expenditures, and households paid for the remaining quarter directly. More than half of household health expenditures went to dental care; the balance was divided roughly equally between spending for private physicians and outlays for medical devices and medications.

The proportion of expenditures paid by households in Israel is among the highest in the European Community (Bin Nun and Ben Ori 1997), and this has far-reaching effects on the equity of availability to the health system. The increase has been primarily due to the government policy of reducing public funding of the health system while allowing sick funds to collect new user charges (e.g., those levied on physicians' visits in 1999) and to increase copayments on medications.

One of the more important objectives of the NHI Law was to financially stabilize the sick funds and eliminate the significant budget deficits that characterized the largest sick fund, the General Health Services, before the law's enactment. The goal of the law was to achieve this objective by setting the cost of the basket services together with an index to update this amount each year. However, this index does not take into account needed adjustments for the costs of new technologies and the growth and aging of the population (Chinitz 1995). For those and other reasons, the amount that the government is required to provide from its general revenues above the health tax to cover health costs has been a source of controversy. In most years, the strategy of the Ministry of Finance to induce the sick funds to become more economical and efficient by reducing the cost of the basket in real terms has been successful; this attests to the central role played by the Ministry of Finance in the determination of the country's health expenditures.

Largely because of the factors described above, the NHI Law failed to reach the objective of financially stabilizing the sick funds' operations in the period from 1995 to 1998. From 1996 on, all sick funds had budget deficits, ranging from very large in 1997 (about 9 percent of the annual budget) to rather small in 1999 and 2000 (from 2 percent to 3 percent of their annual budget). According to calculations made by the Ministry of Health, between 1995 (the first year of the new law) and 2000, the real value of the basic basket of services declined by 16 percent. Several proposals to amend the situation are being discussed by the Knesset, including a proposal to amend the index used to adjust the cost of the basic basket of services.

Health Resources

In 1998, approximately 142,100 people were employed in the country's health system (about 6.8 percent of the working Israeli population) at a ratio of 23 health workers per 1,000 population. As illustrated in Table 12.7, the healthcare workforce is composed of 12 percent physicians, 30 percent nurses, and 58 percent other health occupations. The distribution

TABLE 12.7

Human Resources per 1,000 population

Physicians	3.90
Nurses	6.7
Dentists	1.16
Midwives	.186
Pharmacists	.605

of workers in the health system among primary, secondary, and tertiary medical services has not changed much during the last two decades. About 56 percent of health workers are employed in hospitals, and about 28 percent work in community or other public clinics.

The data on healthcare workers in Israel reflect the number of license holders rather than the number actually working in a specific occupation. According to the Ministry of Health, at the end of 1998, there were 28,656 physicians in Israel, 24,695 of which were younger than 70 years old and presumably still working. Of those still working, 6,012 (24.3 percent) were specialists (excluding specialists in family medicine) and were not employed in primary care (Pilpel et al. 1999). The rate of working physicians (below the age of 70 years) per 1,000 population is among the highest in the world, following those of Italy, Spain, and Norway. In comparison, a shortage of nurses in Israel of only 6.7 per 1,000 population is compared with 9 in the Netherlands and Germany and 17.9 in Norway.

Israel has one of the lowest rates of general hospital beds per 1,000 population in the Western world (OECD 1993), and this is directly related to other indicators of the effectiveness of Israeli general (acute care) hospitals. These indicators include (1) a very short length of stay, averaging 4.3 days in 1997; (2) bed occupancy rates of more than 90 percent; and (3) a hospitalization-days rate per 1,000 population that declined from 1,037 in 1975 to 785 in 1997. Israeli hospitals have undergone a process of streamlining in recent years, with a continuing decrease in the hospital bed rate per 1,000 population from 6.8 in 1975 to 6 in 1996. The decrease was primarily in the general wards (a 28 percent decrease) and psychiatric wards (a 49 percent decrease). The majority of new hospital beds in recent years have been in long-term-care hospitals. These figures indicate that the hospital sector in Israel, in sharp contrast with the situation in a number of advanced European countries, has not been weighed down with surplus hospital beds or unjustifiably long periods of hospitalization. A key issue in the current policy debate on the possible incorporation of government hospitals focuses on the most effective way of maintaining and strengthening these achievements of the hospital sector in Israel.

At the same time, the rate of hospitalization per 1,000 population has risen continuously since the beginning of the 1980s. Between the years

1990 and 1995, it rose by 12 percent, and in 1997 it stood at 182 hospital admissions per 1,000 residents. The number of hospital admissions has increased at a more rapid rate than population growth. This trend is related to the aging of the population and to the introduction of medical technologies that extend the life expectancy of elderly people under intensive-care conditions.

Service Delivery

Sick Funds

Primary and secondary care is provided by four sick funds, which under the NHI Law cover all permanent residents of the country; this means that all permanent residents of the country have access to a relatively wide range of health services through their membership in a sick fund. The NHI Law specified the basic basket of services provided by the sick funds. This basket of health services is quite comprehensive, but it does not include mental health services or chronic or long-term care (which are under the responsibility of the government) or dental care (for which the consumer is financially responsible).

In several respects, the sick funds resemble the staff-model health maintenance organizations of the United States. Under the NHI Law, membership in one of them is compulsory, but a member has full discretion to change his or her enrollment once a year. The sick funds are obliged under the law to accept any new applicant regardless of age, sex, place of residence, or any other criteria. Before the NHI Law came into effect, membership in the sick funds was voluntary, and the sick funds had complete discretion to determine restrictions on the acceptance of new members. The smaller ones restricted acceptance of new members with chronic illness and those above the age of 62 years. Freedom of movement among the funds has been one of the major changes introduced by the NHI Law.

Of the four sick funds, the General Health Services (GHS) is the largest, with about 57 percent of the population belonging to it. It owns and operates a network of public clinics. Most of these clinics are quite large and include general practitioners and specialists, a variety of diagnostic and laboratory equipment, pharmacies, and other primary care curative services. The GHS has been playing a central role in Israel's healthcare delivery system by virtue of its pioneering status, size, and, until 1995, its affiliation with the powerful Histadrut, Israel's federations of trade unions.

However, the competition for members among the four sick funds has changed the role of the GHS in the Israeli healthcare system. Whereas in the past it influenced and shaped the functions and behavior of the other sick funds to a considerable extent, in recent years it has been competing with the smaller sick funds by adopting some of their innovative service features. To illustrate, the GHS has allowed direct access to specialists in several key medical specialties and has supplemented the primary care physicians employed in its clinics by contracting with independent primary care physicians.

The mode of operation of the three smaller sick funds resembles that of the GHS, with two major exceptions. First, the smaller sick funds tend to provide primary care services more through their agreements with private primary care physicians than through clinics employing salaried physicians, as is the prevailing pattern in the GHS. The physicians who sign agreements with the smaller sick funds usually provide care to members in their own clinics. Second, the smaller sick funds do not own and operate hospitals, with one major exception. The Maccabi Health Services, whose members comprise about 22 percent of the country's residents (Bendelac 2000), has in recent years acquired and operated three small hospitals in the country's major urban areas.

Hospitals

The GHS is also the owner and operator of 17 percent of the country's general hospital beds. However, most hospitals are owned by the government (45 percent of all general hospital beds) and by not-for-profit organizations such as Hadassa. The operation of the sick funds in the tertiary sector is augmented by a number of not-for-profit organizations that have established hospitals as well as other medical facilities. An example is the network of hospitals established by certain religious denominations in most cities and especially by several Christian churches in Nazareth.

Elderly people 75 years old and older are heavy consumers of hospital services. In 1996, for every 1,000 elderly people, there were more than 500 hospital admissions per year, half of them in internal medicine wards. Some 20 percent of the population of Israel requires hospitalization each year. For them, hospitals are very important. The claim is sometimes made that some 90 percent of those going to general hospitals receive symptomatic treatment for chronic viral or cancer diseases. At the same time, for the health professions and especially for doctors, hospitals are the source of up-to-date medical knowledge, training, and research. From the point of view of the employee organizations in the system, particularly the doctors' organizations, the hospital and heads of departments represent the backbone of their organizational infrastructure. Accordingly, hospitals are the focus of a number of significant stakeholders' interests that need to be taken into account in any organizational restructuring of general hospitals.

The Ministry of Health

The Ministry of Health has the customary ministerial responsibilities for the planning, regulation, and coordination of the healthcare system; for the general assessment and control of the sick funds' operations; and for the initiation of legislation in these areas. Because of historical circumstances, the Ministry is also the major provider of individual preventive health services, hospital care (including most long-term care), and public health services. The Ministry of Health owns and operates about half of the country's acute care and psychiatric beds and about 20 percent of the long-term-care (geriatric) beds. It regulates the input of labor, technology, and new capital investments in the health sector by licensing physicians, nurses, and health institutions. The Ministry also operates a network of mother-and-child clinics that provide preventive health services to newborn children and prenatal care to mothers. It also provides some individual preventive health services for adults in addition to the public health services.

Responsibility for geriatric, psychiatric, and preventive services has not yet been transferred to the sick funds. In the case of preventive services, this is not a major problem, as the government-run family health clinics function quite well. However, in the geriatric (institutional long-term care) and psychiatric areas, major issues of inadequate financing and equity remain unresolved.

Private Medical Services

Privately operated and consumed medical services are predominant only in dental care. In 1998, private physicians were responsible for about 6 percent of the total expenditure on health, which is indicative of the existence of de facto universal public health insurance through the sick funds.

Utilization of Healthcare Services

Analysis of hospitalization days by age revealed that the highest hospitalization rates were found in the youngest age group (aged 0 to 4) and among adults aged 65 years and over; in these two groups, the most common reasons for hospitalization were respiratory disease and cardiovascular disease, respectively. Data from the 1996–97 Central Bureau of Statistics study of the use of the country's healthcare services reveal that the average annual number of visits to physicians was 6.8 but that significant differences were found across the various age, gender, and ethnic subgroups. Women visit primary care physicians 13 percent more often than men do. Analysis by age shows that the rate of visits to primary care physicians is the highest among those aged 0 to 4 years and among adults aged 65 years and over. Women visit specialists twice as often as men do; among both men and women, the highest rate of specialist visits is in the 75-years-old and older age group, and the lowest is in the 5- to 14-year-old age group. Table 12.8 provides detailed service use rates.

Prospects for the Future

The NHI Law was the first step toward reforming Israel's health system. As we have indicated, the Law was intended to stabilize the system financially, introduce managed competition among the sick funds, allow more

TABLE 12.8
Medical
Service Use
and Rates per
1,000
Population

Total general hospital discharges, 1996	180.5
Total hospital days, 1996	785.4
Visits to specialists, 1996	92 per 100 in six months
Visits to general practitioners, 1996	244 per 100 in six months
Visits to dentists, 1996	132 per 100 in six months

equitable funding of the sick funds, and provide a uniform and comprehensive basket of services. It did achieve a considerable number of its initial goals: providing insurance coverage for the entire population, ensuring freedom of movement among sick funds, and standardizing the way resources are allocated to sick funds. Some of the Law's shortcomings have also been noted, such as its failure to financially stabilize the sick funds. Incentives provided by the Law have encouraged the sick funds to improve the level of services provided to the average member and to develop services in the periphery and for some of the weaker populations. Overall, the law has advanced the equity of service among populations and regions. However, problems such as economic stability and equity gaps remain. These issues, which were not remedied by managed competition, require further reforms in Israel's healthcare system. For example, special allocations can be given for the development of services in the Arab sector or in poor neighborhoods to achieve more equity in access to services.

Despite the NHI Law, the system has yet to attain financial stability and is operating with an ongoing deficit. In addition, disagreement has arisen concerning the system's overall financing level, and the updating processes of the basic basket leaves much to government discretion, as it has in the past. Therefore, the Israeli experience demonstrates that regulating competition and even establishing budgetary caps for the system do not necessarily achieve cost containment because providers can exceed their budget. In the Israeli case, regulating competition did not solve the policy question of the level of resources allocated to health, which was a major issue in the debate leading up to the enactment of the NHI Law. The Ministry of Health and the sick funds lobbied for additional resources to compensate for the aging of the population and technological developments. The Ministry of Finance, on the other hand, insisted that the level of resources should not change in real terms. In itself, managed competition is not an adequate mechanism for determining the level of resource allocation. Allowing price competition could contribute to more efficient operation of healthcare providers by inducing the sick funds to introduce quality improvement and expenditure reduction through efficiency gains. Some health economists suggested that the Law should be amended to allow the sick funds to collect a capped flat-rate premium from their members, thereby introducing price competition among the sick funds. The findings of a comprehensive evaluation of the NHI Law (Gross, Rosen, and Shirom 2001) indicate that some of the sick funds made reductions in expenses per person; however, due to a lack of data, it is not possible to determine to what extent this can be attributed to greater efficiency. Evidence from the literature on market behavior observed in for-profit and not-for-profit providers suggests that providers try to cut back on costs by collaborating among themselves, practicing cream-skimming, marketing aggressively, hiding quality problems, and using other tactics that provide maximum profits for minimal services (Light 1992). In the Israeli case, research on the organizational behavior of sick funds has shown similar competitive methods (Gross and Harrison 2001).

Still other serious issues are not addressed by the NHI Law, among them the organizational structure of the hospital system, labor planning, and the provision of dental care. In 1992, the government attempted to implement reform in the hospital sector, which accounts for about 50 percent of the operating expenses of the sick funds. This attempt to incorporate government acute care hospitals aimed to achieve several objectives, including the introduction of managed competition among the hospitals involved. However, it was aborted when the trade unions representing nurses and administrative employees obtained a court injunction against it, and it was subsequently replaced by an incremental reform allowing government acute care hospitals more autonomy.

The Ministry of Health has not played the major role in quality assurance and information dissemination envisioned in the managed competition model and mandated by the NHI Law. In addition, although one of the NHI Law goals was to release the Ministry of Health from supplying services directly and to strengthen its ministerial functioning, the Ministry still provides preventive, psychiatric, and geriatric services because of doubts about the transfer of these services to sick funds, and it is also still involved in the management of government hospitals. This continues to affect the Ministry's ability to focus on policymaking, priority setting, supervision, and regulation, which are critical functions to the effective implementation of the health system reform.

One of the areas urgently requiring Ministry of Health involvement is the effective regulation of sick funds, hospital development, and the regulation of technological advances; another area concerns regulations designed to prevent unwarranted surgery. In addition, it is important to establish principles for the operation of specialty services to prevent redundancy. Finally, Ministry intervention is urgently required for the distribution of information that allows citizens to make educated decisions (e.g., information about the quality of care in sick funds and hospitals).

As is already known from experience in other countries, health system reform is a long and dynamic process. Up-to-date information is essential in helping policymakers track the process of the reform's implementation and its results and in identifying problems in implementation, as well as unwanted by-products. Based on this information, the reform program can be continuously improved, and problematic components can be adjusted. Therefore, it is important to continue to assess the functioning of the reformed system and to work with policymakers to maximize use of research findings in the decision-making process.

REFERENCES

Bendelac, J. 2000. *Membership in Sick Funds: 1998–1999.* Publication No. 169. Jerusalem: Research and Planning Administration, National Insurance Institute.

Bin Nun, G., and Ben Ori, D. 1997. *Trends in the National Expenditure on Health.* Jerusalem: The Ministry of Health.

Central Bureau of Statistics. 1999. *Statistical Yearbook of Israel, 50.* Jerusalem: Central Bureau of Statistics.

———. 2000. "National Health Expenditures in 1999." *Statistical Bulletin* 60 (5, Suppl.): 15–48.

Chinitz, D. 1995. "Israel's Health Policy Breakthrough: The Politics of Reform and the Reform of Politics." *Journal of Health Politics, Policy and Law* 20: 909–32.

Chinitz, D. P., and Cohen, M. A. (eds.) 1993. *The Changing Roles of Government and the Market in Health Care Systems.* Jerusalem: JDC-Brookdale Institute of Gerontology and Human Development and the Ministry of Health.

Ellencweig, A. Y. 1992. *Analysing Health Systems: A Modular Approach.* Oxford: Oxford University Press.

Gross, R., and Brammli-Greenberg, S. 2001. *Public Opinion on the Level of Service and Functioning of the Health Care System, 1995–1999.* Jerusalem: JDC-Brookdale Institute.

Gross, R., and Harrison, M. 2001. "Implementing Managed Competition in Israel." *Social Science and Medicine* 52: 1219–31.

Gross, R., Rosen, B., and Shirom, A. 2001. "Reforming the Israeli Health System: Finding of a Three Year Evaluation." *Health Policy* 56: 1–20.

Hadassah, The Women's Zionist Organization of America, and The Israel Women's Network. 1999. *Women's Health in Israel, 1999: A Data Book.* Jerusalem: Hadassah and the Israel Center for Disease Control, Ministry of Health.

Kop, Y. (ed.) 1999. *Israel's Social Services: 1998–1999.* Jerusalem: The Center for Social Policy Studies in Israel.

Light, D. 1992. "The Practice and Ethics of Risk-related Health Insurance." *Journal of the American Medical Association* 267: 2503–08.

Organization for Economic Cooperation and Development (OECD). 1990. *Health Care Systems in Transition. The Search for Efficiency.* Social Policy Studies No. 7. Paris: OECD.

———. 1992. *The Reform of Health Care. A Comparative Analysis of Seven OECD Countries.* Paris: OECD.

————. 1993. *OECD Health Systems. Facts and Trends, 1960–1991*. Health Policy Studies No. 3. Vol. 1. Paris: OECD.

Pilpel, D., Shemesh, A. A., Smetannikov, E., and Dor, M. 2000. *The Primary Care Physician in Israel; Primary Physician Workforce and Estimation of Potential Candidates*. Jerusalem: The Ministry of Health, Division of Health Economics and Medical Administration.

Shuval, J. T. 1992. *Social Dimensions of Health. The Israeli Experience*. Westport, CT: Praeger.

State of Israel, Ministry of Health, Division of Planning, Budgets, and Health Economics. 1988. *Indicators for Monitoring Progress Towards Health for All*. Jerusalem: Division of Planning, Budgets, and Health Economics.

State of Israel, Ministry of Health, Israel Center for Disease Control. 1999. *Health Status in Israel 1999*. Publication No. 209. Jerusalem: Israel Center for Disease Control.

Steinberg, G., and Bick, E. 1992. *Resisting Reform: A Policy Analysis of the Israeli Health Care Delivery System*. Lanham, MD: University Press of America.

World Health Organization (WHO). 2000. *The World Health Report 2000*. Geneva: WHO.

13

CANADA

Laurie J. Goldsmith

Background Information

Canada is a highly decentralized federation of ten provinces and three territories.[1] The country was founded with the 1867 British North America Act, under which provincial governments received constitutional responsibility for the financing, management, and delivery of health services. The federal government was given jurisdiction over health protection, disease prevention, and health promotion, as well as responsibility for direct health service delivery to veterans, native Canadians living on reserves, military personnel, inmates of federal penitentiaries, and the Royal Canadian Mounted Police. The federal government eventually assumed a regulatory role in healthcare by assisting with the funding of provincial programs and legislating conditions for receiving federal funding.

The design of the present-day Canadian healthcare system started in the province of Saskatchewan in 1947 with the introduction of a public insurance plan for hospital care. By 1961, all of the provinces and territories covered hospital services in a public insurance plan, and by 1972, all had expanded these public insurance plans to include physician services. As in other countries, economic conditions have influenced the design of, development of, and spending on the healthcare system. Canada's healthcare system is also shaped by the division of governmental power and public opinion. The healthcare system is consistently Canada's most popular social program, and the country's universal health insurance system is often cited as a defining feature of Canada (Evans 2000; Naylor 1999).

Economics

Canada is a wealthy country. In 1999, Canada had a gross domestic product of U.S.$612 billion and a gross national product of U.S.$591.3 billion (World Bank 2000) (Table 13.1). Canada's gross national product was the ninth highest among all countries in 1998. Healthcare spending constituted 9.5 percent of the gross domestic product, which was approximately P.P.P.$2,312 per capita (OECD 2001), making Canada the fifth highest healthcare spender among OECD countries in 1998.

Despite the country's wealth, poverty is an increasing problem. In 1997, 19.8 percent of all children in Canada were living in poverty (Nichols

TABLE 13.1
Selected
Economic
Indicators for
Canada, 1998
and 1999

GNP (U.S.$)	591.3 billion
GDP (U.S.$)	612.0 billion
GNP per capita (U.S.$)	19,320
Percent of GDP spent on health	9.5
Total expenditure on health per capita (P.P.P.$ adjusted; U.S.$)	2,312

NOTE: Gross national product, gross domestic product, and gross national product per capita figures are for 1999; the remaining figures are for 1998.
SOURCE: World Bank (2000); OECD (2001); Canadian Institute for Health Information (2000).

2000). Twenty percent of all individuals were considered to be low income in 1995.[2] Income disparity has also increased. In 1973, the income of the wealthiest Canadian families was 8.5 times the income of the poorest families. By 1996, this disparity figure had increased to 10.2 (Federal, Provincial and Territorial Advisory Committee on Population Health 2000).

Population

Canada is a geographically large but sparsely and differentially populated country. At more than nine million square kilometers in land area, Canada is the second largest country in the world. In 1999, Canada had a population of 30.5 million people and a population density of 3.1 people per square kilometer (Statistics Canada 2000b), with 77 percent of the population living in urban areas (World Bank 2000) (Table 13.2). The population is highly concentrated in the south; almost 90 percent of the population lives within 160 kilometers of the Canada–United States border. Much of the Canadian population lives in the provinces of Ontario (38 percent) and Quebec (24 percent) (Federal, Provincial and Territorial Advisory Committee on Population Health 2000). The province with the largest population (Ontario) has 83 times the population of the province with the smallest population (Prince Edward Island). The three territories, all located in northern Canada, have even smaller populations than Prince Edward Island.

English and French are Canada's two official languages. The majority of Canadians speak English, with the majority of French speakers residing in the province of Quebec (Statistics Canada 2000c). Canada is ethnically diverse, having experienced considerable immigration in the postwar era. In the 1996 census, 11 percent of the population reported being of a visible minority (non-caucasian or non-aboriginal [native Canadians]), and another 3 percent identified themselves with one or more aboriginal groups (Statistics Canada 2000a).

General population trends in Canada include an aging population, a declining birth rate, an increase of children in single-parent families, and a decreasing unemployment rate. In 1996, 12 percent of Canadians were

Population in millions	30.5
Percent urbanized	77
Infant mortality rate per 1,000 live births	5
Under-five mortality rate per 1,000 children	6
Life expectancy at birth (years)	79
Fertility rate	2
Birth rate per 1,000 population	11.2
Percent of population 65 years old and older	12.4

TABLE 13.2
General Demographics for Canada, 1999

SOURCE: Statistics Canada (2000b, 2000d); World Bank (2000).

65 years old or older (Federal, Provincial and Territorial Advisory Committee on Population Health 2000). The 1999 unemployment rate was 7.6 percent (in contrast with a peak of 11.2 percent in 1992), with 66 percent of Canadians 15 years old or older working or actively seeking employment (Statistics Canada 2000).

In the 1996 census, 65 percent of Canadians 15 years old or older reported having completed at least a high school education, although this figure varies considerably across Canada (Federal, Provincial and Territorial Advisory Committee on Population Health 2000). With respect to literacy, Canada compares reasonably well to the ten other developed countries included in the OECD International Adult Literacy Survey. Just under 60 percent of Canadians between the ages of 16 and 65 years achieved the prose, document, and quantitative literacy thresholds (Health Canada 2000).

Measures of health status in Canada are among the world's highest. The World Health Organization (2000) ranked Canada as the twelfth healthiest country in its assessment of health systems around the world. When compared with other OECD countries, Canada also generally ranks highly on specific health measures, with the exception of infant mortality, for which Canada falls roughly in the middle (OECD 2001). In 1999, Canada had an infant mortality rate of five deaths per 1,000 live births and an under-five mortality rate of six deaths per 1,000 children (World Bank 2000). The country's 1999 average fertility rate was 1.6 children per woman of childbearing age (World Bank 2000), which translated into a birth rate of 11.2 children per 1,000 persons (Statistics Canada 2000d). The overall life expectancy of a Canadian at birth is 79 years (World Bank 2000). Canadians in the north (territorial residents and residents of some northern parts of provinces) generally have shorter lives than do those in the south (most provincial residents), with Canadians in southern urban areas living the longest (Nichols 2000a).

Canada is a country with many advantages and resources, although it also has room for improvement. Overall measures of social health reflect this. Canada placed first on the United Nations' Human Development Index[3] six years in a row, from 1994 to 1999. Aboriginal Canadians score significantly lower than other Canadians, having scores more similar to developing countries (Federal, Provincial and Territorial Advisory Committee on Population Health 2000). Canada's social health has been decreasing since the 1980s according to the Index of Social Health, a Canada-specific measure that is more comprehensive than the United Nations' index[4] (Federal, Provincial and Territorial Advisory Committee on Population Health 2000). The decrease in the Index of Social Health has occurred despite the significant increase in Canada's gross domestic product over this time period (Federal, Provincial and Territorial Advisory Committee on Population Health 2000).

Context: Health Needs

Like other industrialized countries, Canada's leading causes of death are from chronic diseases (Table 13.3). Cancer and heart disease are the causes of more than half of all deaths. Lung cancer is the leading cause of cancer death for both men and women (Statistics Canada 2000e). Cancer was also the strongest contributor to potential years of life lost (deaths before age 70) (Federal, Provincial and Territorial Advisory Committee on Population Health 2000).

Most Canadians report a high level of health. Sixty-three percent of Canadians 12 years old and older describe their health as excellent or very good. This is accompanied, however, by unhealthy lifestyle practices by significant numbers of Canadians. Twenty-eight percent of Canadians smoke, 57 percent are inactive, and 48 percent are overweight (having a body mass index of 25 or greater); the percentage of overweight Canadians has increased steadily since 1985. (Federal, Provincial and Territorial Advisory Committee on Population Health 2000).

Aboriginal Canadians have the poorest health of any group in Canada, having a shorter life expectancy and higher rates of health problems and diseases than the Canadian average (MacMillan et al. 1996). For example, aboriginal youth are five to eight times more likely to commit suicide than other Canadian youth; the infant mortality rate for Aboriginal populations is double the Canadian average; and tuberculosis rates are four to seven times higher than the Canadian average (rates differ for off-reservation and on-reservation aboriginal Canadians) (Federal, Provincial and Territorial Advisory Committee on Population Health 2000). Many researchers believe that the poor health of aboriginal Canadians is caused, at least in part, by the deprivation and poverty of aboriginal communities (MacMillan et al. 1996).

Other groups with special health needs include the elderly and

Leading Causes of Death	Percentage of Deaths	Age-standardized Mortality Rate per 100,000 Population
Cancers	27.2	181.5
Diseases of the heart	26.6	173.0
Cerebrovascular diseases	7.4	47.8
Chronic obstructive pulmonary diseases and allied conditions	4.5	29.0
Unintentional injuries	4.0	27.6
Pneumonia and influenza	3.7	23.7
Diabetes mellitus	2.6	17.4
Hereditary and degenerative diseases of the central nervous system	2.3	15.0
Diseases of the arteries, arterioles, and capillaries	2.2	14.3
Psychoses	2.2	13.6
Suicide	1.7	12.0
Nephritis, nephrotic syndrome, and nephrosis	1.2	8.0
Chronic liver disease and cirrhosis	0.9	6.4
Neurotic disorders, personality disorders, and other nonpsychotic mental disorders	0.5	3.5
HIV infection	0.3	2.0

SOURCE: Statistics Canada (2000e).

TABLE 13.3
Leading Causes of Morbidity and Mortality in Canada, 1997

Canadians with low income and low education. The elderly have the highest injury rate of all age groups. They are also the most likely to have long-term activity limitation and the most likely to report taking multiple medications, and they have the longest lengths of stay in the hospital of any age group (Federal, Provincial and Territorial Advisory Committee on Population Health 2000). As has been consistently shown across industrialized countries, most health conditions demonstrate socioeconomic gradients with lower-income and lower-educated people being in worse health; Canada is not an exception to this phenomenon (Federal, Provincial and Territorial Advisory Committee on Population Health 2000).

Organization and Management of the Health System

The Canadian healthcare system is predominantly publicly financed and privately delivered. The defining feature of this system is universal and publicly financed health insurance for medically necessary hospital and physician services. The system is often described as 13 interlocking healthcare systems. Provinces and territories finance and administer their own insurance plans; the federal government provides transfer payments for healthcare and uses this fiscal role to enforce the national principles defined in the Canada Health Act.

The Canada Health Act

According to the Canada Health Act, "the primary objective of Canadian healthcare policy is to protect, promote and restore the physical and mental well-being of residents of Canada and to facilitate reasonable access to health services without financial or other barriers" (Canada House of Commons 1984). This legislation was enacted in 1984 to counteract extra billing by physicians (i.e., charging patients on top of receiving government payments) and the charging of hospital user fees. The five principles of the Canada Health Act—public administration, comprehensiveness, universality, accessibility, and portability—are intended to support this goal (Figure 13.1). Under this act, the federal government may withhold transfer payments from provinces or territories where extra billing or user fees occur.

The principles of comprehensiveness and accessibility have significant system design implications and are subject to varying interpretations. The comprehensiveness concept of "medical necessity" is not defined in the Canada Health Act; in practice, medical necessity has been interpreted to mean different things at different times to different groups (Charles et al. 1997). Although the accessibility principle contains provisions for both financial and nonfinancial barriers, the federal interpretation of this principle has been solely concerned with the removal of extra billing and user charges for insured health services (Birch and Abelson 1993). Anecdotal evidence suggests that patients have been refused care because of premium nonpayment (Rachlis 1995), despite this practice being expressly prohibited by the Canada Health Act (Walker 1999).

Other Government Roles

Although the Canada Health Act only mandates the coverage of physician and hospital services, most provinces and territories also finance dental care, home care, ambulance services, and outpatient drugs, at least for some of their population. Government funding for dental care mainly consists of subsidy programs for the poor. Coverage, financing, eligibility, and copayment mechanisms for home care services vary widely across the country (Dumont-Lemasson, Donovan, and Wylie 1999; Coyte and McKeever

FIGURE 13.1

Principles of
the Canada
Health Act

To be eligible for full federal transfer payments, each provincial or territorial health insurance plan must meet each of the following five principles of the Canada Health Act.

Public Administration

The health insurance plan of a province must be administered and operated on a not-for-profit basis by a public authority accountable to the provincial government.

Universality

Each insurance plan must cover all eligible residents with insured health services on "uniform terms and conditions." All residents of the province are considered eligible residents excluding individuals covered by the federal government (e.g., members of the Royal Canadian Mounted Police) and those who have lived in the province or territory for less than three months.

Portability

Residents are entitled to coverage when they move to another province within Canada or when they travel within Canada or abroad. Limits on out-of-country coverage and insurance plan approval for nonemergency out-of-province or -territory care are allowed.

Comprehensiveness

The plan must insure all medically necessary services provided by hospitals and physicians. The comprehensiveness principle does not require the coverage of drugs outside of the hospital or the coverage of nonphysician providers outside of hospitals. Medical necessity does not include private or semiprivate hospital rooms (unless a patient needs privacy for a medical reason, such as in the case of a patient with a compromised autoimmune system) or accommodation costs for people who permanently reside in a chronic care center.

Accessibility

The plan must provide, on uniform terms and conditions, reasonable access to insured hospital and physician services without barriers. Additional charges to insured patients for insured services are not allowed. No one may be discriminated against on the basis of income, age, and health status. Premiums for public insurance plans are allowed, however, as long as provincial or territorial plans do not deny care based on the nonpayment of premiums.

SOURCE: Health Canada (1999).

2001). Ambulance services, including air ambulances for remote areas, are funded by the provinces and territories, with some copayment mechanisms.

With respect to outpatient drugs, all provinces provide drug insurance for those on social assistance and for the elderly. Some provincial plans for social assistance recipients require deductibles, copayments, or both. All of the drug insurance plans for seniors entail some sort of cost sharing, although some provinces employ different cost-sharing mechanisms based on income. All but two provinces also have drug insurance plans for their general populations. Most of these general population plans have high copayments and deductibles, with some plans only covering specific diseases and therefore primarily serving as catastrophic insurance for the general population (Lindsey and West 1999; Willison, Grootendorst, and Hurley 1998).

The major funding role played by the provincial and territorial governments results in significant management and planning power over the entire healthcare system. Although governments do not interfere with clinical practice, their financing role gives the government indirect control over private providers. Provincial and territorial governments moved hospitals to global budgets in the late 1980s and early 1990s in an effort to control costs, which contributed to an increase in outpatient services. Provinces have attempted to restrict the number of physicians eligible to bill the government in well-serviced areas for cost control and to distribute physicians to medically underserved areas. Provincial governments also reduced the number of first-year medical school slots in public universities (where most higher education occurs) by 10 percent in the 1993–94 academic year in a long-term effort to reduce the number of physicians.

Further decisions about the distribution of public healthcare resources have been used to augment healthcare delivery reform. With the exception of Ontario, all provincial governments have been experimenting with regionalization. The main characteristics of regionalization are the creation of regional governance and management bodies; devolved authority and responsibility for healthcare services from provincial health ministries to regional bodies; the use of global budgets from which regional bodies fund health services (excluding physician services and drugs) and other organizations; and an emphasis on community-based settings (Church and Barker 1998). Some provinces have also experimented with combining funds for healthcare services with those for social services.

Provincial, territorial, and municipal governments provide a variety of public health services. Municipalities are primarily involved in environmental services including garbage disposal, sewage and water management, and building codes. Provinces and territories vary in the public health services provided, but these typically include immunization, dental care, health promotion activities, prenatal classes, and home nursing (Fulton 1993).

Canadian governments also regulate the healthcare system and health-related services, including setting occupational health standards, handling toxic substances, and certifying drugs. Canada is the sole country that regulates the price of patented drugs only; other countries that regulate drug prices do so for both patented and nonpatented drugs (Dingwall 1997). The Patented Medicine Prices Review Board, an independent quasi-judicial body, regulates the prices of patented medicines both by limiting the price of new patented drugs and by limiting the increase in prices of patented drugs already on the market.

Other Funders

Other significant funders in the Canadian healthcare system include private health insurers and individuals. Private health insurance generally exists only for services and providers not covered by public health insurance plans; the majority of the provinces prohibit private health insurance for publicly covered health services (Flood and Archibald 2001). Employers offer some types of supplemental health insurance as part of benefit packages. Benefits provided include drug coverage, dental coverage, semiprivate and private hospital room upgrades, coverage for nonphysician providers (e.g., chiropractors, physical therapists), eyeglasses and other vision care, and supplemental coverage for out-of-the-country emergency care. Many of these extended healthcare plans also cover the recipients' spouse and dependents. Copayments or deductibles may be part of private health insurance plans. Generally, low-paying jobs do not offer supplemental health insurance, while higher paying jobs do offer supplemental health insurance (National Forum on Health 1997). Overall, 22.2 million Canadians had private extended health benefits of some kind in 1999. Almost 15 million of this group had dental care benefits as part of these extended health benefits (Canadian Life and Health Insurance Association Inc. 2000).

Financing

Multiple funding mechanisms are used in the Canadian healthcare system (Figure 13.2). Funds flow from individuals to healthcare services through taxes, health insurance premiums, and out-of-pocket expenditures. Intermediary funders include the federal, provincial, territorial, and municipal governments, regional health authorities, employers, private insurers, and workers' compensation boards. Individuals receive some of their out-of-pocket expenditures back in the form of reimbursements from private insurance companies and tax credits from the federal government for excessive medical expenses.

Individual and corporate taxes paid to federal, provincial, territorial, and municipal governments are the principal source of funds for the public financing of healthcare services; Alberta and British Columbia also levy health insurance premiums. Provincial and territorial governments transfer healthcare funds to municipalities that finance public health and other community health services. The federal government transfers funds to the provincial and territorial governments through the Canada Health and Social Transfer (CHST). The CHST also finances postsecondary education, social assistance, and social services. Provinces and territories may distribute these block funds among these areas as long as they adhere to standards in the Canada Health Act and do not impose minimum residency conditions on social assistance.

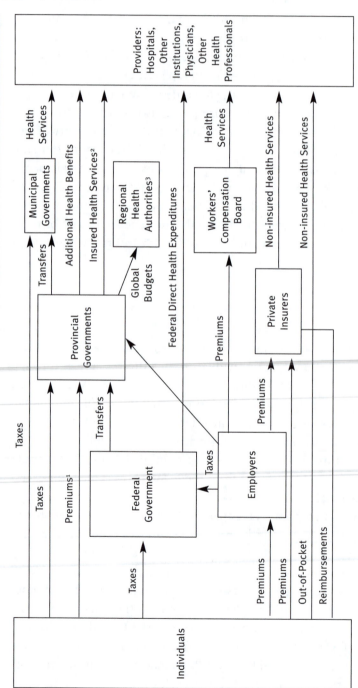

FIGURE 13.2
The Funding
of the
Healthcare
System in
Canada

1. Two provinces, British Columbia and Alberta, levy health premiums.
2. Medically necessary hospital and physician services.
3. Except Ontario.
SOURCE: Adapted from a figure by Health Canada (1999).

Controversy exists about how much of healthcare spending is funded by the federal government through the CHST; the federal government argues that its transfers fund a larger share of healthcare services than the provinces claim. The federal government's ability to ensure the national consistency of provincial and territorial health insurance plans through the fund-withholding power of the Canada Health Act is highly dependent on the actual and perceived magnitude of the federal fiscal transfers. If federal funds represent a small proportion of provincial and territorial spending on health, the provinces and territories can afford to absorb any withholdings for Canada Health Act violations. If the federal government is perceived as not contributing its share of healthcare expenditures, provinces and territories have more political support to refuse to comply with any federal demands. Although federal and provincial governments have disagreed about provincial insurance plan behavior, no provinces or territories have been willing to forgo the federal transfer payments, and all have eventually complied with federal requirements. Financial tensions between the two levels of government reached a standoff when, in September 2000, in response to widespread provincial and territorial government discontent, the federal government increased the CHST by Canadian$21.1 billion over five years. The federal government also committed an additional Canadian$2.3 billion in targeted funding over five years to be used to purchase new medical equipment, adopt health information technologies, and provide funds to accelerate primary healthcare reform.

Health Expenditures

The Canadian healthcare system was established at a time when most expenditures were for hospital and physician services. At present, provincial and territorial governments are single payers for just under half of all health expenditures (Canadian Institute for Health Information 2000) and are dominant funders for healthcare services where they are not the single payer (Table 13.4). Other healthcare expenditures, particularly those for drugs, have been increasing over time. In 1998, hospital services, physician services, and drugs accounted for 32.9 percent, 13.9 percent, and 14.8 percent of all health expenditures, respectively (Canadian Institute for Health Information 2000). The year 1997 marked the first time that drug expenditures exceeded physician expenditures (Canadian Institute for Health Information 2000).

Public spending has decreased as a percentage of all healthcare spending because of the rise in the use of services that are not universally publicly funded and because of more effective cost-control efforts in the public sector. In 1975, 76.4 percent of all healthcare expenditures came from public sources; by 1998, public spending had decreased to 70.1 percent of all health expenditures (Canadian Institute for Health Information 2000). Government spending cutbacks in the 1990s significantly slowed the growth of public-sector health expenditures. The growth in public expenditures

TABLE 13.4
Health
Expenditures
by Use of
Funds in
Canada, 1998

Category of Health Expenditure	Percentage of Health Expenditures	Public:Private Share
Hospitals	32.9	91.1:8.9
Other institutions	9.6	89.7:30.3
Physicians	13.9	98.7:1.3
Other professionals	12.2	10.5:89.5
Drugs	14.8	31.2:68.8
Capital	2.6	81.8:18.2
Other health spending	14.0	83.2:16.8

SOURCE: Canadian Institute for Health Information (2000).

was 4.5 percent from 1985 to 1990 and only 1.2 percent from 1990 to 1996 (Hicks 1999). That trend appears to be reversing: in 1998, public health expenditures grew faster than private health expenditures (Canadian Institute for Health Information 2000).

Private funding consists mainly of individual out-of-pocket expenditures and private health insurance. Out-of-pocket expenditures accounted for 55 percent of private health expenditures in 1996, whereas private health insurance accounted for 35 percent (Canadian Institute for Health Information 2000). The majority of private expenditures in 1996 were for drugs (31 percent) and healthcare professionals other than physicians (e.g., dentists, chiropractors, physical therapists, optometrists) (25 percent) (Health Canada 1997).

Financing Mechanisms

Physician services are largely paid for by provincial and territorial governments on a fee-for-service basis from a negotiated schedule. In the mid-1990s, all provinces had capped global budgets for fee-for-service physician payment (Barer, Lomas, and Sanmartin 1996), although a number of provinces have recently released these caps. The provincial and territorial governments continue to show interest in establishing alternative payment mechanisms for physicians, but most physicians strongly support the fee-for-service status quo.

Most hospitals are paid by provincial and territorial governments using global budgets. Private for-profit hospitals are the exception, receiving payment on a fee-for-service or per-diem basis. Nonphysician providers working in hospitals are paid out of the hospital budgets. Public funds for hospitals are supplemented by private insurance.

Healthcare services delivered by other institutions, such as long-term-care institutions, are generally publicly paid on a per-diem basis. Accommodation costs for these institutions are paid privately, either by the patient or by private insurance. Other providers, such as home-care providers, are paid on a fee-for-service basis using varying combinations of public and private funds. Regional health authorities in various provinces and territories have control over the budgets of some of these institutions and providers.

Health Resources

Human Resources

Table 13.5 shows information about staffing levels in the Canadian health system.

Physicians

The majority of Canadian physicians operate as private practitioners while billing public insurance plans. In 1998, Canada had 185 physicians per 100,000 population, with a slight majority (50.8 percent) in general or family practice (Canadian Institute for Health Information 2000a). Generally, remote areas such as the Canadian North and rural areas have fewer physicians than do urban areas. The sentiment that a physician shortage exists is growing, although the physician-to-population ratio has been relatively stable for the last decade (Canadian Institute for Health Information 2000a).

In contrast with the perception of the physician shortage, most Canadians have recently visited a physician. In the 1996–97 National Population Health Survey, 81 percent reported they had visited a general or family practitioner during the previous year (Federal, Provincial and Territorial Advisory Committee on Population Health 2000). In 1993 and 1994, insured Canadians had an annual average of 6 physician visits as compared with 4.5 physician visits in 1978 and 1979 (Federal, Provincial and Territorial Advisory Committee on Population Health 2000). Thus, there are indications that Canadians are increasing their use of physicians.

Other Health Professionals

Nurses are the largest group of health professionals, with 748 registered nurses and 255 licensed practical nurses per 100,000 population in 1998. These ratios have decreased by 5 percent and 15 percent, respectively, during the last decade (Canadian Institute for Health Information 2000a). Canada was the only country among OECD countries that experienced a decrease in the number of nurses during this time (Anderson 1998), resulting in an acute nursing shortage.

Midwives practice throughout Canada, although only half of the provinces have legislation governing midwives, and only two provinces (Ontario

TABLE 13.5

Human Resources per 100,000 Population in Canada, 1997 and 1998

Physicians, total	185
General practice or family practice physicians	94
Specialist physicians	91
Nurses	
Registered nurses	748
Licensed practical nurses	255
Other medical and treatment services	
Pharmacists	76
Chiropractors	15
Optometrists	12
Dental services	
Dentists	54
Dental hygienists	44
Rehabilitation services	
Physiotherapists	48
Occupational therapists	25
Psychological and social services	
Psychologists	38
Social workers	45

NOTES: Physician and registered nurse figures are for 1998; the remaining figures are for 1997. Figures for physiotherapists, occupational therapists, psychologists, social workers, dental hygienists, and optometrists are estimates.
SOURCE: Canadian Institute for Health Information (2000a); Federal, Provincial and Territorial Advisory Committee on Population Health (2000).

and British Columbia) cover midwifery services under public insurance plans. Ontario had 174 registered midwives in 1999; these midwives attended 3 percent of Ontario's births (College of Midwives of Ontario 1999).

Pharmacists and dentists are the next two largest groups of other healthcare professionals in Canada (76 pharmacists and 54 dentists per 100,000 population) (Canadian Institute for Health Information 2000a). The equality of distribution of other health professionals varies by profession. The most frequently occurring visits to other health professionals included dentists and eye specialists (60 percent and 35 percent of Canadians visited in the year prior to a 1996–97 survey, respectively) (Federal, Provincial and Territorial Advisory Committee on Population Health 2000).

Hospitals

In 1998 and 1999, Canada had 777 hospitals (Table 13.6) with slightly more than 125,000 beds (Canadian Institute for Health Information 2001), which provided 4.1 hospital beds per 1,000 population. Most hospitals are not-for-profit and general service hospitals (96 percent and 86 percent of all hospitals, respectively) (Canadian Institute for Health Information 2001). The distribution of hospitals across Canada generally mirrors the country's population distribution. Hospitals and beds have declined substantially over a brief period of time as part of cost-control and health reform efforts. In 1994 and 1995, for instance, Canada had 978 hospitals and more than 156,000 hospital beds; this was a reduction from 1,224 hospitals and more than 178,000 hospital beds in 1987 (Tully and Saint-Pierre 1997).

Accompanying these hospital closures and bed reductions has been a decrease in the average length of hospital stay. In 1990 and 1991, the average length of a hospital stay was 11.5 days, and the total number of hospital days for all patients was 41.4 million days (Federal, Provincial and Territorial Advisory Committee on Population Health 2000). Comparable 1996 and 1997 statistics found an average length of stay of 10.7 days and total numbers of days stayed of 33.9 million (Statistics Canada 1999). In addition, fewer Canadians were treated in hospital: the 1996 and 1997 hospital separation rate (discharges and deaths) was 10,523 per 100,000 people, which was the lowest separation rate since these data were first collected in 1961 (Statistics Canada 1999). Not surprisingly, the number of outpatient visits increased during this time.

Other Healthcare Facilities and Services

Community Health Centers (CHCs) represent a small but significant mode of delivering ambulatory care in Canada. CHCs are generally multidisciplinary and multifunctional, offering a coordinated team approach to healthcare (Fulton 1993). Canada has 249 CHCs (see Table 13.6), more than half of which are in Quebec (Blair 1999).

Facility Type	Number
Hospitals	777
Community health centers	249
Long-term-care facilities for the elderly	1,167
Other long-term-care facilities	284

TABLE 13.6
Number of Health Services Facilities in Canada, 1999

SOURCE: Canadian Institute for Health Information (2001); Blair (1999); Statistics Canada (2001).

Most of the nursing homes and other long-term-care facilities in Canada are privately run; they may be not-for-profit or for-profit. In 1999, Canada had more than 1,167 long-term-care facilities for the elderly and more than 284 other long-term care facilities (these counts do not include Quebec nursing homes and other long-term-care facilities because Quebec does not report the level of care of facilities) (Statistics Canada 2001).

With respect to home care, most of the provinces and territories employ a single point-of-access system and use their regional health authorities or other regionally based agencies to coordinate the delivery of home-care services (Dumont-Lemasson, Donovan, and Wylie 1999). Provincial and territorial home-care programs served from 825,000 clients to almost 951,000 clients in 1996 and 1997, depending on the data source (Dumont-Lemasson, Donovan, and Wylie 1999).

Service Delivery

At first glance, the Canadian healthcare system seems well set up to ensure equitable access to physician and hospital services. Most importantly, Canadians face no user charges or deductibles for medically necessary physician and hospital services; they simply present their health insurance card. Canadians also have free choice of physicians. Although self-referral to specialists is generally discouraged, this informal gatekeeper model of accessing specialists does not impede access, as the majority of physicians are in general practice. Patients generally can receive nonemergency care at the hospital of their choice, and emergency care can be obtained at any hospital with an emergency department.

A deeper examination of the healthcare system, however, reveals problems with public and providers' satisfaction. Public satisfaction has been decreasing over time; the percentage of Canadians agreeing that only minor changes were needed in the Canadian healthcare system dropped from 56 percent in 1988 to 20 percent in 1998 (Donelan et al. 1999). Canadians are concerned about waiting times, the availability of physicians (particularly specialists) and other healthcare services, quality of care, and decreasing public healthcare funds (Canadian Medical Association 1998; Donelan et al. 1999). In a national survey conducted in 2000 (Marshall 2001), healthcare was considered the most important issue facing Canada today.

What is the evidence surrounding these concerns? Although the number of physicians per capita has been relatively stable, changes in physician practice may explain shortage concerns (Rachlis 1999). Little evidence has been found to support concerns of increases in wait times in Canada or of negative health outcomes because of wait lists (McDonald et al. 1998). When Canadians are asked about their own experiences with receiving healthcare, they generally report positive experiences (Donelan et al. 1999).

The media, however, report negative stories about the effects of funding cuts on service delivery, even when the data cannot demonstrate such problems (Roos 2000).

The Canadian healthcare system also has problems with unequal and inequitable access. Roos and Mustard (1997) systematically examined this issue for residents of Winnipeg, Manitoba, and found that medical need was associated with the receipt of care for part but not all of the healthcare system. These results are supported by other studies (Billings, Anderson, and Newman 1996; Birch, Eyles, and Newbold 1993; Dunlop, Coyte, and McIsaac 2000; Glazier et al. 2000; Katz, Hofer, and Manning 1996; Newbold, Eyles, and Birch 1995; Rivest et al. 1999). The Commonwealth Fund 1998 International Health Policy Survey (Schoen et al. 2000) also documented income-related disparities in accessing healthcare in Canada. Low-income Canadians were more than three times more likely to have not filled a drug prescription during the previous year due to cost, were 2.5 times more likely to have had trouble paying medical bills during the previous year, and were 1.5 times more likely to respond that the Canadian healthcare system needed to be completely rebuilt. The survey found no statistically significant income-related differences in the percentage of Canadian respondents claiming difficulty in obtaining health services or reporting that they received fair or poor care at their most recent doctor visit. In another survey, only 5 percent of Canadians 12 years old or older reported at least one situation during the previous year in which they needed healthcare or advice and did not get it (Federal, Provincial and Territorial Advisory Committee on Population Health 2000).

Rural areas in Canada also generally have impeded access to health services (Fakhoury and Roos 1996; Rivest et al. 1999). Not only do rural areas have fewer providers and healthcare institutions (Buske 2000; Langley, Minkin, and Till 1997; Rivest et al. 1999), but rural residents face additional access barriers such as higher transportation costs (Fakhoury and Roos 1996). As for gender and age differences in accessing care, various studies of specific healthcare services have not found evidence of disparities in the receipt of healthcare services covered under the public system (Ugnat and Naylor 1993). Other studies have found that the elderly have more trouble gaining access to specialists (Schoen et al. 2000a) and are less likely than other age groups to receive specialty care (Verrilli, Brenson, and Katz 1998). For healthcare services not universally covered under the public system, the elderly experience access disparities (Schoen et al. 2000a), with greater access barriers as income decreases.

Prospects for the Future

Canadians are deeply committed to their healthcare system despite their concerns and calls for change. When asked to reflect on the key components and values of the healthcare system, Canadians strongly identify with equality of access and the concept that every person should receive health services according to need (National Forum on Health 1997a). Canadians would like more government investment in healthcare. In a recent survey, 78 percent of respondents supported increased government spending on healthcare with a corresponding decrease in spending in other areas (Marshall 2001). In response to this sentiment, the federal government recently committed more funds for healthcare to the provinces and territories and continues to resist suggestions for user fees and a parallel private system.

Overall, the Canadian healthcare system is doing well, although problems are acknowledged; federal, provincial, and territorial governments appear willing to continue to address these issues. The recently established royal commission on Canada's healthcare system, for example, is charged with developing recommendations for the long-term sustainability of the public healthcare system. Public and private cost control will continue to be an important issue. Future healthcare services and providers will likely be required to work in a more integrated and cooperative way. Indeed, the province of Saskatchewan is currently investigating the use of interdisciplinary primary health service networks to deliver health services in a coordinated way (Fyke 2001). Other changes that will likely occur include improved health information and quality-control mechanisms and the adoption of predominantly non-fee-for-service payment mechanisms for physicians, allowing better alignment of financial incentives with cost control and appropriate healthcare services use. The expected increased demand for healthcare services from an aging population (particularly for home care and drugs) will also require more resources and innovative uses of current resources. Like other industrialized countries around the world, Canada will have to continue to balance increasing costs and increasing demands for healthcare while remaining true to the country's ethos.

Acknowledgments

I am indebted to the work of the Canadian Institute for Health Information, Statistics Canada, and Health Canada. Jerry Hurley, Brian Hutchison, Glenn Wilson, Alba Dicenso, Barbara Gregoire, Toni Newman, and Kathy Brodsky provided helpful comments and suggestions. Thanks to Carolyn Busse for electronically producing Figure 13.2. As usual, despite others' assistance, remaining errors are my own.

Notes

1. The federal government has greater jurisdiction over territories as compared with provinces. Until recently, Canada had only two terri-

tories. The territory of Nunavut was established on April 1, 1999 by subdividing the Northwest Territories.
2. Statistics Canada defines the low-income cutoffs at the points at which families and individuals spend more than 54.7 percent of their income on food, shelter, and clothing.
3. The United Nations Human Development Index uses education, access to healthcare, and average income to rank countries.
4. The Index of Social Health is a composite of 15 indicators of population heath including poverty, unemployment, income inequality, and infant mortality. It was developed by Human Resources Development Canada and Statistics Canada.

REFERENCES

Anderson, G. F. 1998. *Multinational Comparisons of Health Care: Expenditures, Coverage, and Outcomes.* New York: The Commonwealth Fund.

Barer, M., Lomas, J., and Sanmartin, C. 1996. "Re-minding our Ps and Qs: Medical Cost Controls in Canada." *Health Affairs* 15: 216–34.

Billings, J., Anderson, G. M., and Newman, L. S. 1996. "Recent Findings on Preventable Hospitalizations." *Health Affairs* 15: 239–49.

Birch, S., and Abelson, J. 1993. "Is Reasonable Access What We Want? Implications of, and Challenges to, Current Canadian Policy on Equity in Health Care." *International Journal of Health Services* 23: 629–53.

Birch, S., Eyles, J., and Newbold, K. B. 1993. "Equitable Access to Health Care: Methodological Extensions to the Analysis of Physician Utilization in Canada." *Health Economics* 2: 87–101.

Blair, L. 1999. "Cutting and Pasting in Quebec: Community Health Centers and Health Care Reform." *Canadian Family Physician* 45: 261–64.

Buske, L. 2000. "Availability of Services in Rural Areas." *Canadian Medical Association Journal* 162: 1193.

Canada House of Commons. 1984. *Canada Health Act.* Ottawa: Queen's Printer.

Canadian Institute for Health Information. 2000. *National Health Expenditure Trends, 1975–2000.* Ottawa: Canadian Institute for Health Information.

———. 2000a. *Number of Health Professionals Per Capita Drops Over 10-year Period.* Ottawa: Canadian Institute for Health Information.

———. 2001. *Canadian Hospitals by Province, Service Type and Ownership for Fiscal Year 1998–99.* Ottawa: Canadian Institute for Health Information.

Canadian Life and Health Insurance Association Inc. 2000. *Canadian Life and Health Insurance Facts.* Toronto: Canadian Life and Health Insurance Association Inc.

Canadian Medical Association. 1998. *Canadians' Access to Quality Health Care: A System in Crisis.* Ottawa: Canadian Medical Association.

Charles, C., Lomas, J., Giacomini, M., et al. 1997. "Medical Necessity in Canadian Health Policy: Four Meanings and . . . a Funeral?" *Milbank Quarterly* 75: 365–94.

Church, J., and Barker, P. 1998. "Regionalization of Health Services in Canada:

A Critical Perspective." *International Journal of Health Services* 28: 467–86.

College of Midwives of Ontario. 1999. *Midwifery in Ontario, Caseload Data, 1994–1998.* Toronto: College of Midwives of Ontario.

Coyte, P. C., and McKeever, P. 2000. "Home Care in Canada: Passing the Buck." *Canadian Journal of Nursing Research* 33 (2): 11–25.

Dingwall, D. C. 1997. *Drug Costs in Canada.* Ottawa: Health Canada.

Donelan, K., Blendon, R. J., Schoen, C., et al. 1999. "The Cost of Health System Change: Public Discontent in Five Nations." *Health Affairs* 18: 206–16.

Dumont-Lemasson, M., Donovan, C., and Wylie, M. 1999. *Provincial and Territorial Home Care Programs: A Synthesis for Canada.* Ottawa: Health Canada.

Dunlop, S., Coyte, P. C., and McIsaac, W. 2000. "Socio-economic Status and the Utilization of Physicians' Services: Results from the Canadian National Population Health Survey." *Social Science and Medicine* 51: 123–33.

Evans, R. G. 2000. "Canada." *Journal of Health Politics, Policy and Law* 25: 889–97.

Fakhoury, W. K. H., and Roos, L. 1996. "Access to and Use of Physician Resources by the Rural and Urban Populations in Manitoba." *Canadian Journal of Public Health* 87: 248–52.

Federal, Provincial and Territorial Advisory Committee on Population Health. 2000. *Statistical Report on the Health of Canadians.* Ottawa: Health Canada.

Flood, C. M., and Archibald, T. 2001. "The Illegality of Private Health Care in Canada." *Canadian Medical Association Journal* 164: 825–30.

Fulton, M. J. 1993. *Canada's Health System: Bordering on the Possible.* Washington, DC: Faulkner & Gray, Inc.

Fyke, K. J. 2001. *Caring for Medicare: Sustaining a Quality System.* Regina, Saskatchewan: The Commission on Medicare.

Glazier, R. H., Badley, E. M., Gilbert, J. E., et al. 2000. "The Nature of Increased Hospital Use in Poor Neighborhoods: Findings from a Canadian Inner City." *Canadian Journal of Public Health* 91: 268–73.

Health Canada. 1997. *National Health Expenditures in Canada, 1975–1996.* Ottawa: Health Canada.

———. 1999. *Canada's Health Care System.* Ottawa: Health Canada.

———. 2000. *How Does Literacy Affect the Health of Canadians?* Ottawa: Health Canada.

Hicks, V. 1999. *The Evolution of Public and Private Health Care Spending in Canada, 1960 to 1997.* Ottawa: Canadian Institute for Health Information.

Katz, S. J., Hofer, T. P., and Manning, W. G. 1996. "Hospital Utilization in Ontario and the United States: The Impact of Socioeconomic Status and Health Status." *Canadian Journal of Public Health* 87: 253–56.

Langley, G. R., Minkin, S., and Till, J. E. 1997. "Regional Variation in Nonmedical Factors Affecting Family Physicians' Decisions About Referral for Consultation." *Canadian Medical Association Journal* 157: 265–72.

Lindsey, R., and West, D. S. 1999. "National Pharmacare, Reference-Based Pricing, and Drug R&D: A Critique of the National Forum on Health's

Recommendations for Pharmaceutical Policy." *Canadian Public Policy* 25: 1–27.

MacMillan, H. L., MacMillan, A. B., Offord, D. R., et al. 1996. "Aboriginal Health." *Canadian Medical Association Journal* 155: 1569–78.

Marshall, R. 2001. "Paying the Price." *Maclean's* 113 (52): 450–80.

McDonald, P., Shortt, S., Sanmartin, C., et al. 1998. *Waiting Lists and Waiting Times for Health Care in Canada: More Management!! More Money??* Ottawa: Health Canada.

National Forum on Health. 1997. "Directions for a Pharmaceutical Policy in Canada." In National Forum on Health's *Canada Health Action: Building on the Legacy—Volume II—Synthesis Reports and Issue Papers.* Ottawa: Health Canada.

———. 1997a. "Values Working Group Synthesis Report." In National Forum on Health's *Canada Health Action: Building on the Legacy—Volume II—Synthesis Reports and Issue Papers.* Ottawa: Health Canada.

Naylor, C. D. 1999. "Health Care in Canada: Incrementalism Under Fiscal Duress." *Health Affairs* 18: 9–26.

Newbold, K. B., Eyles, J., and Birch, S. 1995. "Equity in Health Care: Methodological Contributions to the Analysis of Hospital Utilization in Canada." *Social Science and Medicine* 40: 1181–92.

Nichols, M. 2000. Children of Poverty. *Maclean's* 113 (26): 46.

———. 2000a. "Northern Perils." *Maclean's* 113 (15): 74–75.

OECD. 2001. "Frequently Asked Data. OECD Health Data 2000." Retrieved 09 April 2001 from www.oecd.org/els/health/software/fad.

Rachlis, M. M. 1995. "The Canadian Experience with Public Health Insurance." In *The Canadian Health Care System: Lessons for the United States*, pp. 143–54, edited by S. Brown Eve, B. Havens, and S. R. Ingman. Lanham, MD: University Press of America, Inc.

———. 1999. "Do We Really Need More Doctors? *The Toronto Star*, August 25, A19.

Rivest, F., Bosse, P., Nedelca, S., et al. 1999. "Access to Physician Services in Quebec: Relative Influence of Household Income and Area of Residence." *Canadian Public Policy* 25: 453–81.

Roos, N. P. 2000. "The Disconnect Between the Data and the Headlines. *Canadian Medical Association Journal* 163: 411–12.

Roos, N. P., and Mustard, C. A. 1997. "Variation in Health and Health Care Use by Socioeconomic Status in Winnipeg, Canada: Does the System Work Well? Yes and No." *Milbank Quarterly* 75: 89–111.

Schoen, C., Davis, K., DesRoches, C., et al. 2000. "Health Insurance Markets and Income Inequality: Findings from an International Health Policy Survey." *Health Policy* 51: 67–85.

Schoen, C. Strumpf, E., Davis, K., et al. 2000a. *The Elderly's Experience with Health Care in Five Nations.* New York: The Commonwealth Fund.

Statistics Canada. 1999. "Hospital Utilization, 1996/97." *The Daily*, February 24.

———. 2000. *Canada at a Glance 2000.* Ottawa: Statistics Canada.

———. 2000a. "Population by Aboriginal Group, 1996 Census. Canadian Statistics." Retrieved 31 July 2000 from www.statcan.ca/english/Pgdb/People/Population/demo39a.htm.

———. 2000b. "Population by Age Group. Canadian Statistics." Retrieved 31 July 2000 from www.statcan.ca/english/Pgdb/People/Population/demo31a.htm.

———. 2000c. "Population by Knowledge of Official Language, 1996 Census. Canadian Statistics." Retrieved 31 July 2000 from www.statcan.ca/english/Pgdb/People/Population/demo19a.htm.

———. 2000d. "Population, Population Density, Births and Deaths for Selected Countries. Canadian Statistics." Retrieved 31 July 2000 from www.statcan.ca/english/Pgdb/People/Population/demo01.htm.

———. 2000e. "Selected Leading Causes of Death by Sex. Canadian Statistics." Retrieved 31 July 2000 from www.statcan.ca/english/Pgdb/People/Health/health36.htm.

———. 2001. "Numbers of Facilities Offering at Least a Type II Level of Care in Canada." Unpublished data. Generated by Richard Trudeau, April 10, 2001. Ottawa, Ontario.

Tully, P., and Saint-Pierre, E. 1997. "Downsizing Canada's Hospitals, 1986/87 to 1994/95." *Health Reports* 8: 33–39.

Ugnat, A.-M., and Naylor, C. D. 1993. "Trends in Coronary Artery Bypass Grafting in Ontario from 1981 to 1989." *Canadian Medical Association Journal* 148: 569–75.

Verrilli, D. K., Brenson, R., and Katz, S. J. 1998. "A Comparison of Cardiovascular Procedure Use Between the United States and Canada." *Health Services Research* 33: 467–87.

Walker, R. 1999. "Doctors Lose when Patients Lack Insurance." *The Medical Post*, April 6, 35 (13).

Willison, D. J., Grootendorst, P. V., and Hurley, J. 1998. *Variation in Pharmacare Coverage Across Canada. Working Paper 98–08.* Hamilton, Ontario: McMaster University Center for Health Economics and Policy Analysis.

World Bank. 2000. "Canada at a Glance. World Development Indicators Database." Retrieved 28 September 2000 from www.worldbank.org.

World Health Organization (WHO). 2000. *The World Health Report 2000: Health Systems: Improving Performance.* Geneva: WHO.

JAPAN

Aki Yoshikawa and Jayanta Bhattacharya

Background Information

Healthcare systems are a product of the unique cultural, political, and economic circumstances in any country, and Japan is no exception. Since the Meiji Restoration, Japanese doctors have primarily practiced Western medicine; the advent of universal health insurance is a more recent phenomenon. The modern Japanese healthcare system has its roots in the 1922 Health Insurance Law, which extended compulsory basic medical benefits to manufacturing and mining employees. This legislation imposed a national fee schedule that Japanese doctors then protested, and this led to the 1938 National Health Insurance Act, which further extended healthcare benefits to the self-employed (mainly fishermen and farmers) and their families and resulted in the formation of national health insurance societies. Japan's involvement in World War II hampered continued expansion of these benefits until 1958, when the National Health Insurance Law was passed and Japanese citizens were guaranteed universal health insurance. The current Japanese system retains the characteristics of its beginnings with a strong emphasis on employer-based financing of healthcare in combination with a nationally set price schedule and fee-for-service billing by medical providers.

The greatest strength of Japan's healthcare system—in addition to its low cost—is guaranteed access to comprehensive medical care for virtually every member of the population. Surveys of Japanese who chose not to seek medical care at one time or another found that an overwhelming majority of the respondents cited reasons other than problems of access and cost. A 1985 national survey by Koseisho (the Ministry of Health and Welfare) showed that only 0.2 percent of the respondents cited problems of access and 0.4 percent cited financial problems. The easy access and the lack of economic burden may explain why the per capita number of physician visits is quite high relative to other nations (Utsunomiya and Yoshikawa 1993).

Japan is a large and geographically diverse island nation of 378,000 square kilometers, a land area slightly greater than that of Germany. Its climate ranges from the colder northern region of Hokkaido to temperate climates in the south. The population of 126 million inhabitants is almost entirely ethnically Japanese with only a small foreign-born population, who are primarily Korean. Japan's population density is relatively high by Western standards, but it varies considerably across the different regions of Japan, and Tokyo is the most densely populated. Like most developed countries, Japan has a near-zero level of population growth, with a total fertility rate well below replacement. Seventeen percent of Japan's population was 65 years old or older in 1998, and this proportion is projected to grow dramatically during the next few decades. Projected growth of the elderly population has enormous implications for the Japanese healthcare system, and financial as well as infrastructure preparations must be made now to accommodate the coming influx of elderly patients. Pertinent demographic statistics are given in Table 14.1.

A dynamo in the 1960s, 1970s, and 1980s, the Japanese economy slumped during the late 1990s. Figure 14.1 illustrates the trend in Japanese gross domestic product and GDP per capita between 1983 and 1998. The spectacular economic growth that Japan experienced during the postwar period came to an abrupt halt in 1996. This, along with the aging population, has put enormous pressure on the Japanese healthcare system.

TABLE 14.1

Demographic Statistics

Total area	378,000 square kilometers
Population in 1998:	
Total	126 million
Foreign-born	900,000
Density	335 per square kilometer
Percent urbanized	79 (concentrated in Tokyo, Osaka, and Nagoya metropolitan areas)
Annual growth rate	0.2%
Age structure (% total population)	
0 to 4 years old	5
5 to 14 years old	10
15 to 64 years old	68
65 years old and older	17
Life expectancy at birth (years)	
Males	77
Females	83.4
Infant mortality rate (% of live births)	0.4
Under-five mortality rate (% of live births)	0.1
Total fertility rate (per women between the ages of 15 and 44 years)	1.48 children

Table 14.2 displays additional pertinent economic statistics. Despite Japan's deep recession, recent inflation has been minimal and the unemployment rate has remained low by Western standards. The working population in 1998 was approximately 54 percent of the total population, which is similar to other developed nations. In addition, the Japanese populace is well-educated, with a literacy rate of nearly 100 percent, a requirement for mandatory secondary education, and a substantial percentage of the population ultimately attaining postsecondary education.

Context: Health Needs

Despite lower health expenditures than many other developed countries, macro-level health statistics reveal that the Japanese population is quite healthy. The infant mortality rate is only 0.4 percent of all live births annually, and Japanese newborns have among the highest life expectancy of any set of newborns in the world, although, as in other countries, females can expect to live nearly 6.5 years longer than males. Table 14.3 shows the leading causes of mortality in 1998. As the population has aged during the past few decades and public health has improved, mortality due to malignancies and heart disease has increased, whereas mortality due to infectious diseases such as tuberculosis has virtually disappeared.

The standard immunization schedule in Japan includes diphtheria-pertussis-tetanus vaccines at 3, 4, and 5 months with boosters at 6 years and 11 to 12 years; a measles vaccine at 12 months; and two doses of an oral polio vaccine between 3 and 7.5 months. Coverage rates for these vaccines in 1996 ranged from 100 percent for diphtheria-pertussis-tetanus to 94 percent for measles, and 98 percent for oral polio vaccine (WHO 2002).

During the past 40 years, a vast improvement has been seen in the availability of safe drinking water in Japan, rising from 53.4 percent of the population having it available in 1960 to 95.5 percent of the population having it today (Koseisho 1997). Although some concern exists regarding

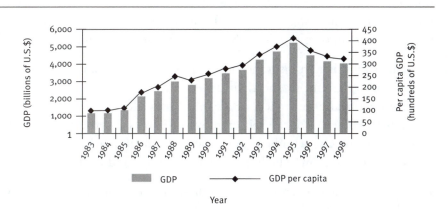

FIGURE 14.1
Japanese GDP and Per Capital GDP, 1983–98

TABLE 14.2
Economic
Statistics

Total labor force (1998), millions	68
Population in labor force, %	53.9
Unemployment rate (1997), %	4.1
GDP (1997)	
Total, millions of U.S.$	4,117,990
Per capita, millions of U.S.$	32,654
GNP (1997)	
Total, millions of U.S.$	4,992,350
Per capita, millions of U.S.$	39,587
Consumer price index (1998) (index 1995 = 100)	102.5
Health spending (1997)	
Total, millions of U.S.$	300,613
Share of total GDP, %	7.3
Per capita annually, U.S.$	2,286

excessive levels of pollutants such as trichloroethylene in the groundwater in some localities (Japanese Ministry of the Environment 2001), modern treatment and purification methods essentially guarantee clean water in virtually all covered areas. The public health infrastructure is well-developed in Japan and includes mechanisms to deal effectively with communicable diseases, promote sanitation, and prevent food contamination.

Organization and Management of the Health System

Japan's universal health insurance system, which covers its entire population, is segmented by workplace. The type of company one works for determines the insurance society to which one belongs and the financial contributions one must make. The three basic groups are as follows:

1. employees' health insurance for employees of firms and other public sector organizations and their dependents
2. national health insurance, or Kokuho (officially known as Kokumin Kenko Hoken), for the self-employed, retirees and their dependents, and anyone else who does not otherwise qualify for health insurance
3. the Roken system, which is a special pooling fund for the elderly

The first group, employees' health insurance, is further broken down into three main categories:

		TABLE 14.3
Malignancies	226.7	Leading Causes of Mortality in Japan (1998)— Deaths per 100,000 Population
Heart disease	114.3	
Cerebrovascular disease	110.0	
Pneumonia	63.8	
Accidents	31.1	
Suicide	25.4	
Unspecified cause ("old age")	17.1	
Renal failure	13.3	
Liver disease	12.9	
Hypertensive diabetes	10.0	

- *Seikan:* government-managed health insurance that covers the employees of small and medium-sized companies and their dependents
- *Kenpo:* society-managed health insurance that covers those employed by larger firms and their dependents (companies such as Toshiba, Honda, and Sony maintain their own Kenpo societies; there are about 1,800 Kenpo associations in Japan)
- *Kyosai:* public employees, both national and local, as well as private school teachers and staff and their dependents, are covered under this system

In an employee health insurance system such as Kenpo, an employee's monthly premium is withheld by the employer from his or her salary. The employer in turn pays a fixed mandated contribution to fund its Kenpo association.

All of the plans have some degree of cost sharing at the point of service. Copayments range between 10 and 30 percent, depending on the insurance society to which an employee belongs. For example, copayment obligations are greater for Kokuho members than for those insured under employees' insurance (e.g., Kenpo, Seikan, and Kyosai). As in the United States, cost sharing through copayments tends to reduce the use of medical services. For example, a 10 percent rate is estimated to reduce the use of services by 2 to 3 percent (Bhattachayra et al. 1996).

Financing

Spending for Japanese healthcare reached ¥28 trillion (roughly U.S.$288 billion) in 1997. Per capita medical spending was ¥230,400 (U.S.$2,286). Healthcare expenditures comprised 7.3 percent of the GDP in 1997.

In fiscal year 1998, Kokuho posted a deficit of ¥102 billion (U.S.$1.01 billion); this represented an increase of about 250 percent from the previous year. Seikan had a similarly dismal performance. Traditionally, it was Kenpo that cross-subsidized the financial losses of Kokuho and Seikan. Various Kenpo associations, set up by large firms to handle health insurance for their employees, have maintained a premium surplus with their young and healthy employees. This macro-level cross-subsidization has been the foundation of Japan's healthcare financing mechanism.

One of the most serious problems facing the Japanese healthcare system today is that, in the declining economy, many Kenpo associations are suffering financial losses. The rapidly aging society and shrinking economy partly explain this phenomenon. Kenpo associations pay nearly 40 percent of their collected premium to cover care for the elderly. Some Kenpo associations have resisted making their "contributions" to the pooling fund for geriatric care despite the tradition of doing so because more than three-quarters of Kenpo associations are currently in debt. Their predicament poses a serious threat to corporate management and the foundation of Japan's healthcare financing mechanism.

The Pooling Fund for Geriatric Care

The health and medical services system for the elderly, Roken, is a pooling fund through which Koseisho has attempted to distribute the burden of paying for geriatric care for all Japanese. Established in 1983, the pooling fund covers those who are more than 70 years old and bedridden people over 65 years old. The fund pools contributions from all insurance schemes.

Under the current system, elderly patients are charged fixed amounts of ¥1,200 per day for hospital care and ¥530 per outpatient visit. Seventy percent of medical costs for the elderly—excluding the portion paid by the recipient—are covered by contributions from health insurance societies for company employees and national health insurance schemes administered by municipalities for nonwage earners. The government shoulders the remaining 30 percent.

The Roken system is a macro-level cost-shifting mechanism. It was created when the employer-based Kenpo associations were fiscally strong and the elderly population was small enough to be supported by a substantial working population. The increasing proportion of elderly people seeking assistance under Roken relative to the number of workers paying into the pooling fund has severely limited the ability of the Japanese government to sustain this financing system, which may be facing imminent collapse.

Nursing Care Insurance

In April 2000, the Japanese government adopted a new nursing care insurance scheme, kaigo hoken, designed to provide assistance to senior citizens certified as needing care and other qualified disabled people. Under the plan, elderly users are assigned to one of six categories on the basis of care needs; the user's assigned category determines the maximum coverage available to the individual. Ceilings exist for the use of two services (care and bathing assistance) provided by visiting home helpers as well as for short stays at nursing care facilities. Whereas all of the elderly were previously covered under health insurance, the new law forces some to be covered under the new nursing care insurance. The key issue in the transition period is whether the elderly who are deemed not eligible for coverage under the new nursing care insurance program will still receive the care they need. Under the new system, the elderly deemed capable of living independently are required to leave government-subsidized nursing homes after a grace period.

Under the new system, 10 percent of the cost of nursing care services is paid by the recipients, half of the remaining 90 percent is publicly financed, and the other half is obtained from mandatory contributions by people 40 years old and older. A typical elderly person in the category of those needing the most intensive care can receive, in one week, about 13 hours of home nursing care, about two hours of home medical care, and one rehabilitation session at home. Depending on physical condition and home environment, the elderly can select from 12 different types of home nursing care service. The premium is calculated on the basis of the fiscal size of the nursing care system and the sum total of the policyholders' incomes. At that rate, a worker 40 years old or older who earns a monthly salary of about ¥330,000 (U.S.$3,274) is asked to contribute ¥3,100 (U.S.$31) each month, although the employer nominally pays half of this premium. Although the elderly only have to pay 10 percent of care expenses within the limits of the categories, they pay the full amount for services exceeding those limits.

Catastrophic Coverage

The High-Cost Medical Care Benefits Law of 1973 was amended in 1984 to introduce a cap on the monthly copayment. The measure established a monthly ceiling for copayments, set as of 1997 to ¥63,600 (U.S.$631) per month. Consequently, the actual daily copayment rate for an inpatient suffering from a major catastrophic illness approaches zero with increasing medical bills.

The Fee Schedule

Under the Japanese system, all medical facilities are reimbursed for medical services according to the official uniform fee schedule (shinryo hoshu). The price list, based on the so-called point system, lists the amount of reimbursement medical facilities receive for individual procedures and pharmaceuticals. This detailed pricing control lists more than 3,000 medical procedures for physicians alone. For example, an initial physician's consultation at a hospital is worth 230 points; currently, each point is worth ¥10.

This fee schedule has proved to be a useful resource for healthcare policymakers because it gives them the power to influence and alter the behavior of healthcare providers and facilities. Manipulation of the fee schedule serves as one of the primary mechanisms by which Koseisho regulates the supply of medical services, utilization rates, and aggregate healthcare expenditures. Low healthcare expenditures have not been realized accidentally: systemic manipulation of the fee schedule has been an effective cost-containment tool. Nevertheless, the imposition of the fee schedule has had some unintended consequences, including excessive prescribing by doctors.

Reimbursement Procedures

All costs incurred by medical facilities are reimbursed on a fee-for-service basis. When patients receive medical services, they are responsible only for their copayment at the point of service. Upon providing medical services to a patient, a hospital prepares a reimbursement claim. The claim, called receputo, is prepared and submitted monthly to receive reimbursement. The receputo itemizes each procedure, including drugs dispensed, for which points are assigned according to the fee schedule.

The receputo is overwhelmingly detailed. Each one contains detailed demographic, diagnostic, and procedure data; there are line items for each billable item, and some receputo go on for tens of pages. The receputo claims are always prepared in paper form. Hospital workers then bundle massive amounts of printed receputo claims with string, put them in boxes, and send these boxes to a clearinghouse.

Over one billion receputo claims, all in paper form, are submitted annually. After receiving the original paper receputo claims from the clearinghouses, an insurance organization (such as the Toyota Kenpo) then calculates the total payment and sends the amount, along with the original receputo, back to the clearinghouse. Minimal oversight or utilization review is performed by the insurance societies. Finally, hospitals receive reimbursement payments from the clearinghouses. The complete process, from submission of a receputo by a hospital to the reimbursement payment, takes approximately two months.

The Official Pharmaceutical Price Schedule

In addition to the official fee schedule is a separate reimbursement schedule for pharmaceuticals. Koseisho sets official medicine prices every two years on the basis of market prices plus a fixed profit margin for hospitals and clinics. Koseisho forecasts that drug expenses will total ¥6.47 trillion during the fiscal year of 2000, which will equal about 23 percent of all medical spending. The existence of yakka saeki (the so-called "doctor's margin")—the difference between the official reimbursement rates for pharmaceuticals and the actual purchasing price that drug companies charge physicians—is a classic example of distortions generated by the price control. Doctors often augment their earnings from regulated medical services by freely prescribing drugs and keeping the doctor's margin. With the existence of yakka saeki, Japanese physicians predictably often opt to sell higher-priced drugs because more expensive drugs result in larger margins.

Health Resources

As we have seen, Japan devotes considerably less of its economic resources to healthcare than do the United States and many other industrialized nations. Given the institutional differences described, that the distribution of health resources across doctors, nurses, and hospitals also differs should come as no surprise. In short, Japan has many more hospital beds, fewer doctors, and fewer nurses than does the United States. The remainder of this section discusses trends in the number of medical personnel and offers a detailed consideration of hospitals in Japan, as they constitute such an important component of the healthcare system.

Medical Personnel

Trends in the number of nurses, dentists, and physicians in Japan are shown in Table 14.4. The supply of doctors in Japan increased slightly between 1990 and 1996 from 1.7 practicing physicians per 1,000 people to 1.8. Despite this small increase, Japan has fewer doctors per patient than the United States (which had 2.4 doctors per 1,000 population in 1996). In contrast, Japan and the United States have roughly the same number of dentists per capita (0.6 dentists per 1,000 population in 1995). Similar to what is found in the United States, however, concern exists that the number of specialist physicians may be excessive relative to generalists.

In comparison with the relative stability of doctors and dentists in Japan during the 1990s, the number of nurses per capita has increased dramatically from 6 nurses per 1,000 population in 1990 to 7.4 in 1996. In part, this increase is in response to a long-standing perceived shortage during the past 20 years (Sawada 1997) as well as a response to the substantial growth in the number of elderly patients. Many hospitals in Japan have wards designated solely for the care of the elderly that serve the same purpose that long-term-care nursing homes serve in the United States. As one might expect, the demand for nurses in these wards has increased with the demand for these wards. Recently, however, results from a 1998 survey conducted by the Japanese Nursing Association (1999) indicate that the growth in the demand for nurses by hospitals is abating. Given the expected growth in the elderly population in Japan during the next 30 years, however, such an abatement seems temporary. Additional human resources information is provided in Table 14.4.

TABLE 14.4
Trends in the
Numbers of
Doctors and
Nurses in
Japan

	1990	1992	1994	1996
Practicing physicians per 1,000 population	1.7	1.7	1.8	1.8
Practicing certified or registered nurses per 1,000 population	6.0	6.4	6.9	7.4
Practicing dentists per 1,000 population	0.6	0.6	0.6	0.7

SOURCE: OECD (1999).

Hospitals

Hospitals are a more important component of healthcare delivery in Japan than they are in the United States. In addition to providing technologically advanced inpatient care, the Japanese hospital is an important site for the provision of outpatient care and even nursing-home-type services. Due to strict price controls, Japanese hospitals compete for patients on the basis of quality. These unique features make an understanding of Japanese hospitals critical to a more complete understanding of the Japanese healthcare system.

In Japan, the definition of a hospital is a medical facility with 20 or more beds; facilities with fewer than 20 beds are classified as clinics. In comparison with other industrialized countries, the number of hospitals and hospital beds in Japan is extremely high. For example, in 1997, the United States reported 6,201 hospitals with roughly 1,062,000 beds, whereas Japan had 9,413 hospitals with 1,660,784 beds in the same year.

Some of the disparity may be attributable to differences in the definitions of hospitals and hospital beds. For example, some of Japan's hospital beds are used as substitutes for long-term geriatric care, making an accurate comparison difficult. However, the large number of hospitals is most likely due to a combined result of the profits that Japanese hospitals can make and Koseisho regulation of hospitals.

Private ownership dominates the Japanese hospital system; private hospitals account for approximately 70 percent of all hospital beds. The iryo-hojin, a form of private hospital, is the most prevalent type of hospital in Japan and has a special legal status as a not-for-profit entity in the medical care sector. Operating healthcare facilities on a for-profit basis is illegal in Japan. An iryo-hojin is prohibited from distributing profits to anyone outside the hospital (e.g., shareholders). Table 14.5 shows trends during the 1990s in the number of hospital beds per capita in Japan by ownership type.

Although the prohibition on distributing profits may lead one to believe that Japanese iryo-hojin private hospitals resemble American not-

	1990	1992	1994	1996	1997
Total inpatient beds per 1,000 population	16.0	16.2	16.2	16.2	16.4
Private hospital beds per 1,000 population	11.3	11.3	11.1	10.8	10.7
Nursing home beds per 1,000 population	0.2	0.4	0.7	1.1	1.3
Psychiatric care beds per 1,000 population	2.9	2.9	2.9	2.9	2.9
Hospital inpatient days per capita	4.1	4.1	4.1	4.1	4.0
ALOS per admission (days)	51	48	46	44	43

TABLE 14.5
Trends in Aggregate Hospital Statistics

SOURCE: OECD (1999).

for-profit hospitals, an iryo-hojin hospital is essentially an entrepreneurial business owned by a doctor or doctors operating under more or less the same financial incentives as for-profit enterprises. Hence, although they may not distribute profits, iryo-hojin hospitals are most analogous to American for-profit hospitals. The Japanese uniform fee schedule provides few incentives to refer a patient to other medical facilities.

Extended Hospital Stays

The average length of stay (ALOS) in Japanese hospitals is far longer than it is in the United States. The ALOS in Japan was 43 days in 1997 as compared with 5.7 days in the United States, and this figure represents a considerable decrease throughout the 1990s. In addition, the average number of in-hospital bed days in Japan—4.1 days per capita—is roughly four times the rate in the United States. These trends for Japan are shown in Table 14.5.

Under the Japanese fee-for-service system, hospitals have a strong incentive to keep their beds occupied; hospitals can earn significant daily reimbursement fees by delaying discharge. Long ALOS in Japan can also be attributed to the fact that Japanese hospitals are often used as geriatric nursing facilities. However, this alone cannot fully explain Japan's long ALOS, because stays are longer in Japan than in the United States even within specific disease categories, including normal pregnancy.

Quality Competition among Hospitals

Under Japanese fee-for-service medicine with the uniform fee schedule, hospitals cannot engage in price competition; under such market conditions, hospitals tend to engage in nonprice competition to attract patients.

With legal restrictions on advertising, a hospital's options are quite limited. Hence, many hospitals may purchase high-technology medical equipment to signal a level of medical sophistication that will attract more patients. Hospitals located in markets with a high level of local competition have an incentive to quickly acquire high-technology medical equipment to compete with their rivals (Vogt et al. 1995).

Two imaging technologies, computed tomography (CT) scanning and magnetic resonance imaging (MRI), have become symbols of high-technology, high-cost medicine and have diffused rapidly in Japan. The dissemination of CT and MRI procedures in Japan has been more extensive than in the United States. In fact, the number of CTs and MRIs in Japan (where the population is slightly less than half that of the United States) rivals that in the United States in absolute numbers.

Interestingly, despite the high rate of diffusion of high-technology medical devices, the rate of surgical procedures per capita has been estimated at under one-quarter of that found in the United States. The estimated number of annual surgeries is 4.8 million in Japan, whereas in the United States that number is 24 million. The estimated annual surgical rates are 27 per 1,000 in Japan and 91 per 1,000 in the United States.

Service Delivery

The greatest strength of the Japanese healthcare system is its provision of guaranteed care to all citizens. However, at least two important demographic and economic trends challenge the ability of the Japanese healthcare system to continue to deliver low-cost services for its entire population. The first challenge arises out of a stark demographic reality: the Japanese population is aging rapidly, and this growth in the elderly population threatens the financing system that keeps the universal healthcare system afloat. The second challenge relates to inequities in service delivery across economic and geographic dimensions.

The Rapidly Aging Society

The number of senior citizens who need care will double to 5.2 million in 2025. Indeed, the proportion of elderly in the Japanese population will increase at a far faster rate than in any other industrialized nation. Table 14.6 provides some international comparisons.

This rapid aging will place substantial burdens on healthcare delivery and financing systems. An older society requires a different healthcare infrastructure than does a younger society, including more nursing homes, more physicians familiar with geriatrics and the diseases of the elderly, and myriad other requirements. These changes will undoubtedly be expensive.

Currently, the ratio of elderly (65 years old and older) to working-age (15 to 64 years old) populations is approximately one to five. By 2025,

Country	Percentage of Population Projected to Be More than 65 Years Old in 2025	Years between 10 Percent of Population Being 65 Years Old or Older and 20 Percent Being 65 Years Old or Older
Japan	27.3	22
Switzerland	23.4	54
Germany	23.2	62
Italy	22.8	48
Sweden	22.4	66
Finland	22.2	45
Holland	21.3	52
Canada	21.2	39
France	20.8	95
United States	19.8	N/A
United Kingdom	19.4	N/A

TABLE 14.6
The Rapidly
Aging Society

it is projected to fall to about one to two. This means that five younger people now financially support each elderly person, whereas in 2025 each person over 65 will have the support of only two working-age people. In the past, care of the elderly was primarily financed by the working-age population via the macro-level cost-sharing mechanisms described above. As the ratio of elderly to workers grows over the next decades, financing elderly care will place a greater burden on the young. The crucial unanswered question is whether Japan, through both the public and private sectors, can prepare quickly enough to accommodate such a rapidly aging population.

Inequities in Service Delivery

On the whole, the Japanese healthcare system equitably serves the Japanese population. Although regional differences exist in the prices paid for doctor visits and inpatient stays (with urban providers receiving the largest fees), these differences are not large. Because charging patients more than is specified by the fee schedule is illegal, doctors receive the same fees for treatments and consultations provided to rich and poor patients alike. Surveys by Koseisho consistently find no correlation between the use of healthcare and income, and financial constraints are rarely mentioned as a cause of avoiding physician visits (Ikegami 1991).

Despite the guarantee of universal access to care, however, sources of inequity remain. First, the concentration of medical personnel in rural areas, especially in the remote northern Hokkaido prefecture, is considerably lower than in the urbanized parts of the country; many characterize this situation as a shortage of doctors in rural areas. This is a problem inherent to any country of sufficiently large geographic size, regardless of the universality of the healthcare system. Efforts to increase the availability of doctors to rural Japanese include the introduction of telemedicine to underserved areas (Jin et al. 2000).

A second important—if ironic—source of inequity in the delivery of health services in Japan arises as an unintended consequence of the uniform fee schedule imposed by Koseisho. As previously discussed, the presence of such a fee schedule implies that hospitals can compete only with quality, not with price. The prohibition on balanced billing means that patients cannot be legally required to bear the extra costs of higher-quality care. The inevitable result is long lines at the highest-quality hospitals, especially the teaching hospitals, for both inpatient and outpatient care. A black market is reported to exist for those who can afford it, complete with large gifts to senior physicians at teaching hospitals in exchange for quicker service (Ikegami 1991). However, this does not necessarily imply that the Japanese are unresponsive to price incentives in their demand for healthcare (Bhattacharya et al. 1996).

Prospects for the Future

Realizing the serious threat to its healthcare financing system, Koseisho has proposed several major reform measures designed to curtail future increases in medical care costs. Many of these fundamental reforms of Japan's health insurance system are strongly opposed by various interest groups, including the Japanese Medical Association (JMA) as well as by patients. The open question is whether Japan can reform its once highly acclaimed healthcare system quickly enough to avoid a crisis; it is by no means clear that the current set of reform proposals will be sufficient. Ironically, the past success of the universal health insurance system is precisely the reason that people are resistant to change today. People have grown accustomed to a high level of care and expect the same high level to continue; healthcare reform is not particularly popular.

Increased Cost Sharing with Patients

Koseisho has introduced a measure to increase the cap on copayments, now uniformly set at ¥63,600 per month, to ¥121,800. In addition to doubling the cap amount, Koseisho is also planning to introduce copayments for elderly care. A proposal has been made for patients over the age of 70 to be responsible for a flat 10 percent of their medical costs rather than the nominal fixed amounts they pay under the current system. According to a set of five proposals developed by a panel advising Koseisho, hospitalized elderly patients would pay 10 percent of the costs, with the maximum copayment raised to a monthly limit of ¥40,800; this would represent a ¥3,600 increase over the present ceiling. Koseisho has also proposed setting a monthly copayment cap for elderly outpatient care between ¥3,000 and ¥5,000.

Increased Autonomy for Kenpo Societies

Many Kenpo executives argue that an important cause of the present financial straits of their health insurance societies is a lack of property rights, which is a result of macro-level cost sharing. Under Japan's fee-for-service system, surplus premiums are claimed by the government as "contributions" to the geriatric pooling fund; Kenpo societies reap no reward for reducing medical expenses via utilization review or other oversight mechanisms. After 40 years with no cost-minimizing incentive, Kenpo executives argue, the associations have lost their entrepreneurial instincts.

Faced with criticism from corporate leaders, Koseisho has announced a plan to yield more autonomy to Kenpo associations. A government panel has recommended that insurance organizations develop a more efficient auditing and utilization review capacity to screen hospital bills and ensure they are getting value for money. The panel also wants Kenpo associations to provide to their members more information about hospitals. Although some view these steps as initial attempts to transform the Kenpo societies into U.S.-style health maintenance organizations, these changes do not address the incentives facing the Kenpo societies. To date, little support exists for more radical reform, such as deregulating the health insurance market entirely and permitting competition.

The Imminent End of Fee-for-Service Medicine

Recently, an advisory panel to Koseisho recommended the introduction of a diagnosis-related group (DRG) payment system similar to the one currently used by the Medicare system in the United States. Under the current Japanese fee-for-service payment scheme, medical institutions can generate higher revenues by increasing prescription drug volume and the number of medical procedures. The proposed system would pay fixed amounts for the treatment of patients with certain diseases, regardless of treatment.

The transition from a fee-for-service to a DRG-type system would trigger a major structural change in Japan's hospital industry. Under a DRG-type payment system, hospitals would no longer receive payment per day of hospital stay, and the ALOS would likely drop drastically. The resulting excess supply of hospital beds would drive many smaller private hospitals out of the market. Not surprisingly, Japanese hospital owners vehemently oppose this reform.

Deregulation of the Hospital Industry

Although deregulation of the hospital industry to allow the entry of private corporations into the market has been discussed, overtures in that direction have met fierce opposition from the JMA. Existing laws protect physicians' interests, and the JMA is quite powerful. For example, when SECOM, the leading home security and burglary protection company in Japan, recently acquired a hospital, the firm was greeted by aggressive opposition organized by the JMA and was quickly forced to sell its acquisition.

In contrast, Koseisho has opened the newly emerging nursing home market to private enterprises to avoid a future shortage of nursing-care service providers. To a large extent, this has proved successful, and various private firms have actively sought new business opportunities in the long-term-care market.

New Information Technology

Policymakers may not be the only ones who influence healthcare reform measures. As previously mentioned, the introduction of telemedicine as a mode of care in rural areas may have an effect. In addition, new information technology may potentially undermine many of today's existing laws and restrictions, and it may trigger a profound and fundamental industrial reorganization.

For instance, the Internet has made serious inroads into the strict regulations governing hospital advertising. Hospital publicity is legally restricted to information on diseases treated, consultation hours, and availability of inpatient care. When Koseisho attempted to revise the law so that factual information such as doctors' backgrounds could be included, the measure was met with fierce opposition from the JMA; the law remains unchanged. However, despite the official prohibition on advertising, a growing number of home pages on the Internet post details about doctors and medical staff, pictures of hospital rooms, treatment approaches and results, and the like. Because restricting web site content is difficult, if not impossible, the law against hospital advertising has been de facto repealed by the Internet, although it may never be removed from the books.

Conclusion

Since its rise from the ashes of World War II, the Japanese healthcare system has produced a number of triumphs, which are a justifiable source of pride for the Japanese. Generally equitable and universal healthcare coverage, a long-lived population, and low infant mortality rates are just three examples. Nevertheless, the Japanese healthcare system faces considerable challenges that make large-scale changes in the near future a virtual certainty.

Although the current structure of the Japanese healthcare system is based on its history, its future direction will undoubtedly be shaped by the demographic and economic challenges faced by the nation. For more than

40 years, the combination of universally mandated coverage and fee-for-service medicine has survived because Japanese workers have financed the care of the elderly and those unable to work. As Japan's population continues to age rapidly into the twenty-first century and the number of workers relative to retirees diminishes, whether the healthcare system can evolve rapidly enough to continue providing universal quality healthcare at a reasonable price remains to be seen.

REFERENCES

Bhattacharya, J., Vogt, W., Yoshikawa, A., and Nakahara, T. 1996. "The Utilization of Outpatient Medical Services in Japan." *Journal of Human Resources* 31 (2): 450–76.

Ikegami, N. 1991. "Japanese Health Care: Low Cost through Regulated Fees." *Health Affairs* 10 (3): 87–109.

Japanese Ministry of the Environment. 2001. "Water Environment Management in Japan," pp. 6–10. Tokyo: Planning Division, Water Environment Department, Environmental Management Bureau, Ministry of the Environment. Retrieved March 2002 from http://www.env.go.jp/en/org/water_pamph/index.html.

Japanese Nursing Association. 1999. "1998 JNA Survey Concerning Hospital Nurse Demand and Supply." *JNA News* 27 (April): 2. Retrieved March 2002 from http://www.nurse.or.jp/jna/english/jnanews/27.pdf.

Jin, C., Ishikawa, A., Sengoku, Y., and Ohyanagi, T. 2000. "A Telehealth Project for Supporting an Isolated Physiotherapist in a Rural Community of Hokkaido." *Journal of Telemedicine and Telecare* 6 (Suppl. 2): S35–S37.

Koseisho. 1997. "Water Japan: Japan's Water Works Yearbook 1996/1997." *Suido Sangyo Shinbun* (Journal of Water Works Industry). Retrieved March 2002 from http://www.mizudb.or.jp/Mizudb/hpj/hpj02.html.

Organization for Economic Cooperation and Development (OECD). 1999. "OECD Health Data 1999: A Comparative Analysis of 30 OECD Countries" CD-ROM data file. Retrieved March 2002 from http://oecdpublications.gfi-nb.com/cgi-bin/OECDBookShop.storefront/1675821381/Product/View/812001073C1.

Primomo, J. 2000. "Nursing Around the World: Japan—Preparing for the Century of the Elderly." *Online Journal of Issues in Nursing* 5 (2): Manuscript 1. Retrieved March 2002 from http://www.nursingworld.org/ojin/topic12/tpc12_1.htm.

Sawada, A. 1997. "The Nursing Shortage Problem in Japan." *Nursing Ethics* 4 (3): 245–52.

Utsunomiya, O., and Yoshikawa, A. 1993. "Health Status and Patients in Japan." In *Japan's Health System: Efficiency and Effectiveness in Universal Care*, pp. 21–44, edited by D. Okimoto and A. Yoshikawa. New York: Faulkner & Gray.

Vogt, W. B., Bhattacharya, J., Kupor, S., Yoshikawa, A., and Nakahara, T. 1995. "The Role of Diagnostic Technology in Competition among Japanese

Hospitals." *International Journal of Technology Management, Series on Management of Technology in Health Care, No. 1.*

World Health Organization (WHO). 2002. "Vaccines, Immunizations, and Biologicals: Statistics and Graphs." Retrieved March 2002 from http://www.who.int/vaccines-surveillance/StatsAndGraphs.htm.

THE UNITED KINGDOM

Laura Marti Dokson Gaydos and Bruce J. Fried

Background

At its zenith, the British Empire stretched over a fourth of the earth's surface. The first half of the twentieth century saw the United Kingdom's (UK) strength seriously depleted in two world wars; the second half witnessed the dismantling of the British Empire and the vision of the UK rebuilding itself into a modern and prosperous European nation.

The present-day UK is a constitutional monarchy comprising Great Britain (England, Scotland, and Wales) and Northern Ireland. The Sovereign acts on the advice of ministers, which cannot be ignored under the constitution. Both the powers of government and the functions of the Sovereign are determined by an unwritten constitution that is based on convention, precedent, and tradition. In most years since 1945, one-party government has been the rule. The UK has been a member of the European Union since 1973.

The landmass of the UK covers 2,449,000 square kilometers, an area slightly smaller than the U.S. state of Oregon. The terrain is mostly rugged hills and low mountains that level to rolling plains in the eastern and southeast regions. The climate is temperate, moderated by prevailing southwest winds over the North Atlantic Current; more than half of the days of the year are overcast. Natural resources of the UK include coal, petroleum, natural gas, tin, limestone, iron ore, salt, clay, chalk, gypsum, lead, and silica.

Although the large majority of the UK population is British, the amalgamation of nations does lead to heterogeneity. Additional ethnic groups include Scottish (9.6 percent); Irish (2.4 percent); Welsh (1.9 percent); Ulster (1.8 percent); and West Indian, Indian, Pakistani, and others (2.8 percent combined). Ethnic minorities are more likely to live in metropolitan areas and in ten local areas (eight in London); minorities account for more than 25 percent of the population. Regardless of ethnic origin, 3.5 percent of the UK population consists of foreigners, mostly from the EU and many of whom are Irish (WHO 1997).

Additional demographic data for the UK are provided in Table 15.1.

Education

In the UK, compulsory education begins at the age of five years; it begins at six in many other EU countries. However, even with this early start, a 1995 Eurostat survey showed that the UK has consistently ranked below

TABLE 15.1
General
Demographics

Population (millions)	58.6
Infant mortality (per 1,000 live births)	6.2
Under-five mortality (per 1,000 live births)	8.5
Life expectancy at birth (years)	76.9
Fertility rate	1.76
Percent urbanized	89

the EU average in the proportion of people with upper-secondary education or higher (Eurostat 1995). The percentage of women with higher education is consistently lower than that of men, although this is less pronounced for the younger population. The literacy rate for the UK is 99 percent. Additional education information is provided in Table 15.2.

The Economy

The UK, a leading trading power and financial center, has an essentially capitalistic economy; it is one of only four trillion-dollar economies in Western Europe. During the past two decades, the government has greatly reduced public ownership and contained the growth of social welfare programs. Agriculture is intensive, highly mechanized, and efficient by European standards, producing about 60 percent of food needs with only 1 percent of the labor force. The UK has large coal, natural gas, and oil reserves; primary energy production accounts for 10 percent of the gross domestic product, which is one of the highest shares of any industrialized nation. Services—particularly banking, insurance, and business—account by far for the largest proportion of GDP, whereas industry continues to decline in importance. Recent structural reforms aimed at stimulating the private and public sectors of the economy for the UK include extensive financial deregulation and a widespread program of privatization. The UK's GDP is about average for the EU nations, and most trade is with other EU countries (Central Intelligence Agency 2000). See Table 15.3 for more economic indicators.

TABLE 15.2
Education
Indicators
(percent)

	Male	Female
Adult literacy rate	99	99
Primary school enrollment	99.9	99.9
Secondary school enrollment	93.2	94.8

TABLE 15.3
Economic
and Social
Indicators

GNP per capita (U.S.$)	$18,110
Real GDP per capita (P.P.P.$), 1994	$17,160
Human Development Index score	14
GDP given to health, %	6.9
GNP given to health, %	7.1

The UK faced a major unemployment problem during the early and mid-1990s, rising from 7 percent in 1990 to almost 10 percent in 1994. Unemployment rates show large regional variations, with high rates in Northern Ireland (14.4 percent) and greater London (13.1 percent) (Eurostat 1995). As of 1999, unemployment rates decreased substantially to approximately 6.1 percent; however, 17 percent of the UK population continues to live below the poverty line (Central Intelligence Agency 2000).

Context: Health Needs

The UK has a strong health system, with nearly 100 percent access to necessary health-enhancing factors such as clean water and sanitation, as shown in Table 15.4.

A comparison of health outcomes in the UK with those of reference countries from within the EU shows that substantial improvements have been achieved during the last ten years. A few of the more important improvements include the following:

- an increase in life expectancy at birth to just below the EU average
- a decline in infant and maternal mortality, although in the case of maternal mortality the UK's relative position in the EU has worsened
- a considerable reduction in mortality from cardiovascular diseases (CVDs) and, among them, from ischemic heart disease and cerebrovascular disease specifically

TABLE 15.4
Access to
Health-
Enhancing
Factors
(percent)

Access to health services	100
Access to safe water	> 99
Access to sanitation	> 99
Immunization levels	92–94

- a decline in the standardized death rates (SDRs) for all cancers, including cancers of the lung, cervix, and breast, but they still remain somewhat higher than the EU average
- a decline in the SDR due to all external causes (e.g., accidental injuries, poisoning, suicide); the UK rate remains the lowest of all of the EU reference nations (WHO 1997)

However, overall population health status measures often mask important differences among population segments, such as those between men and women. In the UK, women tend to have higher morbidity but lower death rates than men; similar differences are observed among social classes. Even in advanced nations like the UK, a newborn's chance of survival varies markedly with his or her father's social class, and a strong social gradient exists with respect to the frequency of many diseases, chronic illnesses, disabilities, and deaths. Death rates also vary from one region to another, with substantially higher rates for overall mortality in the northern regions than in the southern regions (Department of Health 1994). According to latest available comparative OECD data, the UK ranks fifteenth of the 29 OECD countries for infant mortality, thirteenth for male life expectancy, and eighteenth for female life expectancy (OECD 1999).

When asked in the early 1990s to rate their health status, 65 percent of Britons said that their health was "good," 25 percent rated their health as "fair," and 11 percent reported "poor" health. In general, slightly fewer women than men are in good health, and this proportion decreases with age.

As discussed above, life expectancy for men and women differs by about six years at 73 and 79 years of age, respectively. This relatively high average degree of longevity raises the question of whether the quality of life in older age is satisfying or if it is afflicted by a heavy burden of ill health. In attempting to answer this question, a 1992 survey found that expectation of life in good health was 59.7 years for men and 61.9 years for women (81 and 78.2 percent of total life expectancy at birth, respectively) (WHO 1997).

Mortality

Like most developed nations, the major health problems of the UK are chronic in nature and associated with such factors as diet, sedentary lifestyle, and other lifestyle issues. Cancers are the most frequent cause of death in people less than 65 years old, followed by CVDs. However, when the population of more than 65 years of age is included, the situation is reversed, with CVDs as the number one cause of mortality followed closely by cancers. The third leading cause of death in all age groups is external causes, including accidents, poisonings, and suicides. Further mortality data can be found in Table 15.5.

Age- and sex-specific mortality patterns are similar to those of other EU nations; the highest potential for reducing mortality is in the middle-

		TABLE 15.5
Cardiovascular diseases	218.5 per 100,000	Leading
Cancers	151.7 per 100,000	Causes of
Respiratory diseases	79.8 per 100,000	Morbidity and
External causes	26.4 per 100,000	Mortality
Digestive diseases	22.1 per 100,000	
Infectious diseases	4.6 per 100,000	

aged and older populations. This is especially true for mortality from cancers and CVD, and it is more apparent for women than for men. The main features of these patterns are as follows (WHO 1997):

- For those between 1 and 14 years of age, the overall mortality is below the EU averages for both sexes.
- For those between 15 and 34 years of age, the overall mortality is among the lowest in the EU. The SDR for external causes is especially low in this age group.
- For those between the ages of 35 and 64 years, death rates for CVDs are the second highest among the EU countries for women and third highest for men.
- For those 65 years old and older, death rates for respiratory diseases are the second highest observed in the EU for women and the third highest observed for men. Overall death rates for those for CVDs specifically are slightly higher than the EU averages.

Differences in SDRs are also associated with ethnic origin; both men and women from the Indian subcontinent exhibit higher-than-average rates for ischemic heart diseases and cerebrovascular diseases. Rates for ischemic heart disease are lower for people born in Caribbean Commonwealth countries.

Disability

A 1995 comparative study estimated that, in the early 1990s, about 12 percent of the UK population suffered from disabilities that resulted in a handicap in social or socioeconomic terms. Although the proportion of disabled people under the age of 60 is slightly above the EU average, the estimated proportion of people in the same age group entitled to disability pensions (2.8 percent) was the lowest among the EU countries (Eurostat 1995). The percentage of people with long-term illness in the UK has remained steady since 1983, with little difference between men and women. In 1994, one in five unskilled workers suffered a chronic musculoskeletal problem; this was found in only one in ten skilled workers. Similar differences were observed for CVDs and diseases of the endocrine, metabolic, respiratory, and digestive systems (OPCS 1996).

Organization and Management of the Health System

Healthcare in the UK is provided primarily by the National Health Service (NHS), although the private sector is growing. The NHS was established in 1948 to provide healthcare for all citizens on the basis of need rather than ability to pay. The NHS provides universal coverage, and its founding principles of equity, comprehensiveness, and no charge at the point of delivery have remained, with only a few exceptions (dental, ophthalmic, and prescription charges).

The aim of the NHS is to bring about the highest level of physical and mental health for all citizens with the resources available by doing the following:

- promoting health and preventing ill-health
- diagnosing and treating injury and disease
- caring for those with long-term illness and disability who require the services of the NHS (NHS 2001)

In an effort to make the NHS more efficient, it underwent a critical structural reform during the 1990s, which included the introduction of market forces. The key change of the reform was to separate "purchasing" and "providing" (or "buying" and "selling"). In accordance with this change, two major divisions of the NHS emerged: *purchasers,* made up primarily of the District Health Authorities and GP (general practitioner) fund holders, and *providers,* which were mostly self-managed NHS hospital and community trusts and GPs. A competitive "internal market" was introduced that required providers to specify quality and price levels; they are awarded contracts by purchasers on the basis of these. Thus, providers now had to compete with both quality and cost to attract purchasers, who are now free to maintain contracts with providers located outside their traditional geographic boundaries (WHO 1997). Family health services (GPs, dentists, pharmacists, and opticians) continued to work as independent contractors with a national contract. The extensive NHS reforms throughout the 1990s were driven by a desire to keep government expenditures under control and to improve the management of the system.

In 2000, another major change in the NHS resulted from the new Labour government's intention to reduce much of the competition injected into the system by the previous government. The document, *The New NHS: Modern, Dependable,* outlines the government's vision for a healthcare system built around collaboration and partnerships. Among the changes instituted were the dissolution of GP fund holding with primary care groups and the development of interagency collaboration between primary care groups and local social services departments (Robinson and Dixon 1999). The Labour reforms further included the creation of primary care groups, primary care trusts, the Commission for Health Improvement, the National Institute for Clinical Excellence, and the Clinical Governance program.

Financing

The UK operates a low-cost health system as compared with its EU counterparts. It spends 6.7 percent of GDP on health; Germany and France spend about 10 percent, and almost 9 percent is spent in the Netherlands. The proportion of private health insurance remains at 12 percent of total health spending in the UK (Dargie, Dawson, and Garside 2000). Out-of-pocket expenditures are also considerable for such items as private medical care, long-term care, pharmaceutical copayments, and dental and ophthalmic services.

It may be surprising to note that funding levels for healthcare as a percentage of GDP has remained stable over the last 15 years (Dargie, Dawson, and Garside 2000). General taxation remains the primary source of financing; provision of services is mainly through the NHS. In 1996, 81.5 percent of NHS expenditures were from general taxation, and 12.2 percent came from national insurance contributions. The remaining expenditures were accounted for by other sources, including user charges.

The UK has not moved to alternative forms of financing such as social insurance or private insurance. Also, the use of private insurance has not increased significantly, despite rising income levels.

As is the case with other government services, the NHS budget is set annually. Once its budget has been determined, the Department of Health allocates resources between hospital and community health services and family health services. Hospital and community health services include acute and community hospital services; family health services include primary care. In accordance with this distinction, allocations are made to regional health authorities and then to district health authorities. A variety of formulas have been used to make these allocations.

The current Labour government is committed to increased funding for health and education, but levels did not rise after two years in power. However, with the budget in March 2000, the Chancellor, Gordon Brown, announced a 35 percent increase in real-terms spending on health over the following five years. The government now aims to raise UK health funding levels up to the European average by 2006 (Dargie, Dawson, and Garside 2000). An important question for the future is the extent to which the healthcare system will continue to be financed in its present form or whether gradual changes occur that may include increased copayments, medical savings accounts, more widespread use of voluntary health insurance, or a combination of these measures.

Health Resources

The UK has the lowest number of hospital beds per 1,000 inhabitants in comparison with Germany, France, the Netherlands, Austria, Denmark, and Sweden. It also has the lowest average care period in days and the lowest number of doctors per 1,000 inhabitants (Dargie, Dawson, and Garside 2000).

Human Resources

Approximately one million people work in the NHS, which accounts for roughly 1 in 20 of the UK's working population (Dargie, Dawson, and Garside 2000). The core workforce has increased in all professional groups during the 1980s and 1990s, although nursing and midwifery increased more slowly than the rest, and they were reduced as a proportion of the core workforce. Table 15.6 shows current healthcare staffing levels throughout the UK.

Most nurses in the UK work for the NHS. However, the number of private sector nurses is increasing, and so is the number of overseas nurses. Hospital doctors continue to be NHS employees. Hospital physicians have not seen changes to their contractual status, with continuing rights to private practice. GPs still practice as small businesses, having a contractual relationship with the National Health Service. The reforms of the 1980s and 1990s introduced new conditions of service into GP contracts for the first time in the history of the NHS (Lewis 1998).

Over the last two decades, hospital medical staff increased in number, whereas community medical and community dental staff were reduced. Ancillary, works, and maintenance staff were reduced in number because of contracting out (University of Manchester 1996).

Service Delivery

Healthcare activity levels have increased over the last decade, changes in the types of care have appeared. The number of physicians in practice has increased, and so have the number of prescriptions. A small increase in admissions to hospitals and a reduction in elective admissions have been seen. Outpatient treatment has grown significantly, which accounts for the reduction in elective admissions. With the development of outpatient surgeries, reductions in lengths of stay in hospitals, and a rise in the average level of bed occupancy (empty beds being filled more quickly in hospitals),

TABLE 15.6
Human Resources per 1,000 Population by Type

Physicians	1.5
Nurses	4.3
Dentists	.4
Pharmacists	.49

	Number	Per 1,000 Population	
			TABLE 15.7
			Services Use
			and Rates
Hospital admissions	1,072,890	23.1	
Outpatient visits	43,040,699	734.5	

SOURCE: Department of Health (2000/2001).

overall hospital bed numbers have been reduced since 1980 (University of Manchester 1996).

Primary Care

Primary care in the UK is dominated by GPs who act as providers of general medical services and gatekeepers to secondary care. GPs are generally organized in groups or practices and are primarily remunerated by capitation according to the number of patients on their list (about 1,900 patients on average). Every UK citizen has a right to be registered with a GP, and GP clinic visits are free of charge.

Since 1999, GPs have joined together to form "primary care groups" or "primary care trusts" along with other health professionals. This means that the GPs are given the funding to work together to plan and commission health services for their local communities, a role that was previously carried out by health authorities; it also means that decisions about local services are made at the local level by those best placed to make them.

In England and Wales, health authorities identify the health needs of local people and make arrangements for services to be provided by NHS trusts, primary care providers, and other agencies using funding provided by the government. In Scotland, this role is carried out by health boards, and in Northern Ireland, it is the responsibility of the health and social services boards.

A board of executive and nonexecutive directors manages each health authority. The nonexecutive directors are appointed by the government; the executive directors are appointed by the chairperson of the authority, who is a nonexecutive member. Health authorities are monitored by the regional offices of the NHS executive, which manages the NHS for the government.

NHS Direct (a computer and telephone information service) and NHS walk-in centers, which are available for clinical care seven days a week, are also part of the primary care system of the NHS.

Hospital Care

Most hospitals are now separate, self-managed NHS trusts competing for contracts awarded by health authorities of GP fund holders. District health authorities purchase services (mainly via a block contract) on behalf of those people who are not on a GP fund-holding list and some services outside the range of GP fund holders; they are also responsible for purchasing all emergency and long-term-care services.

Hospital trusts are found in most large towns and cities and usually offer a general range of services including general medical and surgical services. Some trusts also act as regional or national centers of expertise for more specialized care, whereas some are attached to universities and help to train health professionals. Trusts can also provide services in the community (e.g., through health centers, clinics, or in people's homes). Except in the case of emergencies, hospital treatment is arranged through the GP. Patients are not charged for appointments and treatment.

Together, NHS trusts employ the majority of the NHS workforce, including nurses, doctors, dentists, pharmacists, midwives, health visitors, and staff from the professions allied to medicine, such as physiotherapists, radiographers, podiatrists, speech and language therapists, counselors, occupational therapists, and psychologists. Other NHS Trust staff may include receptionists, porters, cleaners, IT specialists, managers, engineers, caterers, and domestic and security staff.

Large cities, especially London, are considered to be overprovided with hospital services and, as compared with the rest of the UK, to have relatively weaker primary care provision. Although several reports have emphasized the need for downsizing hospital services in large cities, implementation of the changes has been slow and controversial (WHO 1997).

Private Sector

During the last decade, the private sector has been rapidly developing in all aspects of healthcare (e.g., elective surgery, ambulatory care, dentistry). This growth is due in part to the long waiting times for outpatient consultations and elective surgery. It probably also reflects changing employment conditions, whereby more companies in the UK now offer private health insurance as part of their benefits packages.

The private sector is able to compete with the NHS trusts, offering services that would induce patients to seek private health insurance. Although no national data are available, between 10 and 12 percent of the population is generally believed to now be covered by private insurance. Geographic variations are likely to be significant, although no official estimates exist. Individuals who have private insurance are still entitled to NHS treatment.

Prospects for the Future

The NHS plan, which was published in July 2000, is a radical action plan for the next ten years that describes measures to put patients and people at the heart of the health service and involves a government investment of £19 billion by 2005. The plan promises the following:

- more power and information for patients
- more hospitals and beds
- more doctors and nurses
- much shorter waiting times for hospital and doctor appointments
- cleaner wards and better food and facilities in hospitals
- improved care for older patients
- tougher standards for NHS organizations and better rewards for the best of them

These are the biggest changes to face the NHS since it was established more than 50 years ago. To implement them, the government has to prioritize. It has decided to target the diseases that are the biggest killers, such as cancer and heart disease; to pinpoint the changes that are most urgently needed to improve people's health and well-being; and to deliver the modern, fair, and convenient services people want (NHS 2001).

The Department of Health has established ten taskforces to drive forward the ideas and improvements outlined in the NHS plan. Six of these will focus on specific areas of health service such as coronary heart disease, cancer, mental health, the elderly, child health, waiting times, and access to services. The remaining four will concentrate on how these improvements will be made by focusing on the NHS workforce, quality, reducing inequalities and promoting public health, and investing in facilities and information technology. A new Modernization Agency will play a crucial role in ensuring that the commitments in the plan are translated into reality. The new agency will work with the NHS executive regional offices and NHS trusts to help them redesign their services around the needs and conveniences of patients (NHS 2001).

REFERENCES

Armitage, B., and Scott, M. 1998. "British Labour Force Projections: 1998–2011." *Labour Market Trends* 106 (6): 281–97.

Dargie, C., Dawson, S., and Garside, P. 2000. "Policy Futures for UK Health 2000 Report." Retrieved 12 July 2001 from www.official-documents.co.uk.

Department of Health. 1994. "United Kingdom's Report to the WHO Regional Office for Europe on the 1994 Health for All Monitoring Exercise." Unpublished report.

———. 2001/2002. "Hospital Activity Statistics." Retrieved 12 July 2001 from www.doh.gov.uk/hospitalactivity/statistics.

Lewis, J. 1998. "The Medical Profession and the State: GPs and the GP Contract in the 1960s and the 1990s." *Social Policy and Administration* 32 (2): 132–50.

National Health Service (NHS). 2001. "The NHS Explained." Retrieved 15 March 2001 from www.nhs.uk.

Organization for Economic Cooperation and Development (OECD). 1999. *OECD Health Data 99.* Paris: OECD.

University of Manchester and Conrane Consulting. 1996. *The Future Healthcare Workforce.* Manchester: University of Manchester.

U.S. Central Intelligence Agency (CIA). 2000. *The World Fact Book.* Retrieved 12 March 2001 from www.odci.gov/cia/publications.

World Health Organization (WHO) Regional Office for Europe and the European Commission. 1997. "Highlights on Health in the United Kingdom." Retrieved 15 March 2001 from www.euro.who.int.

POLAND

W. Cezary Wlodarczyk and Monika Zajac

Background Information

Poland has a long and complicated history. Consideration of this past is fundamental to understanding not only the soul of the nation and its destiny but also the ongoing reforms in the structure and provision of health services. The essence of present-day Poland can perhaps be traced to the baptism in 966 of a Slavonic tribal prince and his subjects in Central-Eastern Europe between the Vistula and Odra Rivers. This event is often cited as the beginning of Poland's participation in Western culture and its adoption of Western political processes and structures.

Unfortunately, this Western development was not an easy, linear process. By the end of the eighteenth century, Poland and its territories were partitioned among its adjoining neighbors, Prussia, Russia, and Austria. Poland regained independence in 1918 after World War I as a result of the Versailles Treaty, but lost autonomy again in 1939 upon being invaded by Nazi Germany from the west and the Soviet Union from the east.

The effects of World War II were disastrous for Poland. The country was devastated by the occupation and suffered huge losses in both population and material infrastructure. In addition, upon conclusion of the conflict, Poland was relegated to the Soviet zone by the Yalta Agreement; this pact limited Poland's sovereignty in both domestic and foreign policy. National borders were again moved, and territories to the east of Curzon's line were lost, but a large territorial gain was realized in the west. Such divisions compelled millions of people to move from their familiar surroundings to new ones. The population, which was ethnically diverse before the war, became very homogeneous both in terms of ethnicity and religion during the postwar period. This sequence of events resulted in heightened sensitivity to issues of national independence and a complete unwillingness to compromise with political opponents; any form of concession was viewed as betrayal.

Despite such adversity and in contrast with some other Central European socialist countries, Poland has attempted to develop its national economy, preserve private farming, and maintain a rich and diversified culture. As with many of its geographic neighbors, government has played an important role within Poland; in accordance with the rule of "democratic centralization" (more appropriately termed "domination of the government"), the country has been fully controlled by the Communist party. In light of these political circumstances, real reform of the political, economic, and healthcare systems was not possible until after the "autumn of the nations" in 1989, which signified a period of transformation in Poland and other countries of Central and Eastern Europe (Michta 1997).

The Transition

The fundamental changes that established the context for the evolution of healthcare and its present reform began in 1990 with the implementation of Balcerowicz's Plan, named for the Minister of Finance. This plan included a shift from a centrally planned economy to a market economy. Revisions to national political-economic policy were carried out at various levels of government and included ownership changes (e.g., privatization of previously state-owned property and support of new private initiatives) and development of the financial sector (e.g., the banking system and stock market).

This broad reformation has been largely successful (Wolff-Paweska 1998). Poland has established a stable democratic mechanism to elect people in positions of power while independent courts keep judicial order, resolve jurisdiction disputes between levels of government, and oversee the legality of administrative decisions. On the economic side, the gross domestic product is increasing largely because of growth in the private sector. However, the economic adjustment is not complete. Many old-sector industries such as coal mining, steel works, machinery, and railways have not yet been privatized. Their productivity remains low, but they employ large numbers of workers, many of whom are members of various trade unions. These industries enjoy great political influence and maintain strong resistance to privatization efforts.

Similarly, the agriculture sector has not fully participated in the economic transformation. Many of the private owners of the small farms that make up a large part of the agricultural production of the country cannot afford modern technology to increase efficiency and participate in the market economy. Consequently, they have been largely removed from the larger political and social reform initiatives. In fact, many of the smallest and poorest rural farmers do not take part in the market exchange and produce food only for their own needs.

The decentralization process that led to the reinstitutionalization and strengthening of local self-government was particularly critical to the healthcare reform effort. In general, the national governmental administration now plays an initiating, coordinating, and controlling role, but before 1990, when local government at the gmina (basic level of public administration) was reestablished, this was not always so.

Gminas created locally elected assemblies/boards and provided the infrastructure for substantial changes in healthcare. Additionally, on January 1, 1999, three official levels of territorial government were established:

gmina (county, community), poviat (district), and voivodship (province). The newly formed self-ruling units assumed many of the responsibilities that previously belonged to the central government, including the provision of health services. This administrative structure is presented in Table 16.1.

The creation of self-ruling units was only a part of more complex public administration reforms that altered the scope of responsibility within governmental administration. The government presently operates at two primary levels: the national government, with its ministries in Warsaw, and the 16 voivodships, which are the regional representatives of the national government. The extensive change in functions of voivodships must be emphasized. The number of voivodships was reduced, and new political significance was ascribed to each. Each was given responsibility for the remaining duties not attributed to the national offices and also became a unit of self-ruling administration. These public administration changes are illustrated in Table 16.2.

Population and Demographics

In 1999, the population of Poland numbered slightly more than 38.6 million. Women outnumber men; the imbalance is greater in urban areas and among the older age groups. Overall, more than 60 percent of the population lives in urban areas, but a full 50 percent reside in cities that have more than 100,000 residents. Table 16.3 offers a detailed summary of Poland's demographics.

Poland's family composition traits are beginning to mirror those in Western countries. The average age for marriage has increased progressively, and families remain small. Approximately 60 percent of families have children, but the majority now include only one or two offspring. Also, the rate of children born out of wedlock has increased from 5 to 10 percent since 1994 (Szymborski, Wojtyniak, and Chanska 1996).

As shown above, life expectancy in both sexes is lower than that of most developed countries. At the beginning of the transformation, life expectancy for males was in decline, but improvements have been made recently. Life expectancy has continued to decrease for women.

A constant downward trend in the infant mortality rate has been observed during the past decade after a short and rather minor increase

Level	Governmental Administration	Self-Ruling Administration
Central	Government and ministries	None
Voivodship	Voivod	Marshal
Poviat	None	Starosta
Gmina	None	Woir

TABLE 16.1
Governmental and Self-Ruling Administrations

TABLE 16.2
Administrative
Units Before
and After
Public
Administration
Reform

Level	Units Pre-Reform	Units Post-Reform
Central	1	1
Voivodship	49	16
Poviat	—	373
Gmina	2,489	2,489

during the beginning of the transformation. However, at 8.9 per 1,000 births, it remains high in comparison with international averages.

The Economy

Basic economic indicators, illustrated in Table 16.4, attest to Poland's success in transition. Inflation in the first quarter of 1999 was around 7 percent, whereas ten years ago it was consistently more than 600 percent annually. In recent years, Poland has also had one of the highest growth rates in Europe at around 6 percent. As of the end of 2000, more than half of the state enterprises had been privatized.

Foreign investors have noticed and appreciated Poland's advances. The year 2000 was the second year in which more than half of all foreign investments directed to the states of Central-Eastern Europe have flowed into Poland.

Poland's workforce is one of the youngest in Europe; at the end of 1999, approximately 66 percent of those employed were under the age of 40. Agriculture employs 13.7 percent of the workforce. Industry and services employ 31.5 and 54.8 percent, respectively. In 1999, the public sector employed approximately 29 percent of the total workforce, with 6.1 percent employed in health services and social work.

TABLE 16.3
General
Demographics

Population in millions, 1999	38.654
Infant mortality per 1,000 live births	8.9
Under-five mortality ratio per 1,000 live births, 1998	11
Life expectancy in years at birth, 1999	68.5 (male) 77 (female)
Fertility rate, 1999	1.5
Percent urbanized, 1998	65

SOURCE: GUS (1999); WHO (2000).

		TABLE 16.4
GNP per capita (U.S.$)	3,900	
Real GDP per capita (P.P.P.$)	6,740	
Human Development Index score	0.814 (position 44)	
Percent of GNP to health, 1999	4.15	
Percent of state budget in public outlays on healthcare, 1999	29.6	
ODA inflow/outflow as percent of GNP	0.6	

NOTE: ODA = Official Development Assistance.
SOURCE: World Bank (2000); Ministry of Finance (2000).

The unemployment rate increased from 10.4 percent in 1998 to approximately 14 percent in December 2000. Unemployment has had a negative impact on social and economic life and has remained the main problem in social policy since the beginning of systemic transformation. The unemployment level varies greatly by region, with the highest unemployment rates in the rural areas of northeast Poland. Women comprise nearly 55 percent of the unemployed.

Education

The adult literacy rate both for males and females is 99.7 percent. Primary education is obligatory. Almost 7 percent of people over the age of 15 have a tertiary education; an additional 25 percent succeeded with secondary education. However, differences between urban and rural areas are significant. The majority of rural inhabitants (around 80 percent) have only primary and basic vocational education largely because of the migration of the young population to the urban areas. As a result, rural areas are inhabited by an older and less-educated population that strongly depends on agriculture. Nevertheless, the total percentage of graduates from university and secondary education has been growing significantly over the last few years. Table 16.5 details Poland's educational accomplishments.

Education reform was implemented in September 1999 as a parallel to the other three social reforms: healthcare, administration, and the old-age pension system. The main objective of the education reform is to raise the level of education of the young generation and to equalize educational opportunities across socioeconomic backgrounds. Under the reform, young people are able to acquire knowledge and skills to help them find a good job. Knowledge and qualifications are especially important in the face of Poland's future integration with the European Union.

TABLE 16.5
Education
Indicators

	Male	Female
Adult literacy rate (percentage of those 15 years old and older), 1998	99.7	99.7
Primary school enrollment ratio (%), 1997	99.3	99.3
Secondary school enrollment ratio (%), 1997	84.3	88.5

SOURCE: UNDP (2000).

Context: Health Needs

The primary cause of death among both men and women continues to be cardiovascular disease, which accounts for approximately 50 percent of deaths, although the mortality rate has diminished in recent years. This is followed by an ever-increasing mortality rate due to malignant neoplasm (approximately 20 percent) and deaths caused by accidents and poisoning (approximately 7 percent), the rates of which have remained stable. The most frequent causes of infant deaths are diseases contracted prenatally (more than 50 percent) and congenital birth defects (approximately 30 percent).

In 1996, after recognizing major health problems, the Polish Ministry of Health (MOH) adopted a ten-year National Health Program aimed at disease prevention, health promotion, and health education. The Program's goals include improving early diagnostic capabilities, reducing smoking and alcohol consumption, improving sanitation, and reducing inequalities in health and access to health services (Ministry of Health and Social Welfare 1996).

Poland has a high level of immunization against measles (96 percent) and tuberculosis (94 percent) as compared with the EU countries. Moreover, the infectious diseases control system, which relies on regional sanitary inspectors, works well. Access to running water and sanitation is satisfactory and has improved significantly since the beginning of the program's implementation. However, approximately 1.6 percent of primary schools have no access to running water; this is particularly evident in rural areas. Hospital infections and salmonella poisoning are still present, but the implementation of new standards has brought about a significant decrease in these areas during the last few years.

As life expectancy increases, the Polish society as a whole is growing older. In 1997, 16.2 percent of the population was 60 years old or older, and this number is expected to increase to 24 percent by the year 2020. This aging population will present new medical challenges to the Polish health system.

Among the adult population (those 15 years old or older), 17.5 percent are disabled, and 3 percent of those have a very high degree of disability. For these people, any kind of work is impossible, and they require support from the community. Disability is more frequent among women than men, and the rates are higher in rural areas (20 percent) than in more urban areas (16 percent) (Golinowska 1999).

Disability-adjusted life expectancy in years, understood as the expectation of life lived in equivalent full health for the total Polish population at birth, is estimated at the level of 66.2 years. It varies with gender and is longer for females (70.1 years) than for males (62.3 years).

Among children, 11.2 percent have evident health problems that are most often a consequence of a congenital or developmental defect. Occurrences of childhood illness are more pronounced in urban centers (13 percent) than in rural areas (8.8 percent). However, this difference may also be due to discrepancies in proper documentation.

The inequitable availability of health services across Poland suggests that the past financing arrangements and regional supply capacity have not been adequate to ensure access for low-income earners or the elderly. In addition, the widespread practice of informal out-of-pocket payments tends to work against people with low income because they are unable to participate in this now expected form of payment. The distribution of equipment, beds, and medical personnel across regions is also uneven, and the concentration of resources in large cities is a substantial problem. Patients in rural areas face limited access to hospital care and some specialized health services. Waiting lists have developed for some treatments, especially those that require advanced technology.

Overall, the transformation brought about improvement in the general health status of the Polish population. Much of the progress can be attributed to better diet (the easy availability of fruits, vegetables, and lean meat on the market), improved lifestyles (less use of tobacco products), and ameliorated social and political climates. However, many challenges are still to be met.

Organization and Management of the Health System

Before 1989, healthcare in Poland was based on the Soviet Siemaszko model in which the state maintained a monopoly by creating, financing, and controlling the healthcare system. The rule of universal access, although officially proclaimed, was not an actuality. Problems existed both in the functioning of the system and in access for specific population groups. Nevertheless, access to health services for most was relatively easy although hampered by rigid rules that assigned users to strictly defined providers for all services. Notably, in the decade before the transformation, the health system weakened substantially and became characterized by chaos and a lack of control.

The rapid change in the political system greatly facilitated health-care reformation. The legitimacy of the socialist healthcare system was lost, along with many other arrangements of the previous regime. The new system, which continues to evolve, is defined by three basic factors: a new division of responsibilities for health and healthcare, entitlement to services on the basis of insurance, and contractual agreements among those within the health sector. With this transformation came new stakeholders. For instance, local governments have accepted responsibility for different aspects of healthcare and local health policy, including health promotion and ownership of many health facilities (Wlodarczyk 1998).

Trade unions acting on behalf of large professional groups (e.g., physicians, nurses) at the national level and small parties of employees in health institutions also remain important players in the health system. Historically able to influence major political change, trade unions have become, over time, representatives of both healthcare providers and consumers. Voluntary associations involved in healthcare issues are also playing a more significant role by lobbying insurance providers for expanded benefits. Similarly, various professional organizations, such as physicians', nurses', midwives', and pharmacies' chambers, often have a great impact on the health sector.

On January 1, 1999, sickness funds were established in Poland to complement the insurance system. However, as a major financing tool for healthcare, sickness funds would clearly act as more than a payer agency; they would also control spending, direct funds to services that could be medically justified, and refuse payments for inappropriate care. The introduction of sickness funds is widely regarded as the beginning of healthcare reform in Poland.

The former monopolistic control of healthcare by the central government was replaced with dispersed responsibility among various parties throughout Polish society. Each party has a defined set of obligations, although responsibilities often overlap. For example, sickness funds, local governments, and professional organizations are all extremely interested in issues of access and provision of care. However, many areas of health-care administration, including the planning and financing of new investments, remain unregulated and are not viewed as a priority. As a result, many disturbing gaps remain in the health sector.

Legislative Power

Legislative authority provides a legal framework within which the health system functions. This power was fundamental to the transformation, and its exercise has significantly shaped healthcare policy. Parliamentary decisions concerning allocation of financial resources for healthcare are accomplished in one of two ways:

1. authorization of the budgetary act, which includes allocations for investments, medical education, highly specialized procedures, and specific health programs; and
2. specific legislation regarding public financing of the healthcare system and the establishment of appropriate insurance premium rates.

The Parliament also endorses annual reports of goal fulfillment submitted by the MOH and sickness funds. Rejection of such reports often leads to dismissal of the officials responsible for the failure.

Government Administration

In times of rapid change, the precise classification of governmental activities can be difficult, but the MOH generally assumes the following responsibilities:

*   establishing the criteria for direct funding of services from the central budget as opposed to the services that will be covered by insurance for various population groups (e.g., pregnant women, people suffering from tuberculosis)
*   establishing the list of services that are not covered by insurance (i.e., medical, dental, laboratory tests, orthopedic aids, pharmaceuticals) and that must be paid for, either in part or in full, by the consumer
*   determining the criteria for the development of ambulatory health plans by local self-governments
*   establishing national research and educational institutions including the national health institutes and medical schools and appointing their governing boards

Two central institutions are accountable to the MOH, both of which were part of the MOH until the beginning of 2000. The General Sanitary Inspector attends to health and sanitation conditions; the office of the General Sanitary Inspector addresses water, air, and soil safety; urban sanitation; indoor conditions; food control; disease prevention; and health education. The General Pharmaceutical Inspector is in charge of drug registration and market entrance rules for new drugs.

Although healthcare reform included diminished governmental control, some administrative responsibilities have been retained, including managing some tertiary care facilities, contracting services for highly specialized procedures, and financing specialty programs.

At the voivodship level, the voivod, as the representative of the national government, oversees and coordinates various activities. Responsibilities of the voivod include ensuring the health and safety of the voivodship, collecting health-related data, maintaining a health provider registry, and overseeing sanitation inspections.

Self-Ruling Administration

The health-related tasks of self-ruling administrations cover three areas: general strategy and planning, public health and health promotion, and the management of healthcare institutions. Each level of the local government is responsible for formulating a developmental strategy as appropriate to its territory within the voivodship. Various authorities are responsible for formulating local health policy and establishing priorities on the basis of available financial resources.

Although overall strategy is under the domain of the respective local governments, these governments are not responsible for hospital planning and infrastructure; this duty falls to the MOH. Such a division of responsibility puts local governments in a difficult position; they own the health facilities located in their territories, but they have very little control over their future development. To further complicate the matter, the establishment and management of the ambulatory units are the responsibilities of the self-ruling authority. Healthcare planning in Poland is thus divided as follows:

1. *Gmina:* responsible for the institutions providing primary care
2. *Poviat:* responsible for basic specialties such as internal medicine, pediatrics, surgery, and gynecology and obstetrics
3. *Self-governing voivodship:* responsible for the majority of other specialist services

The tension between these relatively autonomous institutions and the territorial governments that are responsible for them can have varying effects. On one hand, concern that the institutions may pursue their own financial interests at the expense of the community by maximizing profits rather than meeting the health needs of the population creates a precarious situation for local governments, which could lose electorate support. Conversely, too much administrative interference by the local government is feared to result in decreased productivity and institutional bankruptcy.

Financing

Universal Health Insurance

The new Polish health insurance system aims to provide stable and transparent means to raise funds through compulsory, income-based health insurance premiums from the eligible population or from the state for those unable to make such contributions. The insurance premium is set at 7.75 percent of taxable income, which is deductible from personal income tax. Before 1999, healthcare services were funded by social security contributions, which covered all forms of social insurance without a clear demarcation. The insurance program was originally conceived to cover the entire population, and the law provides a list of the many segments of people required to be insured. Such individuals are expected to enter the insurance funds formally and pay premiums or have premiums paid on their behalf by employers.

Health insurance premiums are paid by a wide variety of individuals, organizations, and other legal entities, including entities responsible for paying social or pension benefits. The system covers most groups without employer-based healthcare. The government also pays the cost of coverage for certain groups. The nonpaying sector includes the unemployed, farmers, students, military personnel, veterans, pregnant women, and clergy. As a result, almost everyone is covered, including foreigners with temporary residence cards.

Furthermore, Article 8 of the General Health Insurance Act permits people not otherwise required to be covered, such as the self-employed, to voluntarily insure themselves; most people in this category do choose to be insured. Homeless people are without health insurance coverage; however, social welfare services and local governments are obliged by law to provide healthcare services for this group (Chawla and Kulis 2000).

Only general health insurance coverage allows access to healthcare services contracted with sickness funds. Otherwise, out-of-pocket payments are required. Insurance covers all phases of care: health promotion, preventive services, diagnostics and treatment, rehabilitation, palliative care, and hospice. Medications prescribed in hospitals are free of charge, whereas drugs dispensed in ambulatory care settings are subject to specific payment schedules. Medications considered basic or required for the treatment of "dangerous" illnesses are free or offered at very low cost in any setting. Payments for "supplementary" medications range between 30 and 50 percent of their actual cost. Insurance also covers spa treatments, orthopedic devices, dental prostheses, eyeglasses, and necessary transport, although some copayment may be required for some services.

One of the fundamental tenets of the reformed healthcare system is the separation between payers and service providers; this necessitates contractual arrangements between the two parties. Such agreements include descriptions of allowed services, participating public system providers, and the identification of providers who are authorized to determine resource allocation and service provision. Sickness funds are primarily accountable for reimbursement to providers according to their prearranged agreements. However, the MOH remains responsible for the provision of and reimbursement for a number of specified procedures and health programs, which are covered by the insurance title but not paid by sickness funds.

Payers

For the majority of insured consumers, the health insurance premium is 7.75 percent of their income. Premiums for farmers are calculated separately based on the size of the farming industry and the prices of some agricultural products. People who do not have sufficient income (e.g., the unemployed, mothers on maternity leave, people on social benefits, veterans) can have their premiums paid by a special social security office.

All premiums are collected by the Social Insurance Office and transferred to the sickness funds. A regional sickness fund is operated in each of the 16 voivodships, which are further subdivided into a total of 39 local agencies. One additional branch fund, created to cover employees of the defense, interior, justice, and railways sectors, operates nationwide. The sickness funds have at their disposal the financial resources gathered from their members. As a result, those funds operating in wealthy regions collect much more money than their more disadvantaged counterparts in other areas. In response, an equalization formula has been developed, which considers demographic parameters and their effect on demand for health services.

The equalization fund is designed to address inequalities in income and health risks across individual sickness funds with the objective of making all potential members equally attractive in financial terms. The goal is to ensure that all citizens have similar opportunities to access care by reducing the incentive for sick funds to recruit members selectively. Principally guided by concerns of equity and solidarity, sickness funds retain 60 percent of their collections and set aside the remaining 40 percent for redistribution and equalization across all funds. The risk adjustment formula currently applied only allows for some basic correction for the age and income of the population. The age correction is established for people who are more than 60 years old, and the revenue correction is based on average rather than individual premiums (OECD 2000).

Sickness funds contract services for those they cover. Separate contracts are entered into for ambulatory and hospital services; these contracts specify the type of services that should be provided. If actual treatments differ from those established in the contract, the service provider will not receive payment.

The law does not specify the mechanism by which providers are reimbursed. The parties involved in developing contracts are free to negotiate specific payment terms. However, in a typical payment scheme, specialists receive fee-for-service payments, and hospitals are paid for hospitalized cases. Family physicians are often reimbursed on a capitation basis, but they frequently maintain a surplus of income. Virtually all payment schedules require proper referral and a payment ceiling.

Conceptually and legally, sickness funds enjoy great independence with regard to healthcare priorities and contracting methods. However, some changes in regulation have occurred in the funds' position since they were established. The sickness funds are now overseen by the Health Insurance Supervisory Office, a governmental body located in Warsaw, the chairman of which is nominated by the prime minister and is charged with protecting consumer interests. The office is responsible for the supervision of sickness funds' financial plans, contractual services, and quality control.

In extreme situations of malpractice, the office is further empowered to suspend fund administration and take over direct management for a fixed period.

Private Healthcare Payments

In spite of formal declarations concerning free access to healthcare throughout Poland, private households have experienced continuous growth in out-of-pocket expenditures for medical care. Private spending takes place in two ways. The first involves coinsurance and other expenses related to additional payments for drugs and physician visits. The second is covert spending, which generally happens when a prosthetic device or equipment that would be indispensable during an operation is for some reason not covered by insurance. Many patients also make additional payments to medical personnel. However, whether such actions are voluntary and given by grateful patients as rewards or are extorted by their healthcare providers is unclear.

Since 1995, private expenditures have steadily increased, reaching a transformation-period high in 1999 of 1.8 percent of the GDP (Blaszczak-Przybicinska 1998). This may indicate that personal involvement in the financing of health expenditures is growing as a supplement to public financing.

Health Resources

Health Professional Organizations

The number of practicing health professionals in Poland is almost equal to that found in most highly developed countries, as illustrated in Table 16.6.

Health professionals are organized by mandate into three associations: physicians' chambers, nurses and midwives' chambers, and pharmacists' chambers. All of these organizations have the same structure and are divided into district chambers, and each organization has a head chamber in Warsaw. Each association maintains a court that oversees professional

Physicians	2.4	**TABLE 16.6**
Nurses	5.5	Human Resources per 1,000 Population, 1997
Dentists	0.5	
Pharmacists	0.5	
Administrators	0.01	
Midwives	0.6	
Traditional practitioners	0.03	

SOURCE: National Center for Health System Management (1999).

malpractice claims. These courts have the authority to limit or permanently revoke permission to practice, depending on the situation. The chambers are also responsible for restricting or preventing practice due to mental disease, drug or alcohol abuse, or disability or handicap on the part of the provider. Appeals can be lodged with a higher court in the Warsaw head chamber.

District chambers represent each profession and maintain a register of eligible practitioners and private practices. The chambers also issue licenses to physicians, nurses, and midwives for private practice. If an applicant for a private practice license fulfills all of the necessary educational requirements and has professional experience, the chamber cannot refuse to issue a license. The chamber is only allowed discretionary power with regard to licensing in the case of foreign physicians.

Schools of Medicine

Despite theoretical control by the MOH, the 11 medical universities and academies retain considerable autonomy in the education of medical personnel. Real power belongs to the university senate, which represents the academic community and has a great deal of influence on performance. The senate determines the number of medical students that can be enrolled and offers financial incentives to encourage the university to increase student enrollment. This is based on the rationale that a larger student body qualifies the university for more money from the budget. In addition, continuing education (especially medical specialization) for physicians and nurses is especially lucrative because trainees are obliged to attend a specified set of courses at a medical university. As such, medical academies influence the standards and patterns of medical practice at a level beyond the control of administrative authorities.

Service Providers

Poland has two types of service providers: private medical practices and private or public healthcare institutions. Private practices cover the activities of physicians, nurses and midwives, and psychologists. The majority of such practices offer family medicine services, but some practices also provide specialist care. In 1998, there were only 770 private practices, but an estimated 40 percent of doctors and more than 90 percent of dentists are involved in private practice (GUS 1999). However, many of them also maintain employment in public institutions. Private service providers can be members of individual or group practices.

When private providers sign contracts with sickness funds, they are granted certain privileges associated with public sector practice. These include licenses to prescribe reduced-price pharmaceuticals, free hospitalization referrals, free or lower-priced diagnostic test orders, and authorization to order transportation or issue free or reduced-price orthopedic aids. Furthermore, contractual arrangements with the sickness funds ensure a constant flow of funds for covered services. Private service providers who do not enter into such agreements with sickness funds are deprived of the benefits associated with them.

Healthcare institutions have a much more complex organizational structure. These institutions include hospitals and ambulatory care facilities, both of which must conform to sanitation standards, registration by the voivod, and competency requirements for personnel.

Ownership of the institution determines its status as public or private institution. For example, when an institution is established by a public administration body, the institution is also public. (By exemption, an institution established by the Polish Railway is also considered public by law.) The financial resources of a public institution are derived from contractual agreements with a sickness fund. That is, the institution receives money in exchange for providing contracted services. Public institutions can also provide additional services (e.g., occupational medicine) through contracts with outside payers.

Generally an institution established by an employer for its employees is private; the same may hold true for a church or foundation and its members. Private institutions typically attempt to enter into legal agreements with sick funds to stabilize their financial positions. Contracting is especially vital for private hospitals because few patients can independently cover the costs of inpatient care.

Service Delivery

In 1998, Poland had 5,825 outpatient facilities, 1,087 of which were private. In addition, in 1999 there were 791 general hospitals, 22 of which were private. Highly specialized care is provided by 43 teaching hospitals and 11 research institutes; the number of beds per 1,000 Polish citizens is estimated at 5.5 (National Center for Health System Management 1999).

The first level of outpatient secondary care is provided by the polyclinics that are run by the voivodships and the large gminas. At the second level are district hospitals that provide outpatient care and ambulance services in addition to inpatient care. Specialized secondary care is provided in voivodship hospitals, each of which serves a population of about 800,000. Tertiary care is organized at the regional and national levels into national institutes, which also train specialists and carry out research. Certain government ministries (defense, interior, justice, and transport) also operate parallel healthcare services for some of their employees and dependents. These systems provide both ambulatory and hospital care.

Primary healthcare is organized on a geographic basis, with each primary care doctor covering a population of between 1,200 and 2,500 patients. In rural areas, primary care is provided through small outpatient centers that are usually staffed by an internal medicine specialist, a gynecologist, a pediatrician, a dentist, and a nursing staff (WHO Europe 1999). In urban areas, primary care services are provided in large outpatient clinics, which also house some specialty services and diagnostic facilities. A family medicine model is being organized around individual or group practices that have contracts with a voivodship or gmina or directly with a sickness fund.

Development of primary care with the general practitioner as the gatekeeper and freedom of choice for patients were the basic ideas of the healthcare system reform. Primary care services are provided by physicians and nurses, and they are readily available at no cost to the patient. The patient has free choice of physicians among those contracted with a relevant sickness fund. The patient chooses a general practitioner, usually for a period of one year, although changing general practitioners is possible during this time by paying a minor charge. Twenty-four-hour primary healthcare services are also intended to be provided, but because of lack of institutional and financial arrangements, such coverage is rarely available.

General practitioners are the first point of contact with health services and are meant to act as gatekeepers to the rest of the system; thus, specialty services generally require a referral. Some specialist services are exempt from referral requirements, including obstetrics and gynecology, dentistry, dermatology, infectious disease, psychiatry, and substance abuse treatment. A specialist may be chosen from a list of providers who maintain contracts with the sickness funds. Hospitalization also requires the referral of a primary care physician, with the exceptions of emergencies, routine deliveries, and special circumstances.

Considerable imbalances exist in the supply of hospital facilities throughout the country. Most hospitals are located near urban centers. The highest concentrations of hospitals are found in Katowice (97), Warsaw (48), and Wroclaw (30), whereas the Chelm, Konin, and Przemysl regions have only three to four hospitals each. The supply of hospital beds varies significantly across regions, ranging from 78 beds per 10,000 inhabitants in Wroclaw to 37 beds per 10,000 in Radom, with an average of 55.

Hospitals in Poland are being reclassified as acute care (664), long-term care (81), and palliative care (40), depending on suitability and local need. To meet this goal, the Ministry of Health launched the Program of Restructuring of Health Care in 1999. As a result, an additional 100 palliative and long-term care units were established in 2000. In addition, new accreditation and registration systems implemented under the program are expected to result in the closure of some small hospitals and at least a 10 percent reduction in the number of beds (especially in the areas of gynecology and pediatrics).

For emergency care outside of hospital settings, access problems continue. According to the law, an ambulance or emergency aid may only be requested in justified cases. Although some cases are easy to justify, others are less clearly defined. Consequently, many people are hesitant to request emergency help for fear that they will have to pay the cost themselves.

However, since 1999, the MOH has been financing the Integrated Medical Life Saving Program, which includes the establishment of emergency rooms, the provision of new ambulances, and the training of medical staff in emergency medicine.

Prospects for the Future

Development of the new healthcare system is consistent with one of the most obvious features of current political decision making in Poland: reluctance to compromise. Representatives of the groups most affected by healthcare reform, including professionals, local leaders, employers, and patients, were not consulted throughout the planning process and during implementation of the system. Opinions expressed by the minority party within the governmental coalition were also neglected.

Notably, on the eve of the reform, an overwhelming majority of experts called for a postponement of implementation because the basic concepts had not been fully developed. These dissenters pointed out that previous foundation legislation had not been passed, medical professionals were not prepared, and patients were not informed. Such objections were dismissed because the system was deemed desperately in need of change and any delay would simply exacerbate the situation. This argument was valid, but the rapid pace of the process alienated many interested parties and caused many problems.

As noted previously, the insurance system has significant gaps in coverage, and those who are not legally entitled to its benefits, as well as those who decide not to participate, are excluded. This lack of universality is an issue for further consideration by Polish health authorities.

Sickness funds are generally reluctant to cover contracts for noncurative (preventive) medical services and services targeted at higher-risk and lower-income portions of the population. Consequently, school clinics, which were once a very important component of preventive and emergency care, have virtually disappeared. Many sickness funds argue that providing comparable care by family practitioners is more cost-efficient. Similar problems have arisen for elderly patients in nursing homes, because sickness funds also do not want to contract for this type of care.

Financial stabilization of the health system is precarious. The sickness funds required governmental subsidization in 1999 and at the beginning of 2000. The insurance system has also been compelled to obtain private loans from banks. Reduction in the size of the healthcare system by a minimum of 1,500 physicians and 10,000 nurses may be the only means of addressing these financial troubles. From the professionals' point of view, the most manifest result of healthcare reform is the threat of unemployment. Providers are also vulnerable at the micro level. In the earliest stages of reform, the motto "money follows a patient" was widely followed. However, many providers who increased their patient load have been subject to the limits imposed by sickness funds and face the possibility of bankruptcy.

Mandatory separation of contracts for ambulatory and hospital care encouraged the division of institutions that previously provided an integrated array of services. Large and diverse institutions, which prevailed in the past, have been divided into more homogenous structures that offer only ambulatory care. Newly created outpatient institutions have been further dissolved to establish many small practices for solo-operating doctors, nurses, or midwives. This policy was facilitated in the second half of 1999 and 2000 by both the MOH, which offered inexpensive loans for investments in small practices, and sickness funds, which began signing contracts for very narrow ranges of services.

Increased productivity is expected to result from these divisive measures, but during the interim, the medical community faces growing fragmentation of primary care and increasing difficulty with the coordination of services. The expected improvements are still unrealized.

The following questions must be addressed if further progress is to be made:

- Can the recently created sickness funds function solely in the role of payer, or will they be compelled to assume utilization and quality monitoring responsibilities in an attempt to contain costs?
- Is the health insurance system ready for the implementation of private health plans? What should be the role of private health insurance?
- How will the process of the privatization of healthcare units develop?
- Will both public and private service providers be able to adhere to the cost-efficient policies of the payers, change the volume of services accordingly, and still remain effective?
- Will primary care physicians assume the gatekeeper role? How will this affect service usage?
- Will individual providers employed in public institutions be willing to forego the "under the table" funds that currently supplement their incomes?
- What will be the mechanism of coordination among health promotion, prevention, curative medicine, social services, and planning efforts?
- How will the economy and the healthcare system interact on a macro level?

Understanding and resolving these issues will be difficult and time consuming. An optimistic outlook suggests that the difficulties of the implementation phase will be overcome and that the effectiveness of the system will be improved. Conversely, the reform, which affects the vested interests of influential groups both within and outside the healthcare system, may not sufficiently realize its expected benefits. In both cases, leadership at all levels of society will greatly affect the course of healthcare reform. Moreover, the planning, development, and implementation processes (along with the present turbulent phase) of the reform movement provide the possibility for new learning within the context of Poland's ever-expanding economy and an opportunity to improve the health of the population.

REFERENCES

Blaszczak-Przybicinska. 1998. *Monitoring Household Living Conditions in Poland, 1995–1996. Report Synthesis.* Warsaw: Institute of Public Affairs.

Chawla, M., and Kulis, M. 2000. *An Evaluation of the Financial Sustainability of the Polish Health System Follows the Introduction of Social Health Insurance.* Warsaw: World Bank.

European Observatory on Health Care Systems. 1999. *Health Care Systems in Transition.* Copenhagen: WHO Regional Office for Europe.

Golinowska, S. 1999. "Towards Active and Respectful Aging." In *Ku Godnej i Aktywnej Starosci. Raport o Rozwoju Spolecznym, Polska* (Social Development Report, Poland), Warsaw: UNDP.

GUS. *Rocznik Statystyczny* (Yearbook). 1999. Warsaw: Main Statistical Office.

Michta, A. A. 1997. "Democratic Consolidation in Poland after 1989." In *Consolidation of Democracy in East-Central Europe,* pp. 66–108, edited by K. Dawisha and B. Parrot. Cambridge: Cambridge University Press.

Ministry of Finance. 2000. *State Budget Expenditures in 1999.* Warsaw: Ministry of Finance.

Ministry of Health and Social Welfare. 1996. *National Health Programme 1996–2005.* Warsaw: Ministry of Health and Social Welfare.

National Center for Health System Management. 1999. *Health Care in Numbers 1998.* Warsaw: National Center for Health System Management.

Organization for Economic Cooperation and Development. 2000. *OECD Economic Surveys 1999–2000 Poland.* Paris: OECD.

Szymborski, J., Wojtyniak, B., and Chanska, M. 1996. *Nierownosci w Zdrowiu Dzieci i Mlodziezy w Polsce* (Inequalities in Health in Children and Adolescence in Poland). Warsaw: published by the authors.

United Nations Development Programme (UNDP). 2000. *Human Development Report 2000.* New York, Oxford: Oxford University Press.

Wlodarczyk, C. W. 1998. *Reforma Opieki Zdrowotnej w Polsce. Studium Polityki Zdrowotnej* (Health Care Reform in Poland. Study of Health Politics). Kraków: Uniw. Wyd. Med. "Vesalius."

Wolff-Pawęska. 1998. *Oswojona Rewolucja. Europa Srodkowo-Wschodnia w Procesie Demokratyzacji* (Accommodated Revolution. Central and Eastern Europe in the Process of Democratization). Poznan: Instytut Zachodni.

World Bank. 2000. *Entering the 21st Century. World Development Report 1999/2000.* Oxford: Oxford University Press for the World Bank.

World Health Organization (WHO). 2000. *World Health Report 2000: Health Systems: Improving Performance.* Geneva: WHO.

17

THE RUSSIAN FEDERATION

Pavel Ratmanov

Background Information

The Russian Federation is geographically one of the largest countries in the world, comprising 17 million square kilometers. However, with a population of 145.6 million people in 2000, the country has a very low population density of 8.5 people per square kilometer. During the period from 1992 to 1999, the population fell by 2.8 million people (approximately 2 percent).

The Russian Federation is a federal state with a republican form of government. The country is divided into 89 federal administrative divisions (territories). The territories, in turn, consist of municipal divisions (rural districts and cities), each of which has its own government. A distinguishing feature of the Russian municipal administration is that, unlike many of its Western counterparts, the Russian rural and urban governments are relatively equal in responsibilities and influence. In the mid-1990s, Russia reversed the trend of decentralization and began to reinforce the federal role.

Since 1990, Russia's economy has experienced significant difficulties. During 1999 and 2000, Russia began to recover from an economic crisis that broke out during the latter half of 1998. In recent years, per capita gross domestic product in the Russian Federation was among the highest in newly independent states, but it was still substantially lower than in developed countries. Although health expenditures in European Union countries average more than 8 percent of the GDP and are continuing to increase gradually, health expenditures in Russia are stagnant at around 2.2 percent of the GDP. By some estimates, private spending for medical services—much of it under the table—approached 2 percent of the GDP, which was almost equal to government expenditures for such services. Additional economic information is provided in Table 17.1.

Russia's birth rate fell from 17.2 per 1,000 population in 1986 to 8.4 in 1999, the lowest in the European region. Infant mortality in the Russian Federation, at 16.9 per 1,000 live births in 1999, is lower than in most of the newly independent states, but it is substantially higher than the European average. The fertility rate was low as well in that year, at 1.17 children per woman. According to the latest available data, life expectancy in Russia is also very low, at 65.9 years in 1999. A wide gap in life expectancy exists between males (59.8 years) and females (72.2 years).

TABLE 17.1

Social and Economic Indicators

GDP, P.P.P., in billions of U.S. dollars, 1999	620.3
GDP per capita, P.P.P., U.S. dollars, 1999	4,200
Percent of GNP to health (public share), 1997	2.2
Total labor force in millions, 1997	66
Unemployment rate, %, 1999	12.4

SOURCE: State Statistics Committee (1999).

In 1997, the literacy rate of the adult Russian population was 98.7 percent. Approximately 60 percent of the population over the age of 16 years has completed at least secondary education. See Table 17.2 for more demographic data.

Context: Health Needs

The leading causes of mortality in 1999 are presented in Table 17.3. In Russia, as in most other countries, diseases of the circulatory system are the most frequent cause of death. However, unlike what is found in most

TABLE 17.2

General Demographic and Educational Indicators

Total area (km²)	17,075,400
Population in millions, 1999	145.6
Population growth rate, percent, 1999	−0.49
Age structure as a percentage of total population, 1998	
0–14 years old	19.3
15–64 years old	68.1
65 years old and older	12.6
Population density per square kilometer, 1998	8.5
Life expectancy at birth in years, 1999	
Male	59.8
Female	72.2
Infant mortality per 1,000 live births, 1999	16.9
Total fertility rate as number of live births per woman, 1999	1.17
Literacy rate of the adult population, percent, 1997	98.4

SOURCE: UNDP Office in Russia (1999).

developed nations, a large number of premature deaths (only slightly fewer than those attributed to cardiovascular disease) are due to external causes of injury and poisoning.

The structure of mortality in people 65 years old and older is comparable to the average in Europe, but the share of neoplasms and respiratory diseases in this population sector is significantly lower than the European average. The influence of alcoholism, smoking, transport accidents, and homicides has grown in recent years. Rates of alcohol-induced mental disorders, syphilis, and tuberculosis are also higher, but levels have stabilized.

Organization and Management of the Health System

The Russian Federation inherited the Soviet system of socialized medicine in the early 1990s. The healthcare system in the Soviet Union was characterized by the nominally guaranteed full and free health protection to all citizens, a dual focus on treatment and prevention, and low priority status from the government. At this time, Russia had a huge network of neighborhood and work-site primary care clinics as well as specialized outpatient facilities and large hospitals. All aspects of health services were covered under dedicated national programs. Despite the intended equity of Soviet socialized medicine, the actual system had numerous defects: the quality of services varied significantly, health spending was only 3 to 4 percent of the GDP, and physicians and nurses were badly paid and overloaded with paperwork (American International Health Alliance 1994).

In 1991, Russia was compelled to reform the healthcare system. The primary goals of the reform were to secure constitutional rights to healthcare, to create a multilayered healthcare system with the state remaining as the main provider, and to ensure continuity among healthcare establishments. The reform effort sought to accomplish these goals with two

	Deaths per 100,000	Percent of Total
Cardiovascular diseases	815.7	55.4
Accidents, injury, and poisoning	206.1	14.0
Malignant neoplasms	205.0	13.9
Respiratory system diseases	64.9	4.4
Digestive system diseases	41.9	2.8
Infectious and parasitic diseases	24.5	1.7

TABLE 17.3 Causes of Mortality in Russia, 1999

SOURCE: Ministry of Health (2000).

key mechanisms: decentralization and financial restructuring. Under decentralization, Russian regions gained some independence in decision making and a greater degree of responsibility. In 1993, Russia implemented compulsory social/state medical insurance as an additional source of funding for healthcare (Government of the Russian Federation 1993).

The Ministry of Health of the Russian Federation is the primary actor in the administration of the Russian Health System. The Ministry of Health is directly responsible for both public health and medical care. In addition to these two functions, the Ministry of Health oversees medical education and medical research throughout the country. The sanitary-preventive network in Russia is separate from the curative network and the departments of health.

There are 89 administrative divisions (territories) in the Russian Federation, and every territory has its own department of health. These departments are subordinate both to territory administration and to the federal Ministry of Health. The municipal governments also have departments of health, which are responsible for the organization of medical care in their municipal divisions. The primary goal of this hierarchical governmental structure is to provide comprehensive medical services to the population of the Russian Federation.

The Ministry of Health and the departments of health throughout the Russian Federation own medical facilities and have leverage over the management of all public health facilities. The compulsory medical insurance funds finance only medical institutions. Three layers of healthcare are found in the Russian Federation (Figure 17.1). In rural areas, municipal departments of health run primary care clinics and small hospitals; municipal departments of health oversee the larger, more specialized in-patient and outpatient medical facilities in urban areas. The territory departments of health oversee the large, well-equipped hospitals and consulting clinics that serve the entire population of the territory (including both rural districts and cities). The Ministry of Health manages the medical research centers, federal hospitals, and medical education system.

In addition to the governmental geographic medical care system, an employment-based healthcare system is in place. Besides the military and police, several large industrial and nonindustrial sectors (e.g., railroad and water transport) and enterprises maintain their own clinics and hospitals. Some enterprise medical care institutions are more advanced than the general medical facilities.

Financing

The constitution of the Russian Federation guarantees free medical care to all citizens of the country. However, the federal government does not have the financial resources to ensure this guarantee in full. Since 1998, the gov-

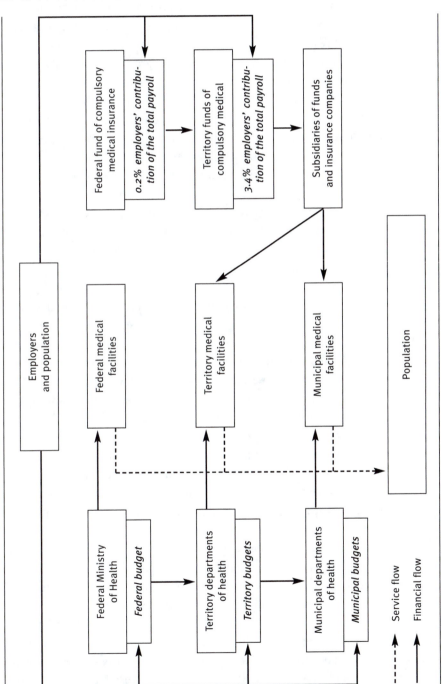

FIGURE 17.1
Service and
Financing
Flows in the
Russian
Healthcare
System

ernment of the Russian Federation has adopted annually the "program of state guarantees" to provide free medical care to its citizens. The program encompasses most healthcare services and indicates which services are provided under the basic program of compulsory medical insurance and which are met from the budgets of the different levels of government.

Guidelines have been established for the volume of medical care (by category), and per capita norms are defined but not quantified. However, some estimates show that the compulsory medical insurance system has financial resources to fund only about 50 percent of the required basic program. To cover 100 percent of the program, the federal government must increase employers' contributions, readjust the territory and municipal governments' contributions for the unemployed, or both.

Decentralization of the health system gave the territories some independence in decision making and a greater degree of responsibility. The federal government now collaborates with the territories in healthcare policymaking. The most important element of this collaboration is the triple agreement, known as the Collaboration in Implementing Government Policy on Developing Health Care, among the Federal Fund of Compulsory Medical Insurance, the Ministry of Health, and the territorial governments of the Russian Federation. The triple agreement is intended to unify healthcare throughout the country.

As of 1 January 1999, 89.2 percent of the total population was insured under compulsory medical insurance agreements. The statutory employers' contribution to this type of insurance amounts to 3.6 percent of the total payroll. In 1997, income from compulsory medical insurance in the Russian Federation covered, on average, 35 percent of health expenditures. Seventy-six percent of this amount was spent directly on the delivery of public medical services; the remainder went to administrative costs. Errors in contribution levels have led to very high administrative costs (Ministry of Health 1998).

Russia has no universal payment system in place today. Under the Soviet system, the Ministry of Health allocated funds on a per-bed basis with little regard to whether beds were occupied or vacant. These funds were also specifically marked so that a certain sum of money was designated for food, salaries, supplies, and other necessities. During the 1990s, other payment schemes appeared: capitation, clinical-statistic group (analogue DRG), per visit, per case, per procedure, per diem (bed-day), and others; many governments and compulsory medical insurance funds continued to use wasteful per-bed budget payments.

It should be noted that the basic program of compulsory medical insurance does not include the cost of outpatient medications. Hospitals do not have enough drugs to ensure the quality of medical care, and most personnel in public medical facilities are poorly paid. Patients are compelled to pay for drugs in most cases and to provide under-the-table payments to physicians for services. Some estimates find that out-of-pocket spending is almost equal to government expenditures on free care. Wide variations also exist in health spending among the territories.

The portion of private (voluntary) medical insurance in the Russian medical market is not significant. This type of insurance exists almost solely in large cities, with dentistry capturing much of the market. Dental clinics typically use fee-for-service payment, but many employment-based dental offices offer free services for employees.

Health Resources

Medical Facilities

Healthcare reform in the Russian Federation is aimed at restructuring and optimizing the work of inpatient and outpatient care facilities. Restructuring led to a decrease in the number of inpatient beds.

In 1999, the Russian Ministry of Health had 10,195 inpatient medical facilities and 17,778 medical establishments with outpatient facilities, including 936 dental clinics. In addition, primary care settings included 3,142 ambulance stations and departments. In 1999, inpatient facilities had 95,064 beds. A general comparison with previous years shows a slight decrease in the number of medical facilities in the Russian Federation. For 1999, the number of hospitals had fallen by 2.5 percent, and the number of clinics fell by 1.3 percent; 1,575,141 inpatient beds were available (Ministry of Health 2000). Table 17.4 provides additional information on health resources.

The number of beds per 10,000 population in 1999 was 108.2, about one-third more than is found in European countries; this number was 111.2 per 100,000 population in 1998. The average duration of inpatient treatment that year was 15.8 days; in 1998, it was 16.3 days. These rates show no clear sign of decreasing as they have in other countries. The average occupancy of each bed in 1999 was 307 days. The average number of outpatient visits per person (including visits to first aid posts and emergency departments) in 1999 was 9.3, one of the highest in Europe.

Human Resources

More than 3 million people work in the Russian health system, making up about 4.2 percent of the total labor force. Primary care physicians in Russia are usually internists who provide a limited number of medical services and, in most cases, refer patients to specialists. Particular attention was paid in the late 1990s to further integrating general practitioners, who can cope with the most common disorders, into the healthcare system.

The number of physicians who work in the Ministry of Health system is about 600,000; the ratio of physicians per 10,000 population was 42.2 in 1999. Again, this is one of the highest ratios in Europe. The number of intermediate-level medical personnel (e.g., nurses, midwives) in 1999

Inpatient care	
Total number of hospitals	10,195
Beds per 10,000 population	108.2
Average length of stay in days	15.8
Outpatient care	
Total number of clinics	17,778
Average number of visits per person per year	9.3
Total number of ambulance stations	3,142
Physicians*	
Total number in thousands	613.5
Number of physicians for every 10,000 of population	42.2
Nurses	
Total number in thousands	1,448.3
Number of nurses for every 10,000 of population	99.5

* The statistical definitions of "physician" and "nurse" differ from those used in the United States.
SOURCE: Ministry of Health (2000).

was 1.4 million, which resulted in a ratio of 99.5 intermediate medical personnel per 10,000 population. The low ratio of physicians to intermediate medical personnel (1:2) is a major problem. Another problem is the retention of medical staff in rural areas; in 1999, rural providers were able to fulfill only 88.8 percent of the estimated needs.

Service Delivery

The 1990s healthcare reform in the Russian Federation was based on a plan approved by the government of the Russian Federation in November 1997. According to the plan, the first approaches to improving the organization of medical care were to be the development of primary healthcare using a basis of municipal healthcare and a shift from inpatient to outpatient care. To accomplish these first goals, the plan focused particularly on the development of the institution of general practitioners and the development of cost-effective technologies.

The Russian health system inherited a geographically based system of care in which a patient's source of treatment is determined largely by his or her address. The smallest unit of the system of the Ministry of

Health is the subdistrict; each of these comprises an average population of about 2,000. In rural areas, each subdistrict is served by an independent clinic; in urban areas, a large clinic (polyclinic) serves several subdistricts. The rural clinics are usually staffed by a feldsher (intermediate-level medical personnel), and a physician oversees the multiple urban clinics. In urban clinics, every subdistrict has an internal medicine physician, and the clinics employ physicians of various specialties. The primary care in rural and urban areas is administered by the municipal department of health and funded by the subsidiaries of compulsory medical insurance funds.

It should be noted that additional primary care networks operate for pediatrics and gynecology, which have similar subdistricts. These networks are administered and financed by the municipal department of health.

On average, a rural municipal division (rayon) in Russia consists of 10 to 15 medical subdistricts. Each municipal government administers a central municipal hospital and is responsible for basic public health services. In urban areas, the city (municipal) government administers a united hospital system. Municipal hospitals are funded by the subsidiaries of compulsory medical insurance funds. Russian patients have little choice of primary care providers at the clinic level. Each patient is assigned to a primary care physician, who provides basic services and refers patients to specialists or facilities. Although clinic personnel are theoretically well-suited to act as gatekeepers, the inpatient settings are quite accessible to individuals without formal referrals. The greatest obstacles to access, however, are not referral patterns or institutional policies but limited diagnostic capabilities in clinics and patients' financial barriers.

The emergency medical system offers another access point to care: each municipal division maintains an ambulance fleet. Most of the ambulances are based at satellite stations, but some are based at hospitals. Patients are transported to a hospital, the choice of which is determined by a combination of the patient's address and the location and specialty of the hospital.

The next administrative unit is at the territory level. Each territory maintains a hospital system that provides all levels of care. In addition to general (multiprofile) hospitals, each territory supports a number of specialty medical centers. In most cases, the territory hospitals and centers are teaching facilities affiliated with medical colleges and universities. Russian hospitals tend to be highly specialized by department, often housing separate specialties in separate buildings. The territory hospital systems are better equipped and staffed and receive more financial support from the government than their municipal counterparts. Consequently, municipal medical facilities refer severely ill patients to the territory hospitals for treatment, surgery, diagnosis, and consultations. Territory hospitals are financed through compulsory medical insurance funds.

The federal medical facilities are the highest level of medical care in the Russian Federation, which is overseen by the Ministry of Health. The system includes highly specialized hospitals, specialty medical research centers, and facilities of medical universities. The Ministry of Health of the Russian Federation directly finances these institutions.

Prospects for the Future

In 2000, the Ministry of Health of the Russian Federation redefined the basic goals of healthcare and medical science development for 2000 through 2004, noting that the healthcare system in Russia needs structural adjustments and managerial and financial reform. To this end, the federal government has been developing a draft federal law regarding sociomedical insurance in the Russian Federation. This law will facilitate the merging of the compulsory medical insurance funds and the "social" insurance fund (which issues sickness benefits) by 2002. This merger will presumably increase spending on and equalize medical care in the territories of the Russian Federation (Ministry of Health 2000a).

Since the late 1990s, the government of the Russian Federation has revisited the issue of centralization. In 2000, the country was divided into seven federal regions, and the Ministry of Health established its own representatives in each region. The primary responsibilities of the representatives are the supervision, coordination, and analysis of healthcare in the supervised territories.

Increasing the quality of medical care and more effectively using available resources should be the main goals of health reform in Russia. The government needs to ensure the real availability of medical care to its citizens by focusing on the following issues:

- balancing state guarantees of free medical care with the available financial resources
- developing a stable "transparent" mechanism of financing healthcare from the different sources
- implementing financial planning and medical care payment schemes that stimulate the effective use of resources

The increased independence of medical facilities is another critical issue for contemporary Russian healthcare. Healthcare managers in the medical institutions should more actively participate in decision making and work to attract nongovernmental financial resources.

Taking into consideration the fact that previous structural adjustments involving decreasing the number of beds and physicians have thus far not succeeded, future reforms should be based on the implementation of new informational and organizational techniques.

REFERENCES

American International Health Alliance. 1994. "Health Care in the New Independent States." Retrieved December 2000 from www.aiha.com.

Government of the Russian Federation. 1993. "Law of the Russian Federation No. 4543-1, dated 24 February 1993, on Establishing a Federal Fund of Compulsory Medical Insurance." Moscow: Government of the Russian Federation.

Ministry of Health. 1998. "Government Report on the Health Status of the Population of the Russian Federation in 1997." Moscow: Ministry of Health.

———. 2000. "Government Report on the Health Status of the Population of the Russian Federation in 1999." Moscow: Ministry of Health.

———. 2000a. "Results of Reforms and Goals of Health Care and Medical Science Development for 2000–2004 and for the Period up to 2010. Report." Moscow: Ministry of Health.

State Statistics Committee (GOSKOMSTAT). 1999. "Information on the Socio-economic Situation in Russia. Demography." Retrieved from www.gks.ru.

United Nations Development Programme (UNDP) Office in Russia. 1999. "Human Development Report 1998. Russian Federation." Retrieved December 2000 from www.undp.org.

World Health Organization (WHO) Regional Office for Europe. 1999. "Highlights on Health in the Russian Federation." Copenhagen: WHO Regional Office for Europe.

CZECH REPUBLIC

Helena Hnilicová

Background Information

[...]zed European country situated in cen-[...]y, Austria, Slovakia, and Poland. The [...] kilometers, with a population of 10.3 [...]nts per square kilometer. The capital [...]ts. As a result of recent public admin-[...] administratively divided into 76 dis-

[...]den era" during the Middle Ages. In [...] Kingdom under the government of [...]anian Emperor, was one of the most [...]e following centuries, the Czechs lost [...]ingdom became part of the Austrian [...]pire. In 1918, after World War I and [...]n Empire, the independent Czecho-[...] merging of the Czech countries and

[...]n, democratic Czechoslovakia was [...]rmany. The Nazis occupied the Czech [...], and Slovakia founded a separate state under the supervision of Germany. In 1945, after World War II, Czechoslovakia as a unified coun-try was recreated. However, as of 1948, Czechoslovakia became part of the Soviet bloc and was under the complete political and economic control of the Union of Soviet Socialist Republics. Accordingly, a totalitarian politi-cal system based on only one "leading" Communist party was introduced; the Communist party basically controlled all spheres of public life in Czechoslovakia.

Political Situation

In 1989, after the collapse of the Soviet satellite system, political pluralism and a market economy were reinstated in Czechoslovakia. In early 1993, Czechoslovakia was divided into two independent, sovereign states: the CR and the Slovak Republic, a feat accomplished remarkably without violence or victimization.

The new CR consists of two parts: Bohemia and Moravia. It is a pluralistic democracy with a government elected by proportional representation. The government as of June 2002 consisted of members of the Social Democratic Party, which won the most recent election, held in 1998. This left-oriented political party came to power after six years of a far-right government.

The CR became the first post-communist country accepted as a member of OECD in 1995. In 1999, the country also attained full membership in the North American Treaty Organization (NATO). At present the main political goal of the CR is acceptance into the European Union, with the earliest date of possible consideration being the year 2003. The goal of EU acceptance has led to an intensive revision of national legislation and many other rules and regulations; reform of the state administration to become compatible with EU standards is also ongoing.

Economic Development

Before World War II, the Czech State was recognized as a developed country. Between the World Wars, Czechoslovakia was also among the 15 most developed countries of the world, although its economic potential was not as high as that of the top countries (Jaroš and Kalina 1998). However, after the implementation of the socialist command economy, Czechoslovakian development worsened, although, notably, it remained at the higher end of Soviet bloc nations.

The CR experienced a great transition in the last decade of the twentieth century. After the political changes in 1989, a market-oriented economy was introduced based on massive privatization of national industries. Heavy industry, which historically made up a very important part of the national economy, has been continuously reduced. The economy as a whole has been structurally reoriented toward consumer industry, which involves small businesses and the development of a tertiary sector. Although it has been viewed as generally positive, this restructuring has created unemployment, which is a new phenomenon after 40 years of absolute employment ensured by the communist regime. In 1995, the unemployment rate was about 3 percent; by the end of 2000, it had reached 8.8 percent (Ministerstvo Financí 2002). Recent data show continued predicted growth in the unemployment trend. Unemployment rates vary significantly among regions; some regions (northern Bohemia and northern Moravia, where steel and mining industries were concentrated) report current rates of unemployment at 15 to 16 percent (Kroupa and Mácha 1999).

The economy has also suffered heavily from an underdeveloped and insufficient banking sector. All Czech banks are overloaded by massive-risk loans due to privatization. Rapid privatization of the national economy, which started at the beginning of the 1990s, was not completely successful. During the last five years, government subsidies were critical to the support of Czech banks, prevention of bankruptcy, and stabilization of the macroeconomic situation; these factors have led to an unfavorable economic situation. At the end of the twentieth century, the gross domestic product of the CR was approximately 3 to 4 percent less than it was in 1989–90. According to the OECD European Comparison Project, in 1998 GDP per capita (using current purchasing power parities) reached the 62 percent level, which was the average for all OECD countries; in 1990, it was about 70 percent (Kroupa and Mácha 1999). Additional economic information is provided in Table 18.1.

In spite of some negative trends, signs of economic potential are also visible. Labor productivity is improving every year, with an increase since 1990 of about 10 percent. Although the economy is lacking, assessments based on the Human Development Index (.833) are much more impressive, largely because of the relatively high level of education of the population (Table 18.2). The CR is among that group of countries with the highest levels of human development: among 174 countries, the CR is ranked number 36 (Kroupa and Mácha 1999).

Demographic Development

The demographic situation in the CR shows the same tendency as other developed countries in Europe: trends include the aging of the population and a significant decrease in the birth rate. Currently, 17 percent of inhabitants are under 15 years old (ÚZIS 1999); the proportion of the population 60 years old and older has remained at 18 percent for the last several years. Additionally, in 1994, the number of births was the lowest recorded since 1785, the year in which births began to be registered. The number of children per 1,000 inhabitants is 8.8 (ÚZIS 1999); total fertility of women is below the margin of simple reproduction (1.2 children per woman of childbearing age). Overall, the population of the CR has decreased annually during the last several years.

Human Development Index, 1994	0.882	**TABLE 18.1**
GPD per person in P.P.P.$, 1999	13,125	Economic and Social Indicators
Inflation rate, 2000	3.9%	
Unemployment, 2000	8.8%	
Immunization coverage, 1996	98%	
Percent of GDP spent on health, 2000	7.2%	

SOURCE: WHO (2000); WHO Regional Office for Europe (2002); Ministerstvo Financí (2002); ÚZIS (2001).

TABLE 18.2

Education

University	7.9%
Secondary general with General Certificate of Secondary Education (GCSE)	4.7%
Secondary technical with GCSE	22.8%
Secondary vocational with GCSE	1.4%
Secondary technical	5.5%
Secondary vocational	33.8%
Compulsory	23.9%

SOURCE: Czech Statistical Office (1999).

Context: Health Needs

Mortality

After World War II, overall mortality decreased, as was the case in other European countries. This trend stopped, however, in the mid-1960s, and the mortality rate during the next 20 years stagnated due to a dramatic explosion of circulatory disorders, especially cardiovascular disorders among middle-aged men. From the 1980s, a slight but continuous decline in mortality can be observed; this decline has accelerated since 1990. In 1998, the standardized mortality rate once again dropped to its lowest level since 1964.

Life expectancy also increased since the end of the 1960s, when life expectancy at birth was comparable to that of neighboring countries such as Germany and Austria. Later, this indicator developed at a rate similar to that of the average for Central and Eastern European countries. Although at the beginning of the 1970s life expectancy at birth was only two years shorter than the EU average, in the mid-1980s, this difference increased to four years (Jaros and Kalina 1998). After 1990, a significant decrease in the crude mortality rate was observed. In the years 1990 through 1996, life expectancy increased by 2.8 years and 1.5 years for males and females, respectively; the increase in this indicator for males was likely the highest in all of Europe. In 1998, life expectancy at birth reached 71.1 years for males and 78.1 years for females. In spite of this positive trend, the CR is not expected to reach average EU values of life expectancy at birth within the next 20 years (ÚZIS 1998).

Infant Mortality

The most notable trend in specific mortality by age was for children who were less than one year old. Since the 1970s, the infant mortality rate in the CR followed EU average levels, and consistent declines in infant mortality in the 1980s and 1990s were one of the most positive movements in CR mortality trends. By 2000, the infant mortality rate had decreased to 4.1 per 1,000 live births, a level comparable with EU standards and half that of the average of Central and Eastern European nations. In that same year, neonatal mortality reached 2.5 per 1,000 live births. Low infant mortality is considered one of the most successful results of the national health policy in the transition period after the political changes of 1989.

Leading Causes of Death

The most common causes of death in the CR are diseases of the circulatory system (55 percent), followed by neoplasms (26 percent). Tied for third most common are injuries and poisoning (6 percent each), followed by respiratory diseases and diseases of the digestive system. These five causes account for approximately 95 percent of all deaths in the CR.

Among cardiovascular diseases, the most frequent causes of death for both genders are ischemic heart disease and cerebrovascular diseases, but women reach male mortality rates five to ten years later. In spite of a recent decrease in deaths due to cardiovascular diseases, mortality from this cause is still twice the EU average (Drbal 1996). According to a World Health Organization project on the monitoring of cardiovascular risks such as smoking, obesity, hypertension, and high blood cholesterol rate (MONItoring of trends and determinants in CArdiovascular disease [MONICA]), the prevalence of these risk factors is extremely high among the Czech population. In a 1985 survey, only 23 percent of men and 31 percent of women were identified as individuals without any of the aforementioned risk factors. The level of blood cholesterol was the highest in Europe, and smoking prevalence for men age 25–64 was 49 percent. Later surveys (1997–2001) indicated significant improvement in blood cholesterol rates and a substantial decrease in the number of males who smoke (Škodová, Cífková, and Lánská 1999; Škodová et al. 2002). Nutritional habits are also an important determinant of health. Czech diets are traditionally based on red meat, animal fats, sausages, bacon, and flour products. The amounts of fish, fruits, and vegetables are still not at recommended levels, but their consumption is gradually increasing (ÚZIS 1998). In recent years, some positive changes in nutritional habits have been observed; vegetable oils are gradually replacing animal fats, and the consumption of vegetables and fruits is increasing.

The prevalence of smoking has been decreasing, but only for men and only in certain age ranges. Men between 45 and 54 years old are the most likely to smoke, and no substantial decreases have been found in this age group. Similarly, smoking levels among women have not decreased. Differences in smoking patterns were found between males and females according to education. Prevalence of smoking is higher for men with lower education; on the contrary, for women, higher education is positively correlated with increased smoking (ÚZIS CR 1995, 2001).

Data on prevalence and incidence of malignant neoplasms (MN) are provided by the National Oncology Registry, which has issued regular reports since 1976. Since 1994, skin cancer has been the most frequent diagnosis, although it is not a cancer with a high fatality rate (1.1 percent). The incidence of MN of the trachea, bronchus, and lung is one of the highest in the world, reaching 101.4 per 100,000 men in 1996 (ÚZIS CR 1996). For women, the incidence is also increasing rapidly, with a growth of 28 percent between 1990 and 1997 (ÚZIS 1999). The fatality rate for MN of the trachea, bronchus, and lung has historically been very high, often close to 100 percent. However, the fatality rate decreased in 1997 to 88 percent for men and 91 percent for women.

The most frequent MN for women is breast cancer. A growth trend is also seen here, with a 25 percent increase reported between 1990 and 1997 (ÚZIS 1999). On a positive note, the incidence of MN of the stomach has decreased consistently in the CR; however, increasing trends in colorectal carcinoma contradicts this positive indicator. Incidence of colorectal MN in the CR is one of the highest in the world, with a prevalence of 76.4 per 100,000 inhabitants reported in 1996. The corresponding number for women is lower, at 59.1 per 100,000 inhabitants. The causes of this situation are unclear, and epidemiological data are not available to address this issue. Screening programs have been in place for nearly 15 years, and a new program is currently being developed.

The third leading causes of death are injuries and poisoning, which include external causes of death such as suicide. Since the 1970s, the mortality trend has decreased slightly for both genders, with the exception of male mortality in 1990. One may only speculate about the impact of the political changes and related issues in 1989 on the accidental deaths of men in this critical year. Over the past 20 years, mortality in this area has fallen by approximately 25 percent, although the difference between the CR and EU countries still remains significant. In 1997, standardized mortality for men (102 per 100,000 inhabitants) was twice as high in the CR as in the EU.

Respiratory diseases are also an important issue because they often affect a patient's ability to work. Approximately 45 percent of all recipients of illness benefits suffered from respiratory diseases.

Organization and Management of the Health System

The history of the Czech healthcare system began when obligatory health insurance for industrial workers was introduced in 1888. From 1919 to 1924, within the newly established first Czechoslovak Republic, mandatory health insurance was extended to the entire salaried population. An insurance contribution of 4.3 percent of wages, split evenly between employer and employee, was required. Approximately 300 health insurance funds provided health insurance for employees of particular industrial sectors or for large companies. Funds covered all employees as well as family members, with healthcare provided by contracted private ambulatory physicians and public hospitals. These funds also compensated workers during illness at a rate of 60 percent of the person's salary; duration of this compensation was 39 weeks. This system was effective until the communist revolution in 1948, when health insurance (coverage of health services and sickness benefits) and social insurance (coverage of pensions) were unified into a mandatory insurance system for all citizens managed by the Central National Insurance Fund. Insurance contributions were paid exclusively by the employer at 6.8 percent of the wage.

In 1951, the insurance-based system was abolished, and a nationalized healthcare system in the Soviet style (according to the Semashko model) was introduced. This system was functional from the 1950s until 1992, and it significantly influenced Czech life in the second half of the twentieth century.

Although the hierarchical structure of the centralized health services provided more or less equal access to health services, the system was unresponsive to economic incentives and did not promote effective management. As mentioned above, the health status of the population declined during the 1970s and 1980s. In 1990, the situation was dubbed "a chronic crisis of health and health care" (Ministry of Health 1990). Additionally, public opinion surveys during the same year showed that Czech citizens were dissatisfied with health services. More than half of respondents (64 percent) agreed with the idea of introducing private physician practices. Respondents believed that privatization of health services was the best way to motivate physician commitment to provide quality care for their patients (IVVM 1990). Healthcare personnel, especially physicians, were also dissatisfied with the system, largely because of chronic underfinancing of the healthcare sector. Total health expenditures in 1989 were about 5 percent of GDP (ÚZIS 1999). In that same year, the highest expenditure category was salaries, which comprised only 39 percent of total expenditures; in the most developed countries, salaries account for more than 60 percent of total expenditures (Massaro, Němec, and Kalman 1994). The above conditions created strong incentives for implementation of basic changes in the health system and were considered the main reasons for a commitment to health system reform.

In 1990, a group of experts presented a draft of a new healthcare system that was then approved by the Czech government (Ministry of Health 1990). This proposal continues to be recognized as the main reform document, although the real reform steps differed somewhat from the original principles. Those principles follow (list adapted from Ministry of Health 1990):

1. The new system of healthcare should be part of a global strategy for health restoration and health promotion.
2. The state will guarantee needed healthcare to all citizens.

3. Health services will be provided in a competitive environment.
4. The community will be responsible for the implementation of health policy in its territory.
5. Citizens will have a right to choose their physicians and health facilities.
6. An obligatory health insurance program will be an integral part of the healthcare system.
7. The monopoly of state ownership in healthcare will be abolished. Provision of healthcare services under a public health insurance scheme will include all providers, regardless of funding source.
8. The basic element of public healthcare will be the autonomous health facility with independent legal status.
9. Healthcare should be focused on primary healthcare. Outpatient care in general should be preferred to inpatient care.
10. Healthcare will be financed from multiple sources such as public health insurance, state budget, community resources, enterprise subsidies, and private sources.

In addition, the Czech Parliament adopted the Charter of Basic Human Rights, which became part of the constitution. The right to needed healthcare without any direct (out-of-pocket) payment for all Czech citizens is included as one of the CR Constitution's basic tenets.

In summary, the key reform strategy was a radical change from the rigid Semashko model of socialized healthcare to a neo-Bismarkian system of pluralistic health services based on mandatory health insurance for the entire population. This choice was not random; it was set in place as a result of the country's positive historical experience with such a system before Communist control in 1948. The decision was also influenced by the fact that a very similar organizational model was working effectively in neighboring Germany; the high economic status and prestige of German physicians provided further incentive for Czech medical professionals. Czech physicians strongly supported this reform strategy (Tobolka 1998). As traditionally very important stakeholders in health policy, physicians substantially influenced the reform agenda (Brussels Conference 1998).

To implement reform principles, three primary changes had to be completed in a very short time period (between 1991 and 1993): a change in healthcare financing, changes in the ownership and structure of health services, and the removal of the monopolization and centralization of health policy.

The introduction of a statutory health insurance system was a key element in healthcare financing reform. Creating completely new health legislation was necessary to implement such major changes. Adoption of the following three laws was of crucial importance:

1. the Public Health Insurance Act (1991)
2. the General Health Insurance Company Act (1991)
3. the Other Health Insurance Companies Act (1992)

New legal conditions enabled the reform process to move forward. Instead of tax-based financing through the state budget, a health insurance fund was established. All Czech employees must participate in the insurance program, but mandated premiums cover only the employee; family members must obtain coverage through their own employment or be eligible for public subsidy. The government pays premiums for state insurees including children, students, mothers on maternity leave, pensioners, the unemployed, the military, prisoners, and recipients of social welfare benefits (with income under the poverty line). These groups represent approximately 55 percent of the entire population (Jaros and Kalina 1998). Insurance premiums are tax deductible and equal to 13.5 percent of wages, with 9 percent paid by the employer and 4.5 percent paid by the employee. The self-employed and those with income from capital pay premiums directly from approximately 35 percent of net profit.

To allocate insurance fees to the health services, the General Health Insurance Fund (Všeobecná Zdravotní Pojišťovna [VZP]) was established with offices in each district. The VZP is the largest of some eight health insurance funds in the CR, covering 75 percent of all Czech citizens. The VZP maintains an exclusive government guarantee in case of emergencies (e.g., epidemics, high inflation rates). All health insurance funds are available to citizens, and they may make changes to their insurance funds once per year.

The Privatization Process

From a legal point of view, privatization was enabled by the adoption of the Act on Health Care Provision in Non-governmental Health Facilities (1992), which caused the decomposition of Regional Institutes of National Health and District Institutes of National Health. Regional Institutes of National Health represented those health facilities in regions that were responsible for providing tertiary health services based on high technologies (e.g., large teaching hospitals, regional hospitals, transfusion stations). District Institutes of National Health represented all health facilities in a district (e.g., district hospital, polyclinics, health centers) except for those belonging to Regional Institutes of National Health.

Through the privatization process, changes in the structure and ownership of healthcare services were implemented and resulted in the division of health facilities into the following three groups:

1. Group A: Free privatization referred to health facilities where no public interest toward the structure of services was explicitly expressed; this included the majority of outpatient facilities
2. Group B: Privatization with a "burden" referred to health facilities where a potential new owner was obliged to provide defined health services for the next ten years; this type of privatization was applied to district hospitals

3. Group C: Health facilities still remaining under state ownership such as all teaching hospitals, clinical research institutes, and educational institutions; the National Institute of Public Health; and district and regional hygiene stations

The process continued for several years, with the key period being from 1993 to 1995, as the number of providers changed dramatically because of the massive privatization of ambulatory care. Instead of the former structure of large institutes of national health, myriad independent health facilities for outpatient and inpatient care were established. Many polyclinics were divided into individual practices, which were also privatized; many other physicians established private practices outside of the former polyclinics. In 1990, before the privatization process, the CR had 140 public autonomous providers. In contrast, in 1995, a single network comprised approximately 23,000 health facilities (ÚZIS 1999), of which three-fourths were completely privatized single-physician practices (general practitioners and ambulatory specialists). Much of the growth resulted from financial incentives offered to ambulatory physicians who turned to private practice; average income after privatization was double the income of state-salaried physicians (Masarro, Němec, and Kalman 1994).

The privatization of hospital care was not so successful. The government's declaration in 1992 of a willingness to privatize a majority of the state-owned district hospitals was not realistic. Because of existing legal and economic conditions, hospital care is much less profitable than ambulatory care. Consequently, of the 67,365 total hospital beds in CR in 1998, only 6,156 (9.1 percent) are currently private (ÚZIS 1999). Private hospitals are usually small hospitals with no significant importance in their regions.

Ambulatory care is currently privatized with the exception of care provided by the outpatient departments of public hospitals (about 25 percent of outpatient care). Substantial parts of hospitals and their capacities, as well as their health equipment, remain public.

Financing

Nearly all health facilities include private providers who maintain contracts with public health insurance funds; thus, services provided by private providers are reimbursed from public sources. From an economic point of view, most health providers must have a relevant contract with the VZP (or other insurance funds). The contract is specific to volume and type of service, and cost-containment measures are explicitly included. Contracts are not mandatory, and a process of public selection of providers to be retained by the public health insurance funds is in place. However, few healthcare providers can survive without a contract with public health insurance funds. Only independent ambulatory stomatologists are paid primarily by private sources; approximately 25 percent of their incomes come from out-of-pocket payment.

Payment of Healthcare Providers

In 1997, the situation surrounding healthcare financing in the CR was critical. The VZP was operating with a substantial deficit (about 5 billion Czech crowns). Before September 1997, insurance companies paid all contractual partners on a fee-for-service basis for all medical care; however, fee-for-service reimbursement had very negative outcomes. All providers, private ambulatory physicians, and hospitals had incentives to provide unnecessary care because their income depended on the number of procedures performed, regardless of actual patient needs or resources available in the public health insurance fund. Therefore, in response to the failing fee-for-service scheme, implementation of the insurance system for healthcare financing on a macro level was initiated. This change was of crucial importance. The attitudes and behavior of physicians and the real extent of healthcare provided have been greatly influenced by this measure.

Primary care physicians are now paid on a capitation basis; ambulatory specialists are still paid on a fee-for-service basis. Hospital financing is based on a global budgeting arrangement, with the actual budget for each hospital set at 75 percent of the expenditure level for the last year of fee-for-service reimbursement. Financing of hospitals through global budgeting is viewed as a temporary measure. On an experimental level, a diagnosis-related-group system of hospital financing has been established by the VZP. The financial value of all medical procedures is expressed by a point assessment in an official document called the List of Medical Procedures (Seznam Výkonůa Jejich Bodové Ohodnocení).

Health Resources

Delivery of health services in the CR is shared among three categories of providers: primary care, specialized ambulatory care, and inpatient care that includes hospitals and highly specialized research and educational institutes.

Freedom of Choice of Healthcare Providers

The Public Health Insurance Act requires that all citizens have complete choice of healthcare providers. Adults and parents can freely choose their primary care doctors, ambulatory specialists, and hospitals. For primary care, individuals are required to register with the doctor of their choice. If they are unsatisfied with the quality of services, they can change their registration after three months. Recently, the government has been discussing the implementation of a gatekeeper function for primary care physicians. However, this idea has not yet been implemented, because the government understands the sensitivity around this issue; gatekeepers were very unpopular under the Communist regime.

Basic Services Covered by Public Health Insurance

Under the Public Health Insurance Act, the insured receive a wide range of therapeutic and preventive services. The basic healthcare package includes "needed medical care," defined as "all therapeutic and diagnostic procedures, long-term care, emergency care, preventive care, rehabilitation including spa treatments, some part of occupational preventive care, pharmaceuticals, health aids, necessary transport to the health facilities, and autopsy (Public Health Insurance Act No. 48/1997 Coll.). Public health insurance also covers emergency healthcare for Czech citizens during short-term stays abroad, but only at the price of such healthcare in the CR. In reality, Czech citizens need additional health insurance for visits to developed countries, where prices for health services are much higher; travel health insurance is offered by all public health insurance companies.

Copayments exist to some extent for outpatient care; most copayments are for drugs used in outpatient care and for dental care. About 25 percent of dental care is paid for out-of-pocket. Coverage of dental care depends on the raw materials used; typically only the cheapest materials are covered by the public health insurance. Similarly, orthodontics is only partly covered by the health insurance. For other services, some copayment is required for health aids, hospital stays are completely free of charge, and no copayment is required for drugs or any other services in the hospital, except for special hotel services.

Pharmaceuticals

In the Czech health system, about one-fourth (25.5 percent) of all expenditures is for pharmaceuticals (ÚZIS CR 1999). The drug market is strictly regulated at the macro level as well as on the level of individual health facilities. A drug can be sold within the CR only under the condition of its registration by the State Institute of Drug Control and after the Ministry of Finance has set a maximum price for it. The government regulates not only prices but their coverage by public insurance. As mentioned above, no copayment is required for drugs in hospitals. However, because hospitals spend almost one-third of their budgets on pharmaceuticals, drug policy in each hospital is a big issue. Hospital administrators, in collaboration with clinicians, have developed their own drug policies based on "positive lists" of recommended drugs; their aim is to improve cost-effectiveness in drug consumption. Prescription patterns as well as total drug consumption in many hospitals are significantly influenced by these lists.

The situation surrounding outpatient therapy is completely different. Ambulatory drug prescriptions are not fully covered by public insurance, resulting in a focus on generic drugs. Drugs consumed in outpatient therapy are divided into three groups: those fully covered by health insurance, those partly covered by health insurance, and those not covered by health insurance.

In each group of generic substances, at least one drug is fully covered by the public health insurance, usually the cheapest one (very often produced by the Czech pharmaceutical industry). Prices of drugs are regulated at the national level through a designated maximum price for each drug, which is defined by the Ministry of Health according to the cost set by the producer of the drug plus a "reasonable" profit. Approximately one-third of total expenditure for drugs is paid out-of-pocket (Jaros and Kalina 1998).

Prospects for the Future

Despite three years of strong financial regulation implemented by third-party payers, the economic situation in the health sector is still unbalanced. The principal issue is a gap between available resources and a package of basic health services guaranteed by the law, which is arguably too comprehensive. Unfavorable economic developments, characterized by the bankruptcies of many large firms and increasing unemployment, have resulted in the inability of many employers to pay health insurance contributions for their employees. Although the VZP tried to implement cost-containment measures by reducing the number of contracted providers, their financial deficit has not diminished; on the contrary, the financial deficit continues to increase. The government tried to resolve this situation by increasing health insurance contributions to 15 percent of wages. However, this proposal was not accepted by the Parliament. Another possible solution seems to be a substantial reduction in the number of services included in the basic health insurance package; this change would bring a significant increase in copayments for patients. Although such an approach is strongly supported by the Czech Medical Chamber, the majority of Czech citizens support copayments only for above-standard services and for drugs, because this kind of copayment is viewed as contradictory to the principle of equal access to needed health services. In light of a lack of popular support, the introduction of additional copayments is extremely problematic.

Also, very acute problems are associated with the low salaries of hospital physicians working in the public sector. Although their salaries are comparable with salaries of all other employees in the state sector, public physician salaries are two to three times lower than those of private ambulatory physicians.

Ambulatory physicians and health personnel are also unhappy with the stringent regulation of care they are allowed to provide; the number of procedures reimbursed per day or per physician is limited. An estimate is determined for the time needed to perform each medical procedure in ambulatory care; physicians can request full reimbursement from public health insurance only for those procedures that can be done in eight to nine working hours. If a physician provides more procedures, some procedures may only be partly covered. At the same time, requiring copayments from patients is not possible. Out-of-pocket payment is only allowed for those procedures provided on a completely private basis, without any public sources. Risks associated with this situation include increased bribes, corruption, and threats of decreased quality of care. Although the media have reported on these effects, the true extent of corruption remains unmeasured.

Future development of the Czech healthcare system depends on the successful social and economic transformation of the entire society. With economic development as limited as it has been in recent years, implementation of substantial restrictions in the coverage of health services will likely be necessary. This would be a fundamental change from a system with traditionally very good accessibility to health services for all citizens.

APPENDIX A

Health Expenditure by Source of Financing (in millions of Czech crowns)

Public health insurance	107.9	81.2%
State budget	13.9	10.5%
Private expenditure	11.1	8.3%
Total	132.9	100%

SOURCE: ÚZIS (1999).

APPENDIX B

Private Expenditures on Healthcare

Pharmaceuticals not covered by insurance	45.6%
Copayment for drugs	11.4%
Medical services not covered by health insurance	20.4%
Orthopedic and other health aids	12.6%
Other	10.0%

SOURCE: ÚZIS ČR (1999, 2000, 2000a, 2000b); ÚZIS (1998).

APPENDIX C

Mortality

Causes of death	Males	Females
Diseases of the circulatory system	51.2%	57%
Malignant neoplasms	27.4%	25.9%
Injuries and poisoning	7.5%	4.9%
Diseases of the respiratory system	4.3%	3.2%
Diseases of the digestive system	4.2%	3.4%
Other	4.0%	5.2%

SOURCE: ÚZIS ČR (1999, 2000, 2000a, 2000b); ÚZIS (1998).

Hospital Beds	Number	Percent
Acute beds	61,460	91
Obstetrics beds	2,395	4
Chronic care beds	3,510	5
Public beds	61,235	90.9
Private beds	6,130	9.1

SOURCE: ÚZIS ČR (1999, 2000, 2000a, 2000b); ÚZIS (1998).

APPENDIX D
Hospital
Beds by
Type of Care

	Per 1,000 Inhabitants	Total
Physicians	3.7	36,855
Nurses	7.1	73,278
Midwives	0.4	4,205

SOURCE: ÚZIS ČR (1999, 2000, 2000a, 2000b); ÚZIS (1998).

APPENDIX E
Health
Providers

Hospital admissions per 1,000 inhabitants	190,400
Hospital occupancy rates (average)	71.3%
Average length of hospital stay	8.6 days
Outpatient examinations per 1,000 inhabitants	14,504

SOURCE: ÚZIS ČR (1999, 2000, 2000a, 2000b); ÚZIS (1998).

APPENDIX F
Service Use in
1998/1999

REFERENCES

Brussels Conference. 1998. "Recent Reforms in Organisation, Financing and Delivery of Health Care in Central and Eastern Europe in Light of Accession to the European Union." Consensus Programme, Contract No. ZZ-9505-01-58. May 24–26.

Cífková, R., and Škodová, Z. 2002. "Změny rizikových faktorův populaci a pokles kardiovaskulární mortality" (Changes of the Risk Factors and Decrease in Cardiovascular Mortality). *Journal of the American College of Cardiology*–CZ 4 (1): 77–80.

Czech Statistical Office. 1999. *Statistical Yearbook of the Czech Republic 1998.* Prague: Czech Statistical Office.

Drbal, C. 1996. *Zdraví a Zdravotní Politika* (Health and Health Policy). Brno: Masarykova Univerzita.

Jaroš, J., and Kalina, K. 1998. *Czech Health Care System. Delivery & Financing.* Organization for Economic Cooperation and Development Study. Prague: Czech Association for Health Services Research.

Kroupa, A., and Mácha, M. 1999. *Zpráva o Lidském Rozvoji. Česká Republika 1999* (Report on Human Development. Czech Republic 1999). Prague: Výzkumný Ústav Práce a Sociálních Věcí.

Massaro, T. A., Němec, J., and Kalman, I. 1994. "Health System Reform in the Czech Republic: Policy Lessons from the Initial Experience of the General Health Insurance Company." *Journal of the American Medical Association* 271: 1870–74.

Ministerstvo Financí. 2002. "Predikce makroekonomického vývoje: Hlavní makroekonomické indikátory" (Prediction of Macroeconomic Development: The Main Macroeconomic Indicators). Retrieved 25 March 2002 from www.mfcr.cz/MakroPre/CZ/2002-1/Komentar htm.

Ministry of Health. 1990. *Reform of Health Care in the Czech Republic.* Prague: Ministry of Health.

Názory Občanůna Zdraví a Zdravotnictví (IVVM). 1990. *Public Opinion Survey on Health and Health Care.* Prague: Institute for Public Opinion Research.

Škodova, Z., Cífková, R., and Lánská, V. 1999. "Dlouhodobý vývoj kardio-vaskulárních onemocnění u obyvatelstva České republiky" (Long-term Development of the Cardiovascular Diseases of the Czech Population). *Forum Medicinae* 1 (3/4): 2–7.

Škodová, Z., Cífková, R., Adámková, V., Jozífková, M., Novozámská, E., Petržílková, Z., Plášková, M., Palouš, D., Peterková, L., Micková-Galovcová, M., and Barátová, M. 2002. "Dlouhodobý vývoj a současný stav kuřáckých zvyklostí obyvatelstva České republiky" (Long-term Development and Current Status of the Smoking Habits of the Czech Population). *Cor Vasa* 44 (2): 81–86.

Tobolka, R. 1998. *České Zdravotnictví v Letech 1989–1997 z Pohledu Sociální Antropologie* (Czech Health Care from the Point of View of Social Anthropology). Prague: Diplomová Práce, Institut Základů Vzdělanosti.

Ústav Zdravotnických Informací a Statistiky (ÚZIS) (Institute of Health Information and Statistics). 2001. *Czech Health Statistics Yearbook 2000.* Prague: ÚZIS.

———. 1999. *Czech Health Statistics Yearbook 1998.* Prague: ÚZIS.

———. 1998. *Czech Health Statistics Yearbook 1997.* Prague: ÚZIS.

Ústav Zdravotnických Informací a Statistiky ČR (ÚZIS ČR) (Institute of Health Information and Statistics of the Czech Republic). 2000. *Ekonomické Informace 1999* (Economic Information 1999). Prague: ÚZIS ČR.

——— 2000a. *Lůžková Péče 1999* (In-Patient Care 1999). Prague: ÚZIS ČR.

——— 2000b. *Zdravotní Stav Obyvatelstva České Republiky 1999* (Health Status of the Czech Population 1999). Prague: ÚZIS ČR.

——— 1999. *Cancer Incidence 1996 in the Czech Republic.* Prague: ÚZIS ČR.

———. 1998. "Sample Surveys of the Health Status of the Czech Population." *HIS CR 96.* Prague: ÚZIS ČR.

———. 1995. "Sample Surveys of the Health Status of the Czech Population." *HIS CR 93.* Prague: ÚZIS ČR.

World Health Organization (WHO). 2000. *WHO Health for All 2000.* Statistical Database (CD-ROM). WHO: Copenhagen.

World Health Organization (WHO) Regional Office for Europe. 2002. "Country Highlights: Czech Republic." Retrieved 26 March 2002 from www.who.dk/Dokument/E73486.pdf.

HUNGARY

Peter Gaál

Background Information

The Hungarian state has a 1,000-year history influenced by both its location in the Carpathian basin of Central Europe and the origin of its people, the Hungarians whose closest relatives can be found in the Finno-Ugric language group. The Hungarian Kingdom—established in 1000 AD when its first king, St. István, was crowned and converted the country into Christianity—was a powerful state throughout the medieval period but suffered difficult times fighting against the Mongols (Genghis Khan), the Turks (the Ottoman Empire), and later against the Habsburg rule. As part of the Austro-Hungarian monarchy, Hungary lost World War I and two-thirds of its territory. During World War II, the Germans and then the Russians occupied the country in turn, and in 1948 a Communist dictatorship was established under the Soviet Union. Hungary regained its independence in 1989 and achieved a quick transition into a multiparty democracy and market economy. The following ten years of freely elected Hungarian governments were characterized by the endeavor to reintegrate the country into the Western world. The Hungarian Republic became a member of NATO in March 1999, and it is among the nations expecting accession to the European Union.

Since 1990, Hungary has been a constitutional democracy with a stable political system. The 386 seats in the unicameral Parliament are filled every four years by a combined majority and proportional electoral system with single-choice voting. Mayors and local government assemblies are also elected for four years, usually a few months after the general elections. The public administration system has three levels: the central government, the local governments of the counties, and the settlements. The 93,000 square kilometers of the country is divided into 19 counties and the capital, Budapest.

Population Demographics

Hungary had 10.1 million inhabitants in 1997. As a result of historical events, an additional five million Hungarians live mostly in neighboring countries as well as some who live overseas. The past decade has witnessed a continual population decrease due to a low fertility rate and high mortality rates, especially in middle-aged men. In 1997, life expectancy at birth was 75.1

years for women and 66.4 for men. More than half of the Hungarian people live in towns with a population of 20,000 or greater, and literacy is nearly 100 percent. Primary education is compulsory, and 86 percent of the youth enroll in secondary schools. Additional demographic and educational information is provided in Tables 19.1 and 19.2.

The Economy

The collapse of central planning and the Communist foreign trade system has made the establishment of a market economy in recent years a challenge. Unemployment rose to 14 percent in 1993, inflation reached 35 percent in 1991 and 28.8 percent in 1995; the gross domestic product of the country diminished year by year until 1994, and real wages fell until 1997. Nevertheless, current macroeconomic indicators show that the negative economic trends have been reversed with an impressive gross domestic product growth rate of 4.4 percent in 1997 and 5.2 percent in 1998. The structural transformation to a stable market economy has also been successful. In 1998, unemployment and inflation fell to 7.7 percent and 14.3 percent, respectively, whereas real wages increased by 3.4 percent. For more economic data, see Table 19.3.

Context: Health Needs

By the early 1970s, chronic, noncommunicable diseases started to dominate health needs in Hungary. This trend has continued throughout the 1980s and 1990s, with cancer and cardiovascular disease dominating mortality. Additional information concerning mortality measurements can be found in Table 19.4.

Notably, health concerns in Hungary are not simply characterized by the problems of an aging society as they are elsewhere in the developed world. During the 1980s, life expectancy in most Western European coun-

TABLE 19.1
General Demographics

Population in millions	10.1
Infant mortality per 1,000 live births	9.9
Under-five mortality per 1,000 live births	11.5
Male life expectancy at birth (years)	66.4
Female life expectancy at birth (years)	75.1
Population change per 1,000 inhabitants	−3.8
Percent urbanized	64

SOURCE: Hungarian Central Statistical Office (1998).

TABLE 19.2
Education

Adult literacy rate	99%
Primary school enrollment	99%
Secondary school enrollment	86%

SOURCE: OECD (1998).

tries continuously improved, but in Hungary it stagnated and started to decrease, especially for men. This trend continued in the first half of the 1990s, reaching its lowest figure of 64.4 years for male life expectancy at birth in 1993 (Hungarian Central Statistical Office 1999). Mortality of middle-aged men is the single most important factor in explaining this sad statistic. In 1994, 16 of 1,000 men between the ages of 40 and 59 years died, a mortality rate that is worse than its counterpart from 1921 (Hungarian Central Statistical Office 1995). Premature mortality due to cardiovascular diseases, cancer, and chronic liver diseases are the most prominent factors contributing to this rate. The number of deaths from suicide and accidents is also among the highest as compared with other European countries (WHO Regional Office for Europe 1999).

One possible explanation for the high mortality rates takes into account the broad context of health and its determinants. Although access to health-enhancing factors including health services does not seem problematic (Table 19.5), lifestyle (e.g., smoking, alcohol consumption, unhealthy diet, lack of exercise) and the changes in the social and economic environment may be contributing factors. Additionally, as Kopp (1999) has pointed out, social cohesion is an important contributor to good health, but it has been seriously eroded in Hungary throughout the past 20 years;

TABLE 19.3
Economic and Social Indicators

Real GDP per capita (P.P.P.$)	$10,968
GDP growth rate (%)	4.4
Public expenditure as percent of GDP	56.8
Annual inflation (CPI)	18.3
Total health expenditure as percentage of GDP	6.5
Inflation in healthcare (%)	18.3
Annual changes of real wages (%)	4.9
Rate of registered unemployment (%)	11.0

NOTE: CPI = consumer price index.
SOURCE: OECD (1998).

TABLE 19.4
Leading
Causes of
Morbidity
and Mortality

Deaths per 1,000 inhabitants	13.7
Mortality of 40- to 59-year-old males per 1,000	15.2
Infant mortality per 1,000 live births	9.9
Maternal mortality per 100,000 live births	20.9
Mortality from communicable diseases per 1,000 inhabitants	0.07
Total number of new AIDS cases	31
Mortality due to accidents per 1,000 inhabitants	0.70
Suicide mortality per 1,000 inhabitants	0.32
Cardiovascular mortality per 1,000 inhabitants	7.0
Cancer mortality per 1,000 inhabitants	3.3
Liver disease mortality per 1,000 inhabitants	0.67

SOURCE: Hungarian Central Statistical Office (1998).

inequalities in income have substantially grown, while the traditional channels of social support have been gradually disappearing.

The role of health services is also worth revisiting. In principle, during the Communist regime, all Hungarian citizens had access to the services they needed; however, the appropriateness and the quality of the service were questionable. The state-socialist system was unable to respond
adequately to the health transition of the population, and the allocation of
resources was subject to political influence. Therefore, service provision
inequalities arose both in terms of geographical locations and specialities.
This factor has to be taken into account as well if health needs and the role
of health services are to be accurately interpreted.

Organization and Management of the Health System

Origin and Reform of the Hungarian Health System

Before World War II, the Hungarian healthcare system was developing
along a Bismarkian path characterized by increased involvement of the state

TABLE 19.5
Access to
Health-
Enhancing
Factors

Access to health services	100%
Access to safe water	84%
Access to sanitation	94%

SOURCE: Hungarian Central Statistical Office (1998).

in both the financing and delivery of health services. Health insurance was beginning to play a major role in the system. However, this path of development was broken by the forced introduction of the Soviet model of healthcare services in 1948. Under the influence of the Union of Soviet Socialist Republics, a communist dictatorship was established in Hungary, and, as with other service sectors, healthcare institutions were nationalized. Health services were provided almost exclusively by the state, which promised free, high-quality, comprehensive care for every citizen.

In its early years, the Soviet system was successful in controlling communicable diseases, and it produced substantial improvement in the health status of the population with public hygiene measures and immunization. However, the system was not able to respond adequately to the health transition of the population, and the favorable trends changed in the 1960s. Despite quantitative improvements in the number of beds and consultation hours, healthcare providers were unable to meet the growing demand, and giving informal payment became widespread.

The need for profound change emerged gradually throughout the 1970s and 1980s, when the crisis of the state-socialist health services became more and more obvious. The first reform plans were developed under the so-called Reform Communist era, which started with the establishment of the Reform Secretariat of the Ministry of Social Affairs and Health in 1987. This period witnessed the first significant steps taken toward a less centralized model of health services. Moving from tax-based financing to social insurance, the Social Insurance Fund was established in 1988, and in 1989, private providers were allowed to reopen their practices.[1]

Between 1990 and 1994, the first freely elected government implemented major structural reforms with considerable decentralization, such as the transfer of ownership of the majority of health providers to local governments. Simultaneously, the government introduced performance-based provider payment methods, started the reform of public health, and gave priority to the development of primary care. In 1992, the Social Insurance Fund was divided into the Health Insurance Fund and the Pension Insurance Fund.[2] The fiscal crisis of 1995 prompted an economic stabilization program that aimed to cut healthcare costs and increase the share of private financing. During the first year of the current government (1998), the policy debate revolved around the adoption of a managed insurance competition model, but the final decision was to preserve the present single-payer system. Nevertheless, further decentralization (privatization) remains on the health policy agenda.

The Current Hungarian Health System

The Constitution of the Republic of Hungary declares health to be a fundamental right, and it makes the state responsible for ensuring this right, among others, through the organization of healthcare institutions and medical care.[3] This responsibility is further clarified by Act CLIV of 1997 on

Health Care, which designates the National Assembly, the government, the Ministry of Health, the National Public Health and Medical Officer Service, local governments, and those who maintain health facilities to be responsible for the organization and control of health services. These main actors have become even more significant as a result of the reform measures of the past 12 years, which replaced previously hierarchical relationships with contractual and quasi-public arrangements. Figure 19.1 summarizes the current organizational structure of Hungarian health services, and Figure 19.2 shows the process of decentralization. Notably, health services in Hungary are still predominantly funded and provided publicly.

The healthcare reforms of the 1990s transformed the system to a model in which the purchaser of services is separated from the providers, and the delivery of services is based on service contracts with the public third-party payer, the National Health Insurance Fund Administration. Although health policy formulation has remained in the sphere of the central government, the formal central planning system of the previous regime has been abandoned; the provision of health services has become the responsibility of local governments.

The prime responsibility of the government and relevant ministries is regulation; other actors such as the Hungarian Medical Chamber, national institutes of health, and the National Public Health and Medical Officer Service are also involved in the process. In Hungary, almost all aspects of the production process are regulated. The quality and the quantity of health personnel are controlled in several ways: the number of students whose education is financed by the government budget is determined centrally; a procedure is in place for the acknowledgment of foreign diplomas; and the Ministry of Education determines the qualification requirements for undergraduate and certain postgraduate training programs and the Ministry of Health oversees compulsory continuing education among health workers.[4] Medical doctors and other qualified health personnel have to register and obtain a license from the Ministry of Health and the relevant professional chambers to start practicing.[5] The employment of health workers is also influenced through the mandatory determination of a minimum wage for public employees.[6]

A registration and licensing system is in operation for control of the quality of pharmaceuticals, medical aids, and equipment. This system is administered by the National Institute of Pharmacy and the National Institute of Hospital and Medical Technology.

Healthcare providers are comprehensively regulated. Act LXIII of 1996 determines the overall capacity (defined by the number of hospital beds and outpatient specialist consultation hours) of publicly funded healthcare providers and their distribution across counties and specialities. According to the Act, service contracts are regulated insofar as the National Health Insurance Fund Administration is obliged to contract for the capac-

FIGURE 19.1

Organizational Structure of the Hungarian Health Services, 1999

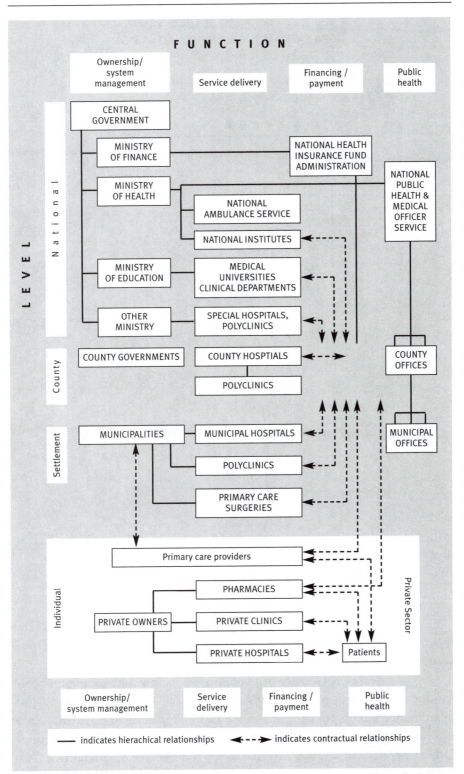

F U N C T I O N

Ownership/system management · Service delivery · Financing / payment · Public health

CENTRAL GOVERNMENT

MINISTRY OF FINANCE

NATIONAL HEALTH INSURANCE FUND ADMINISTRATION

NATIONAL PUBLIC HEALTH & MEDICAL OFFICER SERVICE

MINISTRY OF HEALTH

NATIONAL AMBULANCE SERVICE

NATIONAL INSTITUTES

MINISTRY OF EDUCATION

MEDICAL UNIVERSITIES CLINICAL DEPARTMENTS

OTHER MINISTRY

SPECIAL HOSPITALS, POLYCLINICS

COUNTY GOVERNMENTS

COUNTY HOSPTIALS

COUNTY OFFICES

POLYCLINICS

MUNICIPALITIES

MUNICIPAL HOSPITALS

MUNICIPAL OFFICES

POLYCLINICS

PRIMARY CARE SURGERIES

Primary care providers

PHARMACIES

PRIVATE OWNERS

PRIVATE CLINICS

PRIVATE HOSPITALS

Patients

Private Sector

LEVEL: National · County · Settlement · Individual

Ownership/system management · Service delivery · Financing / payment · Public health

—— indicates hierachical relationships   ◄- - -► indicates contractual relationships

SOURCE: Reprinted with permission, from *Health Care Systems in Transition: Hungary*, published by European Observatory on Health Care Systems, copyright 1999.

FIGURE 19.2

Decentrlization
Reform
Measures in
the Hungarian
Health
Services,
1988–99

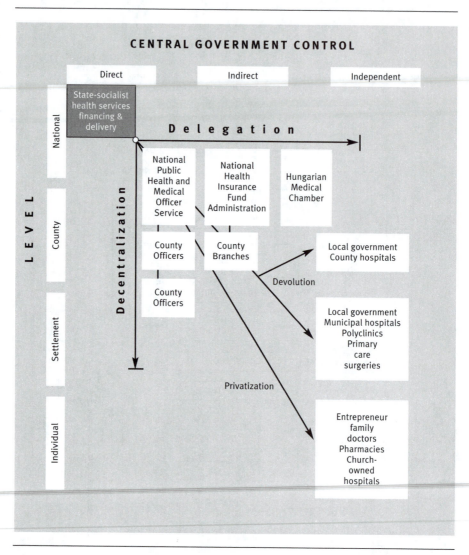

CENTRAL GOVERNMENT CONTROL

SOURCE: Reprinted with permission, from *Health Care Systems in Transition: Hungary*, published by European Observatory on Health Care Systems, copyright 1999.

ities defined by the law, and local governments are responsible for the provision of these capacities.

Healthcare providers must obtain a license to start supplying services for the population. They have to meet certain minimum building and hygienic requirements and personnel and material standards, which are inspected by medical officers of the National Public Health and Medical Officer Service. In addition to the above requirements, special rules are applied to certain services such as fertility treatment, sterilization procedures, and organ transplantation and to the provision of unconventional medical treatment.[7]

Financing

In the Hungarian health system, the dominant sources of finance are public, including statutory health insurance; general taxation; and local taxation. In 1997, public sources made up 75 percent of total healthcare financing, of which the statutory health insurance is the most significant. From the various private alternatives, the role of insurance is negligible; however, out-of-pocket payments in the form of copayments for drugs, medical aids, prostheses, and dental services and informal payments made to public employee doctors make up the remainder of healthcare financing at 25 percent (WHO Regional Office for Europe 1999).

The Tax Office collects the revenue from contributions to the Health Insurance Fund (HIF) by employers and employees. Membership in the statutory health insurance scheme is compulsory. From the total of 14 percent payroll tax collected in 1999, 11 percent was paid by the employer and 3 percent by the employee, with an upper limit for the employee contribution of 4,600 HUF, or approximately U.S.$19, per month.[8] To compensate for noncontributing pensioners, the unemployed, and the indigent, the government collects a lump sum tax called the "healthcare contribution," which is paid into the HIF. This tax was first levied in 1997. Since 1999 it has contained an 11 percent proportional component, levied on income, which has previously been exempt from social insurance contribution.[9] The government is also obliged to cover the deficit incurred by the HIF from general tax revenues.

With regard to expenditures, a special distinction is made between the HIF and other public revenues from general and local taxes. The HIF covers the recurrent costs of curative and some preventive services, whereas owners of healthcare facilities, mainly the local governments, should cover capital costs from its own revenues. However, covering capital costs is often beyond the financial capability of local governments; therefore the central government provides conditional and matching grants via a system of earmarked and targeted subsidies.

Because participation is compulsory, population insurance coverage is virtually universal. Nevertheless, entitlement for services must be proved by the possession of a personal health insurance card and identification number. The scope of benefits offered is very comprehensive, with exclusions limited to ineffective treatments and treatments for aesthetic purposes.[10] Certain high-cost medical technologies (positron emission tomography scans and lung, heart, liver, and pancreas transplantations) are also excluded from the HIF coverage, but they are covered under the government budget.

Most primary, secondary, and tertiary care services can be used free of charge. Copayments for medicines and medical aids make up the largest part of out-of-pocket payments. Ambulatory patients pay 100, 50, 30, 10, or 0 percent of the retail price for drugs or the difference between the price of the medicine and a fixed amount of subsidy.[11] However, a copayment exemption system is in place for the poor, eligibility for which is determined by the local governments. Copayments are also required for (1) chronic care, (2) certain dental services, (3) hospital admissions and outpatient specialist care visits if the official referral system is bypassed, and (4) "extra" hotel services in the hospital.[12]

The budget of the HIF is divided into more than 20 smaller budgets (kassza) according to the type of service. Providers are paid from these smaller budgets according to a variety of payment systems: family physician services are paid by capitation, outpatient specialist services by fee-for-service, acute inpatient care by diagnosis-related groups, and chronic inpatient care by bed-days adjusted for the complexity of the case. These budgets have a national ceiling, and interbudget transfers are not allowed.

Medical doctors and other health workers are mostly public employees and receive salaries according to the pay scale determined by the law, but they are among the lowest paid professionals in Hungary. However, certain specialists like surgeons and obstetricians/gynecologists receive substantial amounts of informal payment directly from the patients (Hungarian Central Statistical Office 1988). The practice of giving informal payment is an important carryover from the Communist regime; it seems to have survived the first 12 years of healthcare reform and probably will be very difficult to remove.

Health Resources

The uneven distribution of health resources is a major difficulty the new government still has to face. The legacy of the state-socialist health services system includes certain regional inequalities of service provision and inequalities between specialties, such as the excess inpatient capacities and the underdevelopment of primary care.

In comparison with European Union averages, Hungary has a large number of medical doctors, particularly specialists, per 1,000 population and a large number of hospital beds. However, Hungary has a shortage of qualified health and nonhealth support staff, including nurses and administrators. In 1997, the ratio between medical doctors and nurses was 1:1. See Table 19.6 for further human resources data.

The level and quality of the training of various health professionals seem less problematic, although the level of nursing education has recently been increased according to the standards of the European Union. The chronic shortages of nurses and other support personnel are more directly related to poor income potential because salaries are still extremely low and informal payments received are considerably less than those found among physicians. Trained nurses can easily find jobs in other industries for higher pay.

Physicians	357	**TABLE 19.6**
Nurses	392	Human
Dentists	42.4	Resources
Pharmacists	47	per 100,000 Population
Midwives	49.5	by Type

SOURCE: WHO Regional Office for Europe (1999).

Some of the reform measures of the past 12 years have tried to address these issues. These include the prioritized development of primary care, the reorganization of traditional public hygiene services according to the modern concept of public health, and the control of healthcare capacities by defining the "needed" number of hospital beds and consultation hours by county and by specialty. The latter measures resulted in a considerable decrease in the number of hospital beds, with a closing of 10,000 beds between 1996 and 1997 (Table 19.7). Nevertheless, the real impact on costs and outputs is still debated.

As a result of the liberalization policy of the Hungarian government, drugs, medical supplies, and medical equipment are readily available. On the other hand, the cost of pharmaceuticals accounts for almost 30 percent of all healthcare expenditures (OECD 1998), and despite the registration and licensing system in operation, the distribution of high-cost medical technologies is not yet under tight control.

Service Delivery

The delivery of healthcare services in Hungary is organized on the basis of geographic area, and since 1990 local governments have been responsible for the provision of services for their local populations. However, the principle of territorial supply obligation does not mean that the local govern-

Hospitals	163	**TABLE 19.7**
Hospital beds per 1,000 population	8.3	Hospital Availability
Hospital admissions per 1,000 population	237	and
Average length of stay	11 days	Utilization

SOURCE: OECD (1998).

ments have to produce the services themselves; contracting out services to private providers is permitted. Service provision is divided between the settlement local governments, which are responsible for primary care, and the county local governments, which are responsible for both inpatient and outpatient specialty care.

Primary care in Hungary includes family physician services, dental care, school health services, and pre- and postnatal care. In certain areas, family doctors provide services for both adults and children. In other areas, especially in cities and their vicinities, family pediatricians care for children. In both cases the physicians have three options. Under the "functional privatization" model, family doctors work as independent entrepreneurs who contract with the local government to provide care for the local residents and also with the National Health Insurance Fund Administration, from which they receive adjusted capitation payments according to the number of individuals registered with them. The local government retains ownership of and control over primary care surgeries and is responsible for covering the capital costs of the facilities, whereas the physician is responsible for covering the running costs from his or her capitation payments. A second option is that the physician has no contract with the local government (i.e., no responsibility for the local population) but receives capitation payments from the National Health Insurance Fund Administration according to the number of people enrolled. Finally, a family doctor may remain a salaried employee of the local government.

Since the introduction of the statutory health insurance model and the new family physician model of primary care, people are allowed to choose their family doctor freely. Each citizen can register at the family doctor of his or her choice using the personal health insurance card; this registration process serves as the basis for capitation payments from the National Health Insurance Fund Administration. Patients are required to have referrals from the family doctor for specialist services with the exception of obstetrics/gynecology; ear, nose, and throat diseases; ophthalmology; general surgery; traumatology; oncology; urology; psychiatric outpatient care; and dermatology.

Local governments are the main providers of specialty health services. By and large, settlement governments own polyclinics and in some cases municipal hospitals, whereas the county governments own large county hospitals. Outpatient specialist services may be provided in any of these health facilities. Municipal hospitals also provide basic secondary inpatient care for the local population. The large county hospitals with more than 1,000 beds provide secondary inpatient care for the population of an entire county in a wide spectrum of specialties such as cardiology and hematology. Highly specialized and expensive tertiary care services are provided on a regional or national basis by county hospitals, medical universities, or national institutes; the latter two are owned by the central government, that is, the Ministry of Education and the Ministry of Health.

Thus far, the private provision of curative services is limited in Hungary except for primary care. In 1997, more than 70 percent of family doctors worked as private entrepreneurs in offices and with equipment still owned by the local government. Most of the pharmacies (91 percent in 1997) are also private (National Health Insurance Fund Administration 1998). Except for a few church-owned hospitals, Hungary currently has only one private hospital and a few private polyclinics.

Prospects for the Future

Despite the considerable reform efforts and achievements of the past 12 years, health services in Hungary are still under major pressure. The imbalance of the structures, financing, and incentives is easily felt, but the direction in which the current government will proceed is not yet known.

The issues that warrant attention in the future can be summarized along the main health policy objectives. From the point of view of sustainability, stable and controllable sources of funding are needed, which implies high willingness to pay. On the other hand, equity in finance should be achieved. In any case, the discrepancy between needs and the available resources calls for more explicit priority setting in a more systematic way, but the feasibility of implementing such a method depends on how much it is accepted by the people. Inequality of access to services is manifested in uneven quality of the provided services moreso than access per se. Major causal factors are the current problems with the healthcare work force and the unresolved issue of covering capital costs. The scope for efficiency gains in purchasing and producing healthcare is not disputed, but less agreement is found on the means by which this can be realized.

Hungary has been a cautious reformer so far, that is, most options for future reform have remained open. Certainly the key issues will be the future sources of funding, especially the roles of social insurance, insurance competition, and taxation. The health policy agenda will not address the adaptation of a managed insurance model in the near future, and the single-purchaser health insurance model will likely be continued, at least during the time that the current government is in place. Currently, the delivery side is the focus of health policy, with plans for further privatization, especially in primary and secondary outpatient services. In the inpatient care sector alternative solutions are proposed for privatization, including the extension of hospital autonomy. Increased managerial freedom and managerial capacities are expected to improve efficiency without changes in ownership.

Notes

1. Act XXI of 1988, Decree No. 113/1989. (XI. 15.) MT of the Ministerial Council, and Decree No. 30/1989. (XI. 15.) SZEM of the Minister of Social Affairs and Health.

2. Act X of 1992.
3. Act XX of 1949 on the Constitution of the Republic of Hungary amended by Act XXXI of 1989.
4. Act LXXX of 1993 and Government Decree No. 72/1998. (IV. 10.) Korm.
5. Act CLIV of 1997 on Health Care.
6. Act XXXIII of 1992 on the Legal Status of Public Employees.
7. Decree No. 21/1998. (VI. 3.) NM of the Minister of Welfare, Government Decree No. 40/1997 (III.5.) Korm. and Decree No. 11/1997. (V. 28.) NM of the Ministry of Welfare.
8. Act LXXX of 1997.
9. Act LXVI of 1998.
10. Decree No. 46/1997 (XII. 17.) NM of the Ministry of Welfare.
11. Government Decree No. 217/1997 (XII. 1.) Korm.
12. Government Decree No. 284/1997 (XII. 23.) Korm.

REFERENCES

Gaál, P., Rékassy, B., and Healy, J. 1999. *Health Care Systems in Transition: Hungary.* Copenhagen: European Observatory on Health Care Systems.

Hungarian Central Statistical Office. 1999. *Magyar Statisztikai Évkönyv, 1998* (Statistical Yearbook of Hungary, 1998). Budapest: Hungarian Central Statistical Office.

———. 1998. *Magyar Statisztikai Évkönyv, 1997* (Statistical Yearbook of Hungary, 1997). Budapest: Hungarian Central Statistical Office.

———. 1995. *Magyar Statisztikai Évkönyv, 1994* (Statistical Yearbook of Hungary, 1994). Budapest: Hungarian Central Statistical Office.

———. 1988. *Vélemények az Egészségügyről és az Egészségügy Igénybevétele* (Opinion on Health Services and the Utilization of Health Services). Budapest: Hungarian Central Statistical Office.

Kopp, M. S. 1999. "A Magyar társadalom egészségi állapota" (The Health Status of the Hungarian Population). *Magyar Szemle* 9–10.

National Health Insurance Fund Administration. 1998. *Statistical Yearbook 1997.* Budapest: National Health Insurance Fund Administration.

Organization of Economic Cooperation and Development (OECD), Centre de Recherche, d'Etude et de Documentation en Economie de la Santé. 1998. *OECD Health Data 98.* Paris: OECD and Credes.

World Health Organization (WHO). 2001. Statistical Information System. Retrieved December 2001 from www.who.int/m/topics/whosis.

World Health Organization (WHO) Regional Office for Europe. 2000. *Highlights on Health in Hungary.* Retrieved December 2001 from www.who.dk.

———. 1999. *Health for All Database.* Copenhagen: WHO Regional Office for Europe.

20

CHINA

Philip C. Williams and Zhou Jian

Background Information

China's land area of 9,596,960 square kilometers is approximately equal to that of the United States. The country is bordered on the north by Kazakhstan, Mongolia, and Russia; on the east by North Korea, the Yellow Sea, and the China Sea; on the south by India, Nepal, Bhutan, Burma, Laos, and Vietnam; and on the west by Pakistan, Tajikistan, and Kyrgyzstan. Its climate ranges from tropical in the south to subarctic in the northern regions. Han Chinese account for 91.9 percent of the population of approximately 1.23 billion people; the remaining 8.1 percent of the population is composed of more than a dozen ethnic groups. Mandarin, Cantonese, Shanghaiese, Fuzhou, and Hokkien-Taiwanese are spoken, as well as a host of minority languages. Table 20.1 provides a demographic overview of present-day China.

China was unified as a nation in 221 BC under the Qin Dynasty. In 1912, after a revolution led by Sun Yat-sen, the last dynasty, Qing, was replaced by a republican government. Another revolution, headed by Mao Ze Dong, resulted in the 1949 establishment of the present Communist state.

During the 1950s, China was isolated from the Western powers, and the Soviet Union was its only powerful ally. To increase China's industrial base, Mao diverted peasants from agricultural work to the development of irrigation systems and new rural industries, which triggered widespread starvation and long-term agricultural displacement. Further disruption occurred during the Cultural Revolution (1966–76), when many educated professionals (including physicians) were persecuted, medical schools and universities were closed, and medical school graduates were required to work in rural areas as "barefoot doctors."

After Mao's death in 1976, his successor, Deng Xiao Ping, ended the Cultural Revolution and began a course of economic reform through a policy of "market socialism." The result has been an enormous expansion of agricultural and industrial production, with an attendant increase in per capita income.

Consequently, China has advanced from its position in the 1970s among the world's poorest countries to take a role as a major economic power. Recently, China's economy has grown at a rate of 8 percent per year,

TABLE 20.1

General
Demographics
(1996)

Population (millions)	1,232
Infant mortality per 1,000 live births	38
Under-five mortality per 1,000 live births	47
Life expectancy at birth (years)	69
Fertility rate	1.8
Percent urbanized	31

SOURCE: UNICEF (1998).

and indicators of social progress have consistently improved (Gurung 1996; World Bank 1998). Literacy rates dramatically improved between 1978, when only one-third of the population could read and write, and 1996, when 90 percent of men and 73 percent of women could do so. Primary school enrollment is now approaching 100 percent, and secondary school enrollment exceeds 50 percent for both men and women. During the same period, the income status of approximately 200 million Chinese rose above the poverty level (World Bank 1998). Tables 20.2 and 20.3 further detail the current economic and social situation in China.

China has several geographic and political subdivisions, including 23 provinces (including Taiwan), five autonomous regions, and three municipalities, each of which maintains its own regional administration subordinate to the central government. The legislative branch of China's central government is the unicameral National People's Congress (NPC), which is composed of members of the Chinese Communist Party who are indirectly elected at county or regional levels. The NPC elects the chief of state (president) for a term of five years and appoints his state council. The head of government (premier) is nominated by the president and confirmed by the NPC.

TABLE 20.2

Economic
and Social
Indicators

GNP per capita (U.S.$)	620
Real GDP per capita (P.P.P.$), 1994	2,800
Percent of health budget in public sector	0 (central government only)
ODA inflow/outflow as percent of GNP	0

NOTE: ODA = official development assistance.
SOURCE: UNICEF (1998); CIA (1998).

	Male	Female
Adult literacy rate	90	73
Primary school enrollment	99	98
Secondary school enrollment	60	51

SOURCE: UNICEF (1998).

TABLE 20.3 Education Indicators (percent)

Context: Health Needs

Immediately following Mao's victory in 1949, infant mortality was estimated at more than 250 deaths per 1,000 live births. Since that time, rates of infant and child mortality have fallen to approximately 38 and 47 deaths per 1,000 live births, respectively. With a per capita gross national product of less than U.S.$700 per year, China's mortality rates and long life expectancy, at 69 years, are surprisingly comparable to those of much richer nations (World Bank 1998).

China has experienced similar improvements in other areas. As a result of preventive efforts implemented by Mao's government in the 1950s, epidemic diseases such as cholera, plague, typhoid, and scarlet fever have essentially been eradicated. By the mid-1980s, the leading causes of death (cancer, cerebrovascular disease, and heart disease) mirrored those found in the industrialized world. However, tuberculosis remains a major health problem, as do hepatitis, malaria, and dysentery. Table 20.4 details rates of access to basic factors of preventative health maintenance.

Current public health priorities in China, some or all of which may be interrelated, include tobacco use, sexually transmitted diseases (including syphilis and HIV/AIDS), poverty, overpopulation, diet, and exercise.

Access to health services	N/A
Access to safe water	67%
Access to sanitation	24%
Immunization levels*	96%

TABLE 20.4 Access to Health Enhancing Factors

* Based on proportion of children fully immunized for diphtheria, measles, and polio by 12 months.
SOURCE: UNICEF (1998).

Tobacco Use

One of every three cigarettes smoked in the world is smoked in China (Tomlinson 1997). Tobacco use is a major cause of death, and risk ratios are similar to those of the United States and the United Kingdom. Thus, in the absence of tobacco-control intervention measures, about half of the 300 million smokers in China will eventually die of tobacco-related diseases. Tobacco now causes approximately 13 percent of all male deaths and 3 percent of all female deaths. Of these, approximately 60 percent result from chronic lung disease and lung cancer (Liu, Peto, and Chen 1998).

Tobacco use in China has followed a pattern similar to that found among adults in the United States, but it is occurring 40 years later. Per capita daily use of cigarettes is now declining in the United States, whereas consumption in China has risen from a rate of one cigarette per adult male in 1952 to four in 1972 and ten in 1992 (Liu, Peto, and Chen 1998). More than 60 percent of Chinese men are smokers, and more than 90 percent of the cigarettes sold in China are smoked by men 20 years old or older; Chinese tobacco mortality is expected to increase from its current rate to about 33 percent of deaths among men in the year 2030 (Niu et al. 1998). Notably, similar smoking patterns are not evident among Chinese women. In fact, smoking rates among women have fallen during the same 40-year period (Liu, Peto, and Chen 1998), although increases have recently been detected among 25- to 29-year-old women.

Efforts by the quasi-governmental Chinese Association on Smoking and Health to persuade people to stop smoking have been largely counteracted by the marketing successes of the state monopoly tobacco industry. However, recent government decisions to ban smoking on China's public transport system and to host the 10th World Conference on Tobacco and Health may signal an increased willingness to forego government profits in exchange for a reduction in tobacco-related risks to public health (Tomlinson 1997).

Sexually Transmitted Diseases

Behind dysentery and hepatitis, sexually transmitted diseases (STDs) are now China's third most common infectious disease category. Gonorrhea is the most common STD in China, but, according to the National STD Control Center, syphilis infections have been rising at a rate of 62 percent per year, and an increasing number of newborns are infected (Agence France Presse 1999). Following a 1987 World Health Organization meeting, the Chinese government announced its support of a global fight against AIDS, although the nation had confirmed only two deaths of Chinese citizens from the disease. By 1998, experts concluded that China was on the verge of a devastating AIDS epidemic, fueled by ignorance about HIV, the growth of prostitution, and a rise in intravenous drug use (ABC News 1998).

Poverty

The World Bank has suggested that, although China has achieved outstanding gains in the overall health status of its population since 1949, this progress may have slowed during the past two decades. According to World Bank reports, the persistence of poverty in rural areas of China has contributed to such stagnation because "poverty leads to ill-health and ill-health leads to poverty" (World Bank Group 1998a). Per capita health expenditure in designated poverty counties is less than half the national average (Agence France Presse 1999). Despite government support of public health programs since the 1970s, China may have experienced a reduction in coverage and quality of health services in poor rural areas.

On the other hand, a large-scale survey of almost 16,000 individuals living in eight provinces (more than half of whom resided in villages rather than cities or suburbs), led Henderson and colleagues to conclude that "China has achieved a very wide distribution of clinics and other services at the local level that are widely used by those who identify need for them" (Henderson et al. 1994). These results indicate that recent reports from China of a decline in health service accessibility for rural and low-income individuals may be erroneous or overstated (Henderson et al. 1994). This should not, however, discount poverty as a persistent public health concern, and the apparent equitable distribution of clinics in China does not necessarily disprove a link between poverty and ill health.

Overpopulation

Mao Ze Dong believed that human resources represented China's greatest defense in a world war, and the population of China rose from 540 million in 1950 to more than 850 million in 1970. However, such growth impeded Deng Xiao Ping's economic reform program and led to the adoption of the "one family, one child" policy in 1979. Since 1984, the policy has been alternately relaxed and enforced, depending on population goals and projections (Hesketh and Zhu 1997).

Among the public health consequences of the "one family, one child" policy are those characterized by Hesketh and Zhu (1997c) as "the good, the bad, and the ugly." "Good" results are obviously China's control of its previously unrestrained population growth and its consequent conservation of natural resources. In addition, the policy frees mothers from the burden of continuous pregnancy and allows more women to enter the workforce, thereby increasing family incomes. "Bad" consequences include the impingement of government policy on fundamental human reproductive rights, the resulting excess of male children due to sex-selective abortions, growing concern about support for the elderly, and the psychological effects on only children, such as the much-publicized "little emperor syndrome." "Ugly" reactions to the limited-family-size policy include female infanticide, forced abortions, and selective abortion of female fetuses.

Perhaps in response to the "bad" and "ugly" aspects of the one-child quota, China has embarked on a joint project with the United Nations to determine the effectiveness of sex education programs as an alternative to mandatory birth limits. This representative, cross-sectional study is being conducted in 32 counties and involves approximately 20 million people. If voluntary family planning measures prove successful, the program may be expanded to other areas of China.

Diet and Exercise

Health behaviors have been influenced by the social and economic transformation of Chinese society since the Cultural Revolution, leading to increasingly unhealthy eating patterns and sedentary lifestyles. The traditional Chinese diet was low in fat, but the proportion of adults who consume a low-fat diet has decreased across all income groups. Among adults between the ages of 20 and 45, the net effect has been a significant decline in the proportion of underweight individuals coupled with a significant increase in the proportion of overweight individuals, except among low-income women (Popkin 1994). According to the Obesity Research Center of the China Health Sciences Institute, more than 70 million Chinese were overweight in 1996, including more than 40 percent of adults living in Beijing (Tomlinson 1997).

As may be expected, a polarizing trend of physical activity patterns among certain groups of people has developed: overweight individuals tend to adopt a more sedentary lifestyle, whereas those who remain in the underweight category maintain or increase their levels of physical activity (Popkin 1994). In response to these unhealthy lifestyle changes, a "grand physical training project" has been proposed by the State Physical Culture and Sports Commission. The initiative includes establishment of "physical training castles" in 20 large cities to provide facilities for swimming, bodybuilding, and general sports activities.

Cancer, stroke, respiratory diseases, and heart disease are by far the leading causes of mortality in China, with significant differences between rural and urban populations. In rural areas, where smoking and the use of bituminous coal for heating are more prevalent, respiratory diseases are the leading cause of death. In urban areas, where conditions and lifestyles more closely approximate those of Western industrialized nations, cancer and stroke are the leading causes of death. Table 20.5 further illustrates mortality and morbidity among rural and urban populations.

Organization and Management of the Health System

Universal healthcare is a basic tenet of Chinese health policy; health services are designed to reach that goal by generating maximum output from the country's limited healthcare workforce. This policy has resulted in a

Leading Causes of Death	Percent of Deaths	
	Urban	Rural
1. Cancer	22.71	17.12
2. Stroke	22.63	17.82
3. Heart diseases	16.77	11.48
4. Respiratory diseases	14.09	23.38
5. Injuries/poisonings	6.18	11.67
6. Digestive system diseases	3.10	4.39

TABLE 20.5
Morbidity and Mortality Measures

SOURCE: Ministry of Health (1997).

systemwide focus on preventive rather than therapeutic medicine since the early 1950s. Preventive health networks are responsible for organizing and mobilizing Great Patriotic Health Campaigns aimed at improving nutrition, sanitation, water quality, and disease prevention (Hesketh and Zhu 1997). The Four Pests Campaign, for example, targeted the elimination of flies, mosquitoes, rats, and sparrows (the last because they eat grain).

Organization and management of the health system have primarily been coordinated through the central government's Ministry of Public Health, but health policy jurisdiction sometimes overlaps with other central government and regional agencies. For example, the Ministry of Finance retains final control over health sector budgets, the Ministry of Labor and Personnel sets occupational health and safety standards, and the Ministry of Environmental Protection oversees air and water pollution and toxic waste control. Jurisdiction is also apportioned among departments of public health, which are located within each province, municipality, and autonomous region, and among county-level subdivisions within each of these departments. At all levels, the Chinese Communist Party plays a dominant role in policy formulation, promotion, and implementation (Gurung 1996).

The central government health organization includes bureaucratic divisions for epidemic prevention, medical administration, science and education, maternal and child health, planning and finance, pharmaceutical administration, and traditional medicine. The National Disease Reporting System collects data on morbidity and mortality associated with communicable diseases and disease outbreaks. The National Disease Surveillance Points comprise a sentinel surveillance network based on cluster random sampling, with a sampling size equal to one percent of the total population. Other public health surveillance and monitoring agencies include regional antiepidemic and hygiene stations, maternal and child health departments, and provincial and local health departments. Data are processed through the Nationwide Anti-epidemic Computer Telecommunication Network, but disease reporting remains a problem in very poor and remote regions of China.

Financing

As a result of the 1982 decision to introduce market factors into the financing of health services in China, the central government's role as the principal funding source has been drastically reduced; central government spending now accounts for less than one percent of total health expenditures (Hsiao 1995). In addition, the collapse of the collective agricultural system resulted in the dissolution of the cooperative medical system, which had administered free healthcare. This combination of reduced funding roles among the central and cooperative systems compelled provincial and county governments to provide "basic" workforce salaries (well below a living wage) for healthcare workers and monies for new capital investments. However, these funds cover only 20 to 30 percent of hospital expenditures (Hsiao 1995); patient contributions on a fee-for-service basis account for the remainder (Hsiao 1996).

Even among employees of state enterprises, less than half the workforce is covered by health insurance, and coverage for dependents is rare. Consequently, better healthcare facilities tend to be located in areas where workers are covered by insurance or where wealthier individuals who can afford the out-of-pocket costs reside.

In theory, prices are set by a central government finance bureau and adjusted at the provincial level according to local conditions, but exceptions to these pricing guidelines are made to allow healthcare providers to operate at a profitable level. For example, hospitals are permitted to adjust the price schedule for Western drugs and technology use. As a result, drug charges now constitute half of all healthcare costs, and the major priority of some local healthcare officials is the acquisition of high-technology medical apparatus such as magnetic resonance imaging, computed tomography, and even "myopia correction" machines, with little regard for the actual health service needs of the community (Hesketh and Zhu 1997b).

Between 1986 and 1993, per capita spending on healthcare increased 11 percent per year, after adjustment for inflation, reaching U.S.$84 in 1993 (Du 1995). For half of the rural population, the cost of one hospitalization exceeds the average annual per capita income. A recent study conducted by seven Chinese medical schools in collaboration with the Harvard School of Public Health found that 28 percent of the population did not seek healthcare when they were ill and 51 percent had refused recommended hospitalization because they could not afford the costs. The study also found that 25 percent of surveyed households had borrowed money to pay for healthcare and that another 6 percent had sold assets (Hsaio 1996).

Regional experiments are underway to address the inequities and inefficiencies in the Chinese healthcare financing system. In the Guandong province, all employers must provide insurance coverage for female workers of childbearing age, whereas in the province of Yunnan, the entire population is required to pay a small insurance premium each month to subsidize childbirth costs for mothers at high risk (Hesketh and Zhu 1997).

Health Resources

During the Cultural Revolution, many professionals (including doctors) were persecuted, and medical schools were closed. Medical school graduates were relocated to the countryside, where many trained local peasants to serve patients as "barefoot doctors," and numerous others were forced to work the land. Medical schools reopened in 1972, but medical training and student selection were subject to political directives, with emphasis on manual labor and conformity to the philosophy of Chairman Mao (Worden, Savada, and Dolan 1987).

In 1992, China had 1.57 physicians, 1.15 pharmacists, and 0.9 nurses per 1,000 Chinese residents. Professional associations do not exist, and professional mobility is tightly controlled by the central government. A study of 180 randomly selected villages in China conducted between 1992 and 1995 determined that 30 percent of the villages had no village doctor (Hsaio 1996). Table 20.6 provides additional details about available human resources within the healthcare system.

The majority of China's hospitals and clinics are state-owned, including those administered by county and provincial governments, municipalities, village resident committees, and the Ministry of Health. The rest, which are mostly clinics rather than hospitals, are owned and operated by collectives, joint ventures, or private entities. The latter category denotes facilities

	Public	Private
Physicians	1,440,921	64,421
Nurses	1,182,784	15,444
Administrators	445,827	2,220
Traditional practitioners	297,414	48,319

TABLE 20.6
Human Resources

SOURCE: Ministry of Health (1997).

established by doctors who have retired or resigned from the workforce. The number of private hospitals in China is assumed to be insignificant. The availability of the various medical facilities is shown in Table 20.7.

Types and functions of health facilities in China depend on location and level of sophistication within a three-tiered service delivery structure. In urban China, the three tiers include lane health stations, street health stations, and district hospitals. In rural China, the levels are village health stations, township health centers, and county hospitals.

China's hospital facilities have been described as continuously deteriorating and of poor quality, with a large number built before the 1949 revolution or, in the case of rural hospitals, during the 1950s. Hospital equipment tends to fall within one of two categories: outdated resources that are not regulated for quality or ill-fitting Western technology that has been purchased for the primary purpose of circumventing provincial pricing guidelines and increasing hospital revenues (World Bank 1992).

Approximately 28 percent of Chinese hospitals are devoted to the practice of traditional medicine (Rosenthal 1987). More than 20 percent of China's doctors practice only traditional medicine; this figure does not include those practitioners of modern medicine who adopt one or more traditional methods into their practice (Gurung 1996).

China is self-sufficient for its supply of traditional and modern drugs and is, in fact, an exporter of both. Approximately 800 pharmaceutical plants produce modern drugs, whereas 480 factories produce traditional herbal supplements. The government does regulate drug safety, efficacy, and effectiveness, but no regulatory cost evaluation of pharmaceuticals takes place.

Service Delivery

At the First National Health Congress in 1950, four guidelines were formulated for the organization of healthcare in China (Hesketh and Zhu 1997):

TABLE 20.7
Number and Types of Health Services Facilities by Population*

	Number	Per 1,000 Population
Hospitals	89,543	0.073
Health centers/clinics	225,490	0.183
Specialty facilities**	6,652	0.005

* Based on 1,232 million population.
** Specialty facilities are predominately hospitals but also include a few specialty clinics.
SOURCE: Ministry of Health (1997).

1. Medicine should serve the workers, peasants, and soldiers.
2. Preventive medicine should take precedence over therapeutic medicine.
3. Traditional Chinese medicine should be integrated with Western scientific medicine.
4. Health work should be combined with mass movements.

Vestiges of this organizational structure can still be found in rural China, where the administration of healthcare services is organized according to the three tiers. In rural areas, the village health station offers rudimentary preventive and primary care (mostly first aid and pediatric) services practiced by a village doctor who is assisted by one or more midwives or health aids. The township health center, which is the second tier, offers similar services, but it is staffed by a more highly trained physician who supervises assistant doctors, village doctors, and nurses. The third tier, the county hospital, is managed by a team of still more highly educated physicians and is equipped to offer inpatient and outpatient services through a staff of assistant doctors, nurses, and technicians. The two lower tiers comprise the "rural collective health system" that provides most of China's rural medical care; the third tier is reserved for the most seriously ill patients.

Evidence suggests that, although China has achieved a broad distribution of clinics and other services at the local level and developed a system widely used by those who identify a need for those services, health facilities in rural areas are planned and staffed in response to central government directives; no mechanism appears to be in place for ensuring the allocation of resources according to health priorities. Health facilities at the three rural administrative tiers have conflicting referral and supervisory relationships and often function in competition with one another (World Bank 1997).

In urban areas, the first two tiers (the lane and street health stations) are staffed by mid-level medical clinicians with training that is equivalent in most cases to that received in the West by physician assistants and nurse practitioners. These facilities are equipped to offer immunizations, family planning advice, and other preventive services. District hospitals offer a full range of inpatient and outpatient medical services. One consequence of the three-tiered system in urban areas has been a form of system gaming, which enables people employed by powerful state enterprises or government agencies to circumvent the paramedical stages and seek care directly from district or municipal hospitals (Zeckhauser 1996). Table 20.8 further details use of health facilities and services.

Prospects for the Future

The future direction of China's health system will depend in part on the outcome of system experiments currently underway. For example, the World Bank recently announced the China Basic Health Services Project, which

TABLE 20.8
Service Use

	Number (millions)	Per 1,000 Population*
Hospital admissions	50.44	41
Hospital days	545.92	443
Outpatient/clinic visits	2,157	1,751

* Calculated on 1,232 million population.
SOURCE: Ministry of Health (1997).

is designed to improve the management of rural health resources, upgrade rural health facilities, improve the quality of health services, and increase affordability of essential healthcare in ten poor provinces and the municipality of Chongqing. The six-year, U.S.$127.6 million project was initiated in 1999. The project's success will be assessed on the basis of improvements in health facilities and services for the region's estimated 48 million people; presumably, a successful outcome will result in the extension of the project to other regions. Similarly, success or failure of the United Nations' sex education and family planning program as an alternative to mandatory birth limits could determine the central government's willingness to relax the mandatory "one family, one child" policy.

Over the past three decades, the burden of healthcare financing has shifted from the Chinese central government and collective enterprises toward individual fee-for-service payment. Such action lays the foundation for a hodgepodge of regional and private insurance arrangements. Current developments in healthcare financing at the provincial level suggest that regional differences may proliferate and expand over time; this may give rise to a patchwork system of healthcare financing that could evolve into a mixture of central, provincial, and private financing arrangements not unlike those that currently exist in Germany and the United States. Results from the experiments in the Guandong and Yunnan provinces will determine the extent to which other provinces imitate, customize, or reject similar measures.

China's current healthcare structure, which was completely reorganized during the 1950s, is again undergoing rapid change. This time, however, the direction and goals of the transformation are less clearly defined and will depend heavily on the effects of political, historical, and social forces.

REFERENCES

ABC News. 1998. "China on Verge of AIDS Outbreak." Retrieved 30 November 2000 from http://www.abcnews.com:80/sections/world/DailyNews/chinaaids981130.html.

Agence France Presse. 1999. "Suspected Killer 'Spirit Doctor' Arrested for

Murdering 190." Retrieved 18 January 2001 from http://www.insid-echina.com/china/news/99011806.html.

———. 1998. "Syphilis, Other STDs on the Rise." Retrieved 08 December 2000 from http://www.insidechina.com/china/news/98120811.html.

———. 1998a. "WHO Calls for Universal Health Care." Retrieved 23 November 2000 from http://www.insidechina.com/china/news/98112314.html.

Du, L., and Yin, W. 1995. "Health Care Costs and Financing Patterns in China 1970–1993." Proceedings of the International Health Care Seminar, Beijing, China, October 8–10 1995. Beijing: Chinese National Institute of Health Economics (in Chinese, cited by Hsiao 1996 below).

Gurung, D. K. 1996. "Health Care Systems: A Comparison Between China and the United States." Unpublished working paper (October 1996). Clemson, SC: Clemson University, Department of Agricultural and Applied Economics.

Henderson, G. E., Akin, J. S., Li, Z. M., et al. 1994. "Equity and the Utilization of Health Services: Report of an Eight-Province Survey in China." Social Science and Medicine 39 (5): 687–99.

Hesketh, T., and Zhu, W. X. 1997. "Health in China: From Mao to Market Reform." British Medical Journal 314: 1543–48.

———. 1997a. "Health in China: Maternal and Child Health in China." British Medical Journal 314: 1898–04.

———. 1997b. "Health in China: The Healthcare Market." British Medical Journal 314: 1616–22.

———. 1997c. "Health in China: The One Child One Family Policy: The Good, the Bad, and the Ugly." British Medical Journal 314: 1685–90.

Hsiao, W. C. L. 1995. "The Chinese Healthcare System: Lessons for Other Nations." Social Science and Medicine 41: 1047–55.

Hsiao, W. C. L., and Liu, Y. 1996. "Economic Reform and Health: Lessons from China (Editorial)." New England Journal of Medicine 335 (6): 430–32.

Liu, B. Q., Peto, R., and Chen, Z. M. 1998. "Emerging Tobacco Hazards in China: 1. Retrospective Proportional Mortality Study of One Million Deaths." British Medical Journal 317: 1411–22.

Ministry of Health. 1997. National Health Statistics Annual 1997. People's Republic of China (in Chinese).

Niu, S. R., Yang, G. H., Chen, Z. M. et al. 1998. "Emerging Tobacco Hazards in China: 2. Early Mortality Results from a Prospective Study." British Medical Journal 317: 1423–24.

Popkin, B. M. 1994. "Social Change and Its Nutritional Impact: The China Health and Nutrition Survey." China Exchange News 22 (2): 9–11.

Rosenthal, M. M. 1987. "Health Care in the People's Republic of China: Moving Toward Modernization." Westview Special Studies in China. Boulder: Westview Press.

Tomlinson, R. 1997. "China Bans Smoking on Trains and Buses (News article)." British Medical Journal 314: 769.

UNICEF. 1998. "The State of the World's Children." Retrieved 01 December 2001 from http://www.unicef.org/sowc98/tab1.htm.

U.S. Central Intelligence Agency (CIA). 1998. The World Factbook 1998.

Retrieved 01 December 2000 from http://www.odci.gov/cia/ publications/factbook/ch.html.

Worden, R. L., Savada, A. M., and Dolan, R. E. (eds.) 1987. "Health Care." In *China: A Country Study.* Washington, DC: Federal Research Division, Library of Congress.

World Bank Group. 1998. "Country Brief: The World Bank and China." Retrieved 01 December 2000 from http://www.worldbank.org/html/ extdr/offrep/eap/cn2.htm.

———. 1998a. *Loan & Credit Summary: China Basic Health Services Project.* Washington, DC: World Bank.

———. 1997. "Reducing Poverty in China: World Bank Loans US$180 million for Qinba Mountains Project." News Release No. 97/1375/EAP. Washington, DC: World Bank.

———. 1992. *China: Long Term Issues and Options in the Health Transition.* Washington, DC: World Bank.

Zeckhauser, R. J. 1996. "Comment: Government Intervention in Markets for Education and Health Care." In *Individual and Social Responsibility: Child Care, Education, Medical Care, and Long-Term Care in America,* edited by V. Fuchs. Chicago: The University of Chicago Press.

TURKEY

Aysıt Tansel

Background Information

The Republic of Turkey was founded in 1923 by Mustafa Kemal Atatürk, who was also its first president. Straddling the Straits of Bosphorous, Turkey is bordered by Bulgaria and Greece on the west; Georgia, Armenia, Azerbaijan, and Iran on the east; and Iraq and Syria on the south, and it covers an area of 775,000 square kilometers. Turkey is governed by a parliamentary democracy. The country is divided into 81 provinces, each of which is administered by a governor appointed by the Ministry of Interior and responsible to the central government.

The Republic of Turkey did not inherit a coherent structure for the provision of health services. After the founding of the Republic, the public sector made major investments in health systems in terms of both personnel training and facility construction. Programs to control malaria, tuberculosis, and other infectious diseases received particular attention, and over time, public hospitals increased in number. The first social security system was established in 1945 to provide health and retirement benefits to workers. During the early 1960s, major reforms were undertaken with the goal of making health services universally accessible; the expected results were never considered by observers to be achieved.

On January 24, 1980, structural adjustment and stabilization programs were implemented, marking the beginning of a period of major economic policy changes. Interest rate ceilings were abolished, the exchange rate was allowed to float, and the foreign trade regime was liberalized; private investment in the healthcare sector was also encouraged.

Since the late 1980s, several proposals to reform the Turkish healthcare system have been proposed because the current system is considered unsatisfactory by many in terms of both quality and quantity; regional differences and rural-urban differences are both major concerns. Health system reform is ranked high on the government agenda.

Turkey's per capita income in 1998 was U.S.$3,160. The labor force was 30 million in 1998; it grew by an average of 3.3 percent annually during the period from 1990 to 1998. Women made up 37 percent of the labor force in 1998, a figure that has remained relatively stable. The unemployment rate in 1998 was about 12 percent; the combined unemployment/underemployment rate was about 18 percent. The inflation rate has remained quite high; in 1998, the inflation rate as measured by the consumer price index was 70 percent. To combat this, a major disinflation program was initiated in 1999. Table 21.1 provides further details about Turkey's economic and social indicators.

Turkey's population reached 63.5 million in 1998. Population density—although still not high by European standards—has also increased from 58 per square kilometer in 1980 to 82 per square kilometer in 1998. The average annual growth rate of the population was 1.8 percent during the 1990 to 1998 period, the same growth seen during the period from 1980 to 1990.

Turkey's population is relatively young; children under 15 comprise about one-third of the total population. Although it is not currently very large, the elderly population is projected to rise in coming decades; this trend will have significant effects on the country's healthcare needs. Life expectancy at birth in 1997 was 67 years for men and 72 years for women. The fertility rate was 4.3 births per woman in 1980, and this declined to 2.7 in 1997. Urbanization has been rapid, with 73 percent of the total population living in urban areas in 1998.

Mortality rates have declined significantly over the last two decades, but current levels are still very high by European standards. The infant mortality rate per 1,000 live births was 109 in 1980, declining to 40 in 1997. The under-five mortality rate per thousand was 133 in 1980, declin-

TABLE 21.1
Economic and Social Indicators

Total area (thousand km²)	775
GDP per capita (U.S.$)	3,160
Real GDP per capita (P.P.P.$)	6,350
Human Development Index score (%)	72.80
Human Development Index rank	86
Labor force:	
Total (millions)	30
Average annual growth rate (%), 1990–98	3.3
Female (% of labor force)	37
Unemployment rate (%)	12.3
Underemployment rate (%)	5.8
Average annual rate of inflation (%)	69.7
Health spending: share, public in GDP (%)	2.7

SOURCE: World Bank (2000); UNDP (1999); State Institute of Statistics (1998a).

ing to 50 in 1997. Ten percent of children under five suffered from malnutrition. The maternal mortality rate per 100,000 live births was 180 during the 1990s. According to the 1998 Turkish Demographic and Health Survey, about 80 percent of births are attended by health personnel (Ministry of Health 1998). Table 21.2 provides further demographic details.

The 1997 adult illiteracy rate was 26 percent for women and 8 percent for men. Illiteracy is a particularly difficult problem for women in Turkey. The proportion of the relevant age group enrolled in primary school is high, and the gender gap is small at this level. However, female enrollment levels lag far behind those of males at the middle school and higher education levels. A major educational reform was initiated in August 1997 extending compulsory primary schooling from five to eight years, thereby covering the middle school years. Considerable regional differentials in educational attainment have persisted over time. Educational indicators are detailed in Table 21.3.

According to the 1995 Multiple Indicator Cluster Survey, 62 percent of dwellings in urban areas had piped water, whereas only 28 percent of dwellings in rural areas had piped water. Eighty percent of urban dwellings had flush-toilet-to-sewage-system sanitation facilities; only 19 percent of rural dwellings were so equipped. Table 21.4 shows vaccination rates for children between the ages of 12 and 23 months at any time. No significant differences between genders are found, but coverage in rural areas is lower than that found in urban areas.

		TABLE 21.2
Population (millions), 1998	63.5	Selected
Population per square kilometer, 1998	82	Demographic
Population growth rate (%), 1990–98	1.8	Indicators
Infant mortality rate (per 1,000 live births), 1997	40	
Under-five mortality rate (per 1,000), 1997	50	
Maternal mortality rate (per 100,000 live births)	180	
Prevalence of child malnutrition (%)	10	
Total fertility rate, 1997	2.7	
Percent of population urbanized, 1998	73	
Life expectancy at birth (years), 1997		
Female	72	
Male	68	

SOURCE: World Bank (2000); State Institute of Statistics (1998).

TABLE 21.3
Education
Indicators

	Female	Male
Adult illiteracy rate, 1997	26	8
Enrollment ratio, 1994–95		
Primary school	89	93
Middle school	54	76
High school	39	59
Tertiary level	14	21

SOURCE: World Bank (2000); State Institute of Statistics computations.

Context: Health Needs

Epidemiological data in Turkey are not very reliable, particularly for rural areas. However, data indicate the following leading causes of mortality in Turkey (State Institute of Statistics 1999):

- infancy: infectious diseases
- children between the ages of 1 and 5: infectious diseases and complications associated with malnutrition
- adolescents and young adults: accidents
- people between the ages of 25 and 44: heart disease and accidents
- people between the ages of 45 and 64: heart disease and neoplasms

Under-five mortality accounts for 50 percent of all deaths. Child health is thus one of the most significant health problems in the country. Currently, infant mortality is 40 per 1,000 live births and the under-five mortality rate is 50 per 1,000. Both of these figures are higher in rural areas than in cities.

Infectious diseases (particularly malaria, tuberculosis, and measles) are also a significant focus of concern. After years of malaria eradication

TABLE 21.4
Access to
Health-
Enhancing
Factors

	Urban	Rural
Access to safe (piped) water (%)	62	28
Access to sanitation (flush-to-sewage-system) (%)	87	19
Child immunization levels (all vaccinations) (%)	74	64

SOURCE: State Institute of Statistics and UNICEF (1996).

campaigns, malaria infection was reduced to only 1,263 cases in 1970. However, since the mid-1970s, agricultural development programs in southern and southeastern Turkey created favorable conditions for the proliferation of malaria vectors, resulting in 36,842 cases of malaria in 1998. In addition, in 1998, Turkey had 20,222 cases of tuberculosis and 27,120 cases of measles (Ministry of Health 1998). In contrast, only 235 AIDS cases and 416 HIV-positive carriers were reported in 1997 (Ministry of Health 1997).

Organization and Management of the Health System

Health expenditures as a percentage of the gross domestic product in 1997 amounted to 2.7 percent (World Bank 2000), which is lower than most countries in the same income group. Health expenditures as a percentage of gross national product were 3.71 percent in 1996 as compared with the OECD average of 7.2 percent (Tokat 1998). The share of Ministry of Health expenditures in the general budget was 2.81 percent in 1999 (Ministry of Health 1998). In 1996, an estimated 43 percent of total health expenditures came from the general budget, 25 percent came from premiums, and the remaining 32 percent came from direct household expenditures. Thus, the public sector (general budget and premiums) is responsible for 68 percent of all health expenditures in Turkey (Tokat 1998). In 1996, per capita health expenditures were U.S.$108 in Turkey, whereas the OECD average was U.S.$1,828 (Tokat 1998).

Under the Law on Socialization of Health Services, enacted in 1961, the government is required to provide preventive and curative services, especially in rural areas. The State Planning Organization is responsible for planning healthcare services, and it drafts objectives and policies in the Five Year Development Plans. The Ministry of Health develops and implements operational plans. Once its budget is approved by the Parliament, the Ministry decides on resource allocation for recurrent and capital expenditures. Health directorates at the provincial level administer health services. Provincial health directorates are administered by the Ministry of Health, but they are accountable to the provincial governors. In 1998, Turkey had 1,180 hospitals. The Ministry of Health operates 732 hospitals, which accounts for more than half of the hospital beds in the country. These hospitals had an average occupancy rate of 55 percent. Hospital services are also provided by the Ministry of Defense, universities, the Social Security Organization, state-owned enterprises, and the private sector. The Social Security Organization provides services in 118 hospitals, which contain about 16 percent of the hospital beds. The 36 university hospitals account for about 14 percent of beds. Table 21.5 provides further details about health facility availability.

TABLE 21.5
Health
Facilities

Health posts	11,881
Health centers	5,538
Hospitals	1,180
Hospital beds	164,887
Bed occupancy rate	59%

SOURCE: Ministry of Health (1998a).

Financing

Turkey's healthcare financing system is quite complex and involves a number of organizations, including the following:

1. *Ministry of Health:* The Ministry of Health is financed by taxation through the general budget. Ministry of Health hospitals also have revolving funds, which have become increasingly important. Revolving funds include fees paid by insurers and individual users and tax revenues derived from the sale of fuel, new cars, petroleum, and cigarettes.

2. *University hospitals:* The two main funding sources for university hospitals are the general budget through the Higher Education Board and revolving funds. The Ministry of Finance controls recurrent expenditures of the university hospitals, and the State Planning Organization controls capital expenditures. As is the case with Ministry of Health hospitals, fees paid by insurers and individual users constitute the main sources of revolving funds.

3. *Social Insurance Organization (SSK):* SSK is a social security organization for private sector wage earners and blue-collar workers of state-owned enterprises. It provides retirement and healthcare services, but it does not provide or pay for preventive healthcare. Members use SSK services in addition to Ministry of Health and university hospitals. SSK health services are funded by the premiums paid by employers and employees. Fees paid by nonmembers using SSK services (e.g., Bağ-Kur members as discussed below) and the 20 percent copayment for drugs paid by outpatients are relatively minor funding sources. SSK has difficulty collecting premiums from employers, and it has been experiencing financial difficulties. Of those people whose healthcare was paid for by the SSK, health expenditures per insured person were U.S.$41 in 1996 (Tokat 1998).

4. *Bağ-Kur:* Bağ-Kur, established in 1972, is the insurance organization for the self-employed. Its original function was to provide retirement benefits; healthcare services were not provided until 1985. Bağ-Kur has no health facilities of its own; it contracts with healthcare providers

and reimburses them at standard rates. Currently about 14 million people are covered by Bağ-Kur. Subscription to Bağ-Kur health insurance is rather low, with only about three million active members in 1999 including both agricultural and nonagricultural members. Active members have a copayment of 20 percent for drug purchases, whereas retired members pay a 10 percent copayment. Bağ-Kur experiences difficulties in collecting premiums. Its health expenditures were U.S.$23 per person in 1996 (Tokat 1998).

5. *Government Employees Retirement Fund (Emekli Sandığı [ES]):* ES is a pension fund providing retirement and health benefits for retired civil servants that is financed by contributions from active civil servants and government employers. However, neither active civil servants nor retirees pay any specific health insurance premium. ES contracts with providers (usually Ministry of Health facilities) and pays for all healthcare services for retired civil servants based on amounts charged by the providers. ES is managed by the Ministry of Finance and often operates at a deficit, which is covered by transfers from the general budget. ES health expenditure per person was U.S.$188 in 1996 (Tokat 1998).

6. *Active civil servants:* Most government organizations have healthcare units that provide at least primary healthcare services for their employees. For secondary or tertiary healthcare, civil servants are referred to other healthcare providers. All expenses are covered by their organizations through specific state budget allocations, and a 20 percent copayment is assessed for drug expenses.

7. *Private health insurance:* In 1995, about 30 private health insurance companies covered about 500,000 people, primarily employees of banks, insurance companies, computer companies, chambers of commerce, and the like. Most subscribers purchase private insurance in addition to their membership in the SSK. Private employers often pay the private insurance premium in addition to their statutory obligation of SSK premiums. Active civil servants or ES members may also purchase private insurance.

8. *Green card holders:* A green card is issued to poor citizens who are unable to pay for health services; applicants are required to provide information about family income, assets, and insurance status. Green card holders get free treatment at any government health center including Ministry of Health hospitals and university hospitals; the Ministry of Health pays the entire cost. Green cards have been issued since 1992. In 1997, 6.7 million people held green cards, which accounted for about 10 percent of the population (Ministry of Health 1998).

Table 21.6 shows the proportions of the population covered by different insurance schemes. SSK has the largest membership among the insurance schemes, covering almost 40 percent of the population. Retired civil servants constitute the smallest insured group. About 66 percent of the population is covered by mandatory public insurance. However, 34 percent have no insurance coverage.

As observed in Table 21.6, health expenditures per insured person in 1996 in U.S. dollars were highest for retired civil servants and lowest for Bağ-Kur members. This confirms the widely held belief that Emekli Sandığı provides the best healthcare services.

Health Resources

Table 21.7 provides information about health facilities and human resources. In spite of significant improvements over time, the availability of basic health services is inadequate, and substantial regional differences are seen in accessibility to care.

Service Delivery

The health post (sağlık evi) is the smallest health unit. Each post, which serves a population of 2,500 to 3,000 in rural areas, is typically staffed by a midwife. In 1998, Turkey had 11,881 health posts. At the next level, health centers (sağlık ocağı) typically serve a population of 5,000 to 10,000. Health center staff typically consists of a physician, a nurse, a midwife, a

TABLE 21.6 Health Insurance Coverage by Type and Percent of Persons Covered	Number (thousands)	Percent of Population	Health Expenditures (U.S.$)
Public mandatory insurance			
Emekli sandiği (retired civil servants)	2,000	3.2	188
SSK (workers)	24,000	38.5	41
BağKur (self-employed)	9,000	14.4	23
Active civil servants	6,000	9.6	—
Not covered	21,400	34.3	—
Private insurance	—	< 1	—
Total	62,400	100	—

SOURCE: Ministry of Health (1998a); Tokat (1998).

Physicians	73,659	**TABLE 21.7**
Nurses	67,265	Human
Midwives	40,230	Resources,
Dentists	12,737	1998
Pharmacists	20,557	
Health officers and technicians	39,659	

SOURCE: Ministry of Health (1998).

health technician, and a medical secretary. Health centers have multiple patient care functions, including prevention and treatment of communicable diseases, immunizations, and provision of maternal and child health services including family planning. They are also charged with conducting public health education, implementing environmental health programs, and collecting statistical data. In 1998, the number of health centers was 5,538. Turkey also has a variety of specialty dispensaries: 283 maternal, child health, and family planning centers; 271 tuberculosis dispensaries; 12 venereal diseases dispensaries; 5 leprosy dispensaries; and 1 mental health dispensary were in operation in 1998.

Turkey had 1,180 hospitals in 1998. Sixty-two percent are operated by the Ministry of Health; 10 percent are SSK hospitals; 18 percent are private hospitals; 4 percent are Ministry of Defense hospitals; and 3 percent are university hospitals.

In 1997, there was one physician per 853 people and one nurse for every 935 people. Among physicians, 44 percent were specialists and 56 percent were general practitioners. Midwives and health officers provide most primary care, whereas nurses work in secondary and tertiary care. Physicians, dentists, and pharmacists are all university-educated. Although some nurses and midwives are university-educated, the majority are graduates of health vocational high schools.

Although most physicians work at least part time in the public sector, dentists, pharmacists, and specialist physicians usually have private practices; many specialist physicians combine a part-time job in a public hospital with a private practice. In 1996, 86 percent of physicians worked in the public sector either full time or part time (Tokat 1998). Other health personnel, including nurses, midwives, technicians, and general practitioners, are typically employed in the public sector. Ministry of Health personnel are civil servants and are paid accordingly; their pay scale is based on education and years of public service with cost-of-living adjustments made twice a year. As civil servants, public sector health personnel are guaranteed lifetime employment and have few incentives to improve their performance.

Provincial health directorates and hospital managers have little autonomy and little authority to manage their own staff. A head physician and an administrator are responsible for each Ministry of Health hospital. The head physician typically is not expected to be charged with administrative duties (Kılıçdaroğlu 1998).

The geographic distribution of health personnel is unbalanced. Shortages of all kinds of health personnel are seen in the eastern part of the country and in rural areas. Compulsory service in the less-developed regions for specialist and nonspecialist physicians was introduced in the early 1980s; problems in service quality and job satisfaction resulted in the discontinuation of the program in 1994. There are no incentives to work in these regions.

Prospects for the Future

Several of Turkey's health indicators are not considered satisfactory by most observers. Authorities contend that the most common causes of mortality and morbidity are preventable and controllable. Population growth, demographic changes, and technological developments have also placed increasing demands on limited healthcare resources. Resources are widely believed to be wasted despite their short supply; service quality is poor and inefficient.

The current healthcare system also presents problems of equity. Only insured people and green card holders are entitled to free access to healthcare services. Only 66 percent of the population is covered by a social insurance scheme; 34 percent (about 21 million people) are uninsured (see Table 21.6). Generally, low-income urban workers in the informal sector (those workers who do not have social security coverage) and rural inhabitants lack health insurance coverage.

Inequitable rural-urban distribution of benefits is of special concern. High-income people with insurance coverage benefit more from the government subsidy than low-income uninsured people. According to the results of a recent survey, people living in urban settlements in western Turkey use health services more frequently than those in rural areas in eastern Turkey. The main cause of this inequity is the government subsidy of institutions—which are most frequently located in urban areas—rather than individuals (Engiz 1996).

Preventive services and health promotion services are also inadequate. The Ministry of Health is the only provider of preventive services, and in 1996, only 3 percent of total resources were allocated to preventive care (Tokat 1998). Primary healthcare clearly has not been emphasized. For this reason, health services are hospital-centered. Hospitals are overused by patients who should be served at primary care units, and, as a result, hospital waiting times constitute a major cause of dissatisfaction. Excess use and waste of drugs is another major problem in the Turkish health system (Kılıçdaroğlu 1998).

These considerations have led the government to look for alternative financing and delivery models. The Ministry of Health started a comprehensive health reform project in 1990 and organized National Health Congresses in 1992 and in 1993. The goals of these developments were to improve accessibility of primary healthcare services by establishing a family physician system, to reduce inequality in health status and access to basic health services, and to allocate more resources to environmental and preventive health services by introducing a health insurance scheme for the uninsured population.

The following attributes were anticipated in this scheme:

- Compulsory membership and premium payments, adjusted according to household earnings, would be required to receive health services under the system.
- The government would contribute to the premium from general tax revenues. Premiums were to be based on the cost of a standard benefit package that included primary health services and hospital curative services.
- Insured citizens would be referred to hospitals by first-level medical staff. Hospitals were to be reorganized as competitively operating health enterprises.

The new system was intended to be phased in gradually in different parts of the country. Nationwide coverage was to take several years.

This reform project has not been implemented because required legislative changes have not been adopted. Legislative drafts were prepared by the Ministry of Health and submitted to the Parliament in 1995 and 1998. However, for various reasons, these laws did not pass. Currently the Ministry of Health has new reform projects in preparation, which it expects to submit to the legislative body in the near future.

REFERENCES

Engiz, O. 1996. "Türkiye'de Sağlık Finansman Sorunu ve Çözüm Arayışları" (Problems of Financing Health Expenditures in Turkey and the Search for Solutions). *Toplum ve Hekim* 11 (72): 22–31.

Kılıçdaroğlu, K. 1998. *Türkiye'nin Sağlık Sorunları ve Çözüm Önerileri* (Health Problems in Turkey and Proposals for Solution). Ankara: Former General Director of Social Insurance Organization.

Ministry of Health. 1998. *Health Statistics, 1998*. Ankara: Ministry of Health, Research Planning and Coordination Council.

———. 1998a. *Kişisel Sağlık Sigortasi Sistemi* (Individual Health Insurance

System). Unpublished document. Ankara: Sağlık Bakanlığı, SaĞlık Projesi Genel KoordinatörlüĞü.

——. 1997. *Health Sector Reforms in Turkey, 1997*. Ankara: Ministry of Health, Health Project General Coordination Unit.

State Institute of Statistics (SIS). 1999. *Death Statistics from Provincial and District Centers*. Ankara: SIS.

——. 1998. *Statistical Yearbook of Turkey 1997*. Ankara: SIS.

——. 1998a. *Household Labor Force Survey Results*. April and October. Ankara: SIS.

State Institute of Statistics (SIS) and UNICEF. 1996. *Multiple Indicator Cluster Survey, Turkey 1995*. Ankara: SIS and UNICEF.

Tokat, M. 1998. *Türkiye Sağlık Harcamaları ve Finansmani, 1992–1996* (Health Expenditures and Their Financing in Turkey, 1992–1996). Ankara: Sağlık Bakanlığı, Sağlık Projesi Genel Koordinatörlüğü.

United Nations Development Programme (UNDP). 1999. *Human Development Report, 1999*. New York: Oxford University Press.

World Bank. 2000. *World Development Report 1999/2000: Entering the 21st Century*. Oxford: Oxford University Press.

SOUTH AFRICA

Eric Buch and Carel B. Ijsselmuiden

Background

South Africa is now in its eighth year of parliamentary democracy; this follows nearly 50 years of apartheid rule, which were preceded by 50 more years of racial segregation and another 100 of colonial rule. A constitution now provides the basis for governance (Constitutional Assembly 1996).

Nonracial and democratically elected national and provincial governments have replaced the segregated white, colored (a specific term used in South Africa to denote individuals of mixed race), and Indian parliaments, the ten bantustan (homeland) "governments" for Africans, and the four white-controlled provinces of the apartheid system.[1] The president is elected by Parliament and chooses his or her ministers from among its members. The nine provincial legislatures likewise elect a premier who appoints members to his or her executive council.

Under apartheid, cities and towns were racially segregated and separately managed. The poorly serviced black townships were physically separated from the "main" white towns. Political integration followed with the local government elections of 1995. However, the local authorities, which totaled more than 1,000, did not provide the economies required, and they did not cover the entire country. Under new local government laws, the country has been divided into fewer contiguous district and metropolitan councils. Other changes in municipal government have resulted in the emergence of executive mayors; this will complete the split in all three tiers of government between the executive and legislative authorities, who in turn are separate from the judiciary authorities.

South Africa covers 1,223,201 square kilometers at the southern end of the African continent. It has a population density of 34.4 people per square kilometer, which varies from 2.3 people per square kilometer in the Northern Cape to 448.4 in Gauteng because of the large tracts of uninhabitable land, urbanization, and other factors (Statistics South Africa 1998). The density in most provinces is between 20 and 40 people per square kilometer.

The country has three major physiographic features: the interior plateau, the escarpment, and the land from that to the coast. The subtropical location has warm, temperate conditions and a belt of high pressure, resulting in an average (but unpredictable) annual rainfall of only 464 millimeters. Thus, although the country is well-endowed with natural resources, water is potentially limited.

The South African economy was traditionally built on mining (gold, minerals, and coal) and agriculture, but industrial and commercial development have been steadily increasing their share of the gross domestic product. The GDP stood at U.S.$109 billion (approximately U.S.$2,500 per capita) in 2000 (Burger 2000), making South Africa a lower-middle income country. Real GDP has grown since the country became a democracy, following negative growth between 1990 and 1992. It grew by 3.2 percent in 1995, 3.4 percent in 1996, and 1.7 percent in 1997, but it did not grow in 1998. Government spending for 1999 was set at U.S.$31.4 billion (31 percent of the GDP), of which U.S.$6.9 billion was to repay debt (Burger 2000). The unemployment rate is 36.2 percent.

The 2000 mid-year population was just over 43.7 million, growing at just over 2 percent per year (Statistics South Africa 2000). Urbanization is ongoing as a result of a number of economic forces and the removal of apartheid restrictions on people's movement. Currently 53.7 percent of the population are urban dwellers; this includes large numbers of people living in informal settlements with levels of poverty similar to that of the rural poor.

The crude death rate was estimated at 12.8 per 1,000 in 2001 (Bradshaw 2001). A 1998 National Demographic and Health Survey found an infant mortality rate of 45.4 per 1,000 live births, an under-five mortality rate of 59.4 per 1,000 live births, a total fertility rate of 2.9, and a teenage birth rate of 13.2 (South Africa Medical Research Council 1998). The 1999 October Household Survey found that 38.8 percent of households had piped water, 53 percent used electricity for cooking (Crisp and Ntuli 2000), and 66 percent of adults were literate.

The above gross statistics for the country hide the significant disparities in socioeconomic well-being among South Africa's people. In general terms, rates for Africans are worse than those for coloreds, followed by those of Indians, with whites experiencing the best living conditions; this is an accurate reflection of the country's history. This pattern, which is driven by history but being altered by transformation and democracy, is also evident in the health of and healthcare for South Africans.

Health Status

Overall, the health of South Africans is poorer than it should be for the country's socioeconomic status, although the national picture hides differentials in burden of disease by race. These are reflections of socioeconomic disparity, of a health system that historically neglected to focus on improving health, and now also of the AIDS epidemic (WHO 2000).

Early evidence of improvements in health that have been emerging as a result of the efforts of the new government have rapidly been masked by the impact of the HIV epidemic; the epidemic has eclipsed all other health problems in the country. On the basis of the findings of a national antenatal survey, an estimated 4.7 million South Africans (approximately 1 in 9) are HIV positive. Table 22.1 shows the rapid growth in HIV seroprevalence in antenatal clinic clients to its current level of 24.5 percent, and Table 22.2 shows the high prevalence in youth. Approximately 7.3 percent of South African women tested positive for syphilis; this figure reflects the high overall prevalence of sexually transmitted diseases.

Tuberculosis rates have always been high, particularly in the Western Cape, but the picture is rapidly worsening as a result of AIDS. The incidence of tuberculosis is estimated, on the basis of surveys, at 392 per 100,000 (Ntuli and Crisp 2001). The notification rate of 169 per 100,000 is accepted as an underestimate as a result of inadequate case finding and notification. Malaria is also undernotified at 160 per 100,000, but South Africa has to some extent managed to keep malaria resurgence under control. However, in 1999, 50,939 cases of malaria were confirmed. Hepatitis A is endemic in rural areas, and hepatitis B is common. Schistosomiasis is endemic in eastward-flowing rivers. In the summer of 2000 through 2001 a cholera epidemic was concentrated in KwaZulu-Natal, with 93,456 cases reported.

Acute gastroenteritis and respiratory infections remain major causes of child mortality. Measles has dropped from 22,798 notified cases in 1992 to less than 1,000 in 2000 (Ntuli and Crisp 2001), and few cases of other vaccine-preventable conditions are now found. In 1994, 2.6 percent of children between 6 months and 6 years were wasted, 22.9 percent were stunted, and 9 percent were underweight (Ntuli and Crisp 2001). School feeding programs were introduced in 1994, and their effects are expected to be reflected in improvements in nutritional status.

Chronic diseases of lifestyle are a major cause of morbidity and mortality in South Africa. Whites, coloreds, and Indians have among the highest levels of myocardial infarction in the world. It is also an emerging problem in Africans, who already have high rates of hypertension and cerebrovascular accidents. Seemingly paradoxically, African women have a

TABLE 22.1 HIV Prevalence in Antenatal Clinic Attendees*

Year	1990	1991	1992	1993	1994	1995	1996	1997	1998	1999†	2000
Prevalence	0.7	1.7	2.2	4.0	7.6	10.4	14.2	17.0	22.8	22.4	24.5

* These data are based on a national sample of antenatal clinic attendees.
† These 1999 data are considered by some to be an underestimate due to methodology.
SOURCE: National Department of Health (2001).

TABLE 22.2

HIV Prevalence by Age in Antenatal Clinic Attendees

Age	1998 Percent HIV Positive	95% CI†	1999 Percent HIV Positive	2000* Percent HIV Positive
20 years old or younger	21.0	18.4–23.8	16.5	16.1
20 to 24 years	26.1	24.1–28.1	25.6	29.1
25 to 29 years	26.9	24.7–29.0	26.4	30.6
30 to 34 years	19.1	17.1–21.1	21.7	23.3
35 to 39 years	13.4	11.2–15.6	16.2	15.8
40 to 44 years†	10.5	6.8–14.1	12.0	10.2
45 to 49 years†	10.2	0.4–20.0	7.5	13.1

* The reduction in the 20 years old or younger age group and in fact the impression that the epidemic curve is flattening is considered to be methodological consequences rather than prevalence changes.
† Confidence intervals (CI) are shown for 1998 to reflect the sampling effect, including the small sample size in the section of the population that is 40 years old or older. The pattern for 1999 and 2000 is similar.
SOURCE: National Department of Health (2001).

high rate of obesity (34 percent). High levels of alcohol- and smoking-related diseases (42 percent of males and 11 percent of females [South African Medical Research Council 1998]) and domestic and criminal violence all add unnecessarily to the burden of disease, as do motor vehicle accidents. Approximately 55,000 motor vehicle accidents occur each year, resulting in death in 8 percent of cases, with an additional 17 percent of victims suffering serious injuries (Hospital Association of South Africa 2001).

Cancer is a major cause of adult mortality, with a lifetime risk of about 1 in 6 for men and 1 in 7 for women (Cancer Association of South Africa 2000). Comparatively high levels of esophageal cancer (1 in 59 lifetime risk) and liver/bile duct cancer (1 in 227) occur in African men (Cancer Association of South Africa 2000). Disability and mental health problems also increase South Africa's healthcare burden.

Poor water and sanitation still pose major environmental health hazards in rural areas and in the urban informal settlements that have grown rapidly during the past 15 years. Respiratory disease was extremely high in townships due to indoor pollution; however, the improvements in the number of households with electricity have reduced the incidence of respiratory infections.

Air pollution from coal-fired power stations remains a problem in the Eastern Highveld. This is also a cause of acid rain, and the use of dichlorodiphenyltrichloroethane (better known as DDT) for malaria control and deforestation adds to environmental health risks. At the household level, burns from open fires used for cooking and warmth and a chemical pneumonitis in children from accidental paraffin ingestion are common (paraffin is often stored in Coca-Cola® bottles).

Legislation requires that hazardous wastes be disposed of in approved sites and that pesticide is controlled, although laws are not always adhered to and enforcement is limited. However, a number of environmental laws and programs are slowly changing the picture. Occupational health laws have also been tightened to impose a responsibility on owners to protect the health and safety of their workforce. However, much remains to be done. Conditions in the mines have improved, but silicosis and asbestosis acquired from prior exposure are still problems.

Organization and Management of the Health System

South Africa has in effect dual public and private health systems that largely run parallel to each other. The former serves mainly the poor majority of South Africans, and the latter serves those with health insurance.

Comprehensive legislation is expected to be passed in 2002, despite its slow progress, to replace the 1977 Health Act. A combination of individual pieces of legislation, commitment to change, and the new constitution have allowed a number of important changes to be made to the health system. Key legislative changes since 1994 have affected medical schemes, pharmaceuticals, termination of pregnancy, and tobacco. Powerful interest groups have also influenced new laws.

Overall, health policy for the country is set at regular meetings of the Minstry of Health and the provincial members of the Executive Council for Health (dubbed the MINMEC). Much of what is presented at the MINMEC has been reviewed by a meeting of the administrative heads (public servants) of the national and provincial Departments of Health, whose meeting agenda is developed from the work of members of their staff, at times with the use of outside consultants. The provinces have extended autonomy and can set policies for provincial matters outside of the decisions made at the MINMEC, but the consultative process means that this seldom happens in practice on substantive matters.

The public sector has moved away from its racial and geographic fragmentation and toward an integrated system. The constitution requires cooperation in governance between the national, provincial, and local tiers of government.

The national ministry is responsible for overall policy and coordination of the health sector, including legislation governing the health professions and the private sector. The provinces are responsible for the provision of public health services, the running of 343 hospitals (Crisp and Ntuli 2000), and most curative primary healthcare, whereas local authorities provide preventive and environmental health services. In reshaping the primary healthcare system, a decision was made to work within a district health model. The process toward this seemingly simple decision is quite complex and will entail the transfer of a number of provincial staff to local government and service contracts between the provinces, which will provide the majority of the funding, and the municipality.

Public sector hospitals are divided into district, regional (which aim to have medical specialists in the basic disciplines), and ten central hospitals. Central hospitals provide highly specialized care comparable with that found in highly industrialized countries; they also serve as the base for medical education. Hospital management and all staff are employed by and accountable to the provincial ministry, although an openness toward the contracting out of noncore services, such as laundry and food, is emerging.

The organization and management of the public health system under apartheid reflected its priority of supporting a system driven by politics rather than one driven by efficiency. In addition, a highly centralized bureaucracy was in place that included all of its associated inefficiencies. The values of access, equity, and efficiency are now paramount and have been reflected in the growth of clinics in historically disadvantaged communities and in the goal of making primary healthcare free for all. Efficiency is improving as the process of managerial transformation truly gets underway. Decentralization, performance management, and accountability are key words that reflect the direction. A move is being made to appoint chief executive officers of hospitals and to give them substantial management autonomy, although progress in this regard has been slow.

The private sector operates, within overarching legislation, largely as a free market made up of medical aid schemes, medical insurance administrators, private hospital groups, some private primary healthcare groups, and private health professionals. The private hospital sector is largely controlled by three listed companies: Afrox Healthcare, Netcare, and Medi-Clinic Holdings. They employ nurses, whereas other health professionals work independently in private practices. A large number of private general practitioners also operate individually or in small groups, among which are an ever-increasing number of African doctors. The mining industry provides care for its staff in its own hospitals.

Tentative but not yet successful attempts have been made to introduce managed healthcare into South Africa. The business sector has also started up primary healthcare clinic groups, but their penetration of the market has been slow.

The involvement of nongovernmental organizations (including the church) in the health sector is small. However, a large number of health and welfare organizations are active in health matters in the community, and they tend to focus on a specific health problem (e.g., cancer, tuberculosis, AIDS, mental health, disability) rather than on broader health services. The professed commitment of the government to the development of nongovernmental organizations has not been matched by a sufficiently enabling environment or appropriate funding.

Advocacy as an influence on policy is now much more that of a democratic society. Government has national and other consultation forums with all stakeholders, but these have not proved to be truly effective means of consultation. Hospital boards and clinic committees are playing a useful role in many areas, whereas district health advisory bodies are envisaged.

International organizations like the World Health Organization have returned to South Africa. They and donors play a positive supportive role in the country, largely through government. South Africa has not taken substantial loans from the World Bank, so the World Bank's sometimes controversial policies have not been factors in the country.

Financing

South Africa is considered to spend approximately U.S.$210 per capita per annum (8.4 percent of GDP) on healthcare. However, these figures do not tell the full story. Because of comparatively high public-sector salaries, a dollar does not buy the same volume of care in South Africa as it would in other African countries, so expenditure is skewed. More than half of the money is spent in the private sector on only about 20 percent of the population. Total private health expenditure is above U.S.$5 billion annually, including private medical aid expenditure of approximately U.S.$2.9 billion (Council for Medical Schemes 2000). The bulk of the remaining expenditure is comprised of medical scheme copayments, out-of-pocket expenditure, company health services (including mine hospitals), workmen's compensation, and the Road Accident Fund.

Approximately U.S.$3.6 billion was spent in the public sector in 2000 (Whelan 2001). Expenditure by the National Department is comparatively small, because most expenditure is incurred by provincial health departments on the basis of budgets presented to provincial legislatures. The main source of funding is from allocations made by the central treasury to provinces and from conditional grants from the National Ministry, which are largely to fund the ten central hospitals and for health professional training. A small amount comes from provincial licensing fees and gambling taxes, whereas hospital fees provide minimal income. Primary healthcare is free, but public-sector hospital fees are set into four categories based on income. The poor management of revenue has recently led to the incentive whereby hospitals can retain the revenue they collect above a set target.

Local authority health departments provide limited services that are funded largely through provincial grants, local taxes, and profits from utilities. Private medical aid expenditure is far from efficiently used, with inflation well above the prevailing national rate. The inefficiency is rooted in the sector's financial structure. The bulk of private users are members of not-for-profit employer medical schemes. The employer generally contributes half or more of the membership fee, which is tax deductible. The member seeks care at the place of his or her choice and then submits the claim to the administration company. This system of guaranteed third-party payment to fee-for-service providers by administration companies, whose profit is linked to turnover, has been at the root of extensive overuse of services. A lack of sophisticated professional controls, limited litigation, and passive and poorly informed consumers have further fueled the problem. Risk management and other cost-containment techniques are arriving gradually.

Just before handing over power, the apartheid government changed legislation to deregulate medical schemes. This led to a number of changes in the market, particularly with regard to risk rating. As a result, companies started to offer low premiums and diverse packages to the employed, young, and healthy, thereby abandoning the cross-subsidization of the elderly and ill that had been the core principle until then. It also led to additional charges for the elderly, and many of these companies no longer covered chronic illnesses. The government has amended the Medical Schemes Act in 1999, and it now requires open membership and comprehensive hospital and expensive chronic disease coverage. A result of this is less dumping of patients onto the public sector. Schemes now have more restricted coverage of primary healthcare services.

About 16.1 percent (seven million) of South Africans enjoy private medical coverage (Council for Medical Schemes 2000); the expenditure pattern is presented in Table 22.3. Until the advent of the Sullivan and European Union Codes of Conduct for businesses operating in apartheid South Africa, in line with general discrimination in the country, there was little black membership of medical aids. Although black membership has grown, it is still only a fraction of white membership. Dreaded disease coverage through the insurance industry is estimated to add another U.S.$63 million to health expenditure.

Out-of-pocket payments make up a smaller proportion of expenditure. This portion goes largely to the member's portion of medical aid claims, for payment for nonprescription drugs, and to general practitioners serving poorer communities. The latter tend to charge a flat rate for the consultation, including medication. An unknown amount is spent outside the formal health sector on traditional healers and other forms of alternative medicine.

Donor funding has tended to support infrastructure and systems development in the public sector, although some continues to go to nongovernmental organizations. These organizations also stand to benefit from the newly introduced national lottery and other efforts from the government to support the revitalization and refocusing of this sector.

Category	Percent of Total Expenditure*
General practitioners	9.5
Medical specialists	19
Dentists	5.9
Dental specialists	0.9
Hospitals	29
Medicines	27
Other	9
Total (U.S.$)	2.9 billion

TABLE 22.3
Breakdown of Medical Scheme Expenditure by Category, 1999

* This does not include copayments and other costs borne by members.
SOURCE: Adapted from the Report of the Registrar of Medical Schemes (Council of Medical Schemes 2000).

Health Resources

Human Resources

South Africa produces a large number of health professionals who are trained to a high standard and who often have expectations of high income. A consequence of this is excessive emigration and movement to the private sector. Not surprisingly, there are still more white and Indian health professionals than African health professionals. The overall picture is presented in Tables 22.4 and 22.5.

Category	Private Sector*		Public Sector		Total	
	Number	Ratio	Number	Ratio	Number	Ratio
Dentists	3,868	1:2004	324	1:104,653	4,192	1:9,938
Doctors	19,935	1:389	7,616	1:4,452	27,551	1:1,512
Nurses†	71,447	1:109	102,200	1:332	173,647	1:240
Pharmacists	8,531	1:909	1,184	1:28,638	9,715	1:4,288

TABLE 22.4
Health Professionals in South Africa, 1998

* Based on 18 percent of the population dependent on the private sector and 82 percent on the public sector, the former based on membership of medical aids.
† Includes both professional nurses and nursing auxiliaries.
SOURCE: van Rensburg and van Rensburg (2000).

TABLE 22.5

Provincial Distribution by Number and Ratio of Selected Health Professionals

Province	Population Size/ Percent of Population	Dentists	Doctors	Professional Nurses	Pharmacists
Eastern Cape	6,469,754 15.5 percent	229 1:28,252	1,983 1:3,296	11,659 1:555	829 1:7,804
Free State	2,703,381 6.5 percent	163 1:16,585	1,528 1:1,769	6,864 1:394	467 1:5,789
Gauteng	7,543,404 18.1 percent	1,828 1:4,127	10,214 1:739	26,676 1:283	4,127 1:1,828
KwaZulu Natal	8,640,356 20.7 percent	539 1:16,030	4,699 1:1,839	16,575 1:521	1,478 1:5,846
Mpumalanga	2,875,024 6.9 percent	159 1:18,082	966 1:2,976	3,706 1:77.6	373 1:7,708
Northern Cape	862,618 2.1 percent	54 1:15,974	371 1:2,325	1,638 1:527	108 1:7,987
Northern Province	5,060,162 12.1 percent	103 1:49,128	750 1:6,747	5,587 1:906	251 1:20,160
North West	3,443,841 8.3 percent	144 1:23,916	846 1:4,071	5,697 1:605	444 1:7,756
Western Cape	4,061,866 9.7 percent	973 1:4,175	6,217 1:654	12,584 1:323	1,638 1:2,480
South Africa	41,660,406 100 percent	4,192 1:9,938	27,551 1:1,512	90,986 1:458	9,715 1:4,288

SOURCE: van Rensburg and van Rensburg (2000).

Eight universities train doctors in South Africa. Access for African medical students is still below what it should be, with only the two historically black institutions training the majority of African doctors. Curricula shifts toward generalists and local relevance are slow in coming, whereas problem-based curricula are emerging. Most training still takes place in a tertiary hospital setting.

Training of nurses largely takes place in nursing colleges under the provincial health departments, which now have university affiliations. The four-year professional nursing course includes midwifery. There is quality training in all the specialized areas of nursing, including the training of nurse clinicians (primary healthcare nurses), but demand for their skill in the private sector (and abroad) makes it hard to retain them in the public sector. For a time, it appeared that the two-year enrolled nurse course would be phased out, but it and the one-year nursing assistant training seem set to continue, albeit in a revised fashion. Enrolled nurses can complete a two-year course to qualify as professional nurses.

The costs of health-professional training are largely borne by the state, with tuition fees covering less than a quarter of real costs. Six fledgling schools of public health have emerged in the country since democracy, but they still need to reach a critical mass. Although national targets for training and deployment have not yet been set, the main problem is not in the numbers but in their distribution. Tables 22.4 and 22.5 reflect the strong private sector and urban bias. The urban distribution is itself biased toward the suburbs and away from rural areas and informal settlements; this led to the introduction of a year of community service for newly qualified doctors. The first group was deployed in 2000, and the trend will continue for other health professionals. Although these professionals receive a full salary, they must work where the need is. The uneven distribution has also led to consideration of the registration of new private practices only where a need has been identified.

Again, with its focus on the needs of the elite, few auxiliary or village health worker programs were developed under apartheid. In fact, the latter emerged as a means whereby the apartheid state could provide cheap, second-class care for the poor rather than providing them with an appropriate range of care in a well-supported environment as an affordable extension of the health service. Under democracy, little movement has been seen on the question of auxiliaries, and the use of village health workers was left to provinces to decide. One province has recently given a large contract to nongovermental organizations to train and manage a substantial village health worker program.

Professional practice is governed by Health Professions, Nursing, and Pharmaceutical Councils, which are made up of elected members and ministerial nominees; there are moves to combine these councils. Personnel in the sector are highly organized into unions, and professionals are generally members of professional associations.

Health Facilities

There are 102,300 public hospital beds, 24,800 private beds, 6,000 beds in mine hospitals, and 14,500 beds contracted by the state for chronic care (e.g., mental health, tuberculosis) (Hospital Association of South Africa 2001). Of the public hospital beds, 15 percent are in central hospitals, 26 percent are in regional hospitals, and 38 percent are in district hospitals. The remaining 22 percent principally reflects beds for mental health care and tuberculosis (Ntuli and Crisp 2001).

The definition of a central hospital is one that provides tertiary-level care, although not all of its beds are used for this purpose. Similarly, a regional hospital should have the facilities for general specialist care (i.e., anesthetics, obstetrics and gynecology, internal medicine, orthopedics, pediatrics, radiology, surgery). Chronic mental health care is provided in designated public and contracted psychiatric hospitals; there are moves to deinstitutionalize patients.

There are 2.67 public beds per 1,000 population, or 3.27 per 1,000 if one considers public-sector users only. Although this appears to be a reasonably satisfactory state of affairs, there is concern that this number of beds is unaffordable. One province that was well-endowed with beds has already closed eight hospitals (2,000 beds) to enhance occupancy levels and offset the duplication of a black and a white hospital serving the same town.

The global picture also hides the skewed distribution of beds. Table 22.6 shows the comparative number of beds per population per province. Almost all of the public-sector tertiary beds are concentrated in the four most developed provinces, and the same is true of the greatest proportion of secondary beds. This has resulted in inequitable access and the referral of patients over long distances. There is now active implementation of plans to develop specialist-level care in five hospitals in each of the underdeveloped provinces; this idea is supported by a special redistribution grant taken from the central hospital grant.

Private hospitals, which are already concentrated in the cities, have started to move away from inner-city areas, and single-specialty hospitals have emerged. Some private hospitals have been built in what were the

TABLE 22.6

Beds per Population per Province in 2000

Province	Public Sector		Private Sector	
	Public Population	Beds per 1,000 Public Population	Private Population	Beds per 1,000 Private Population
Eastern Cape	6,112,093	3.09	679,121	1.74
Free State	2,270,771	2.56	498,109	3.22
Gauteng	4,786,748	3.49	3,191,445	3.40
KwaZulu Natal	7,928,553	3.44	1,185,383	2.85
Mpumalanga	2,647,988	1.82	431,403	1.63
Northern Cape	701,356	2.27	186,662	2.07
Northern Province	5,052,045	2.00	439,583	0.61
North West	3,129,812	2.08	509,790	2.58
Western Cape	3,017,762	3.54	1,232,578	3.95
South Africa	35,647,128	2.87	8,354,074	2.94

SOURCE: Boulle, Blecher, and Burn (2001).

black townships, particularly as a result of the willingness on the part of emerging black entrepreneurs to take such a risk. These new private hospitals also threaten to draw staff out of the public sector.

Private hospitals typically have state-of-the-art equipment; in fact, because so many of these hospitals do have such equipment, the State has begun to think about the need for licensing the most expensive pieces. This may seem an intrusion on the private market, but it is seen by many to be a necessary move to curb oversupply and consequent overuse. Financial incentives for physicians to refer patients for radiological and pathology services have recently come under scrutiny, and so has physician ownership of shares in hospitals.

The state of private health facilities often contrasts sharply with that of many public facilities. Historically, black hospitals tend to be in the worst state. Some need a facelift just to resemble a place of care, because apartheid architects or budgets often took shortcuts in areas such as lighting, ablutions, and space. However, many of the apparently better, historically white hospitals are also in need of major repair. A national audit has shown a backlog of beyond U.S.$1 billion in the maintenance and repair of public hospitals.

Commodities

Drugs must be registered with the Medicines Control Council, which classifies drugs into schedules that determine certain properties of the drug (e.g., whether or not a prescription is required). All of the major international drug companies are active in the South African market, and the latest drugs are available.

The public sector obtains its drugs and medical supplies at lower rates through a national public tender, although patented drugs without a generic equivalent remain a costly problem. In general, public health facilities have sufficient drugs and medical supplies, although the pressure to reduce budgets has created some difficulties. The tendency of academic hospital staff to want to use expensive drugs that are not on the tender more often than is clinically necessary has also been an issue; although in itself this is not of primary importance, it reflects wider changes that are required in clinical practice. Evidence-based medicine is not yet a strong force, but essential drug lists for primary and hospital care have been prepared by expert panels and are being effectively implemented.

The drug bill in the private sector continues to grow excessively, even after accounting for the costs of the latest discoveries and the weakening of the South African Rand (the local currency). Factors driving costs upward include the incentive marketing techniques of the industry, private pharmacists gaining income from the mark-up of drugs rather than a professional fee for their service, and the emergence of doctors who sell the drugs that they prescribe. The state is considering options to use to deal with this situation, including controls on advertising, professional fees for pharmacists, and restricting dispensing doctors. Not surprisingly, these moves have generated controversy among those with vested interests. However, most controversial was the promulgation of legislation (considered to be within international trade agreements) to offset patient rights against the national interest of making expensive essential drugs affordable. The multinational pharmaceutical companies brought a case against the Department of Health to block implementation of this act but subsequently withdrew it following a massive national and international outcry. Negotiations are continuing between the two parties.

Public sector information and management systems are archaic and inefficient. There is a positive national effort to redress this, and most provinces are investing in information technology. On a positive note, private sector systems that focus on financial management are quite strong.

Service Delivery

Public sector primary healthcare is provided through a clinic system. In urban areas, clinics are usually larger and have clinical care nurses supported by doctors. Clinics are quite widely distributed, but access in rural areas is still sometimes difficult. Ambulance services to poorer areas have improved as greater equity has been achieved, but generally services are still too thin to achieve desired response times.

Tertiary care is centered in the more urbanized provinces, but once in the tertiary hospitals, care is not incomparable to that of advanced countries, although loads on staff are greater, equipment is older, and queues—even for urgent surgery—are longer. Efforts to provide basic specialty (secondary-level) care in all provinces are bearing fruit. Occupancy rates in public hospitals are generally high.

The strong commitment to equity, availability, and access in the public sector has seen new clinics built in historically underserved areas and the beginning of a shift of funds out of the academic hospitals. Nonetheless, substantial rural-urban and formal-informal settlement differentials are still to be addressed.

One real difficulty in strengthening service provision has been financial pressure. Although there was real growth (albeit small) in the health budget during the first few years after 1994, substantial salary increases given in 1997 resulted in a de facto loss of buying power of U.S.$200 million. This, together with other bargaining chamber agreements (e.g., that there would be no retrenchments), put services under great pressure and threatened a number of advances. It also put the spotlight even more strongly on the tertiary care/primary care balance.

If quality of care is used in its broadest sense, much can be found in South Africa that is positive. There is, however, much concern about certain aspects of quality of care. In the public sector, this relates to issues like queues, linen, and food. In addition, there is a deeper concern that the patient care ethos has suffered and with it the level of caring and respect for patients; this shift remains one of the enigmas of transformation in South Africa. A health charter is one of a number of steps taken to deal with this problem, and quality of care is one of ten major areas of focus in the government's five-year health plan (Department of Health 1999).

The current aim is to offer comprehensive primary care, with health centers offering a larger range of services than clinics. A primary care package has been defined, but its affordability remains a concern. A number of national initiatives are integrated into these services, including the AIDS and syndrome-based sexually transmitted disease care programs, the Directly Observed Treatment Short Course (DOTS) for tuberculosis, and the Extended Program on Immunization (EPI) (which still faces an unsatisfactory level of 63 percent of infants having received all their immunizations by the age of one year) (Ntuli and Crisp 2001). Integrated management of childhood illnesses is taking off slowly, and a number of women's health initiatives are progressing steadily, including addressing maternal mortality (150 out of 100,000 in 1998) (Equity Gauge 2000), increasing antenatal care (some 94 percent receive some), and offering termination of pregnancy, which has reduced the number of admissions for septic abortions. Mental health and disability care have shown some useful developments since 1994, but much remains to be done.

Overall there is still much to be done in the arena of service delivery, not the least of which includes fighting the AIDS epidemic. In general, service delivery will need to strengthen chronic care and develop measures to protect and promote health.

Prospects for the Future

The health sector has undergone significant changes since 1994, not the least of which has been the removal of structural racism. As can be seen throughout this chapter, the process of transformation of the health sector is still ongoing. Because of this, the next few years will be focused on consolidating the implementation of developments and on coping with the full force of the AIDS epidemic. Questions of financing, affordability, and quality will also force a further wave of policy developments.

Disease Changes, Particularly AIDS and Tuberculosis

The main disease change will be the full impact of AIDS and the associated escalation in tuberculosis. Many AIDS deaths still occur in hospitals, and there are not yet that many AIDS orphans. However, this picture will change rapidly in the next few years, and new strategies will be required. These strategies are not currently being adequately prepared in the country; this is underlined by the fact that already approximately a quarter of adult medical and pediatric beds in many hospitals are used for AIDS patients.

Although AIDS eclipses all other problems, it is hoped that, as a result of government strategies, trauma and violence morbidity and malnutrition will be reduced. However, although the economy is doing well overall, the benefits of development are not reaching the poor fast enough. It is generally thought that non-AIDS-related gastroenteritis and pneumonia are decreasing due to improvements in water supply and electricity, but empirical evidence is lacking. Chronic diseases of lifestyle are increasing as the lifestyle changes of the past few decades have an impact on the health of the aged, whose proportion of the population is growing.

Affordability

Even if optimal efficiency in the health sector is achieved, the hard truth is that the GDP is not commensurate with the expectations of the community regarding access to expensive high-technology treatments. Rationing was previously based on the unethical grounds of race and geography; now there are simply not enough public facilities to offer renal dialysis to all who might benefit, even if they fit the national criteria for admission to the program. These pressures are likely to result in further efficiency measures such as the use of microsurgery, high care instead of intensive care (one nurse for every two beds instead of one per bed), wider use of auxiliaries, and more home and community care; it may also result in the curtailing of certain services.

The Public Sector

Progress toward equity, redistribution, and cost control are likely to be consolidated, and big changes will be made in public sector management. These will include decentralization and performance agreements, changes in management style, and contracting out of non-core services in line with the global mood of a market economy. Although the private sector is gearing up to be a private provider of care for public-funded hospital and ambulatory patients, there is little government support for this.

The primary-tertiary healthcare balance is still a matter of great debate. In comparison with developed countries, South African academics are expected to spend two-thirds of their time on patient care and one-third on academia and to manage larger patient loads. Ongoing pressures for academic practice to be more efficient (e.g., in the choice of drugs and volumes of laboratory tests) are expected.

Social Health Insurance

Because it has been recognized that efficiency and limits to care must play their parts, more funds will need to be spent on public sector patients and preventive measures to achieve the health and healthcare levels that are desired. These funds are unlikely to be obtained from a greater slice of tax money, because the government has set a tax ceiling, and there are already many demands on funds. This has led to the emergence of support for what is loosely called "social health insurance." Whether this will take the form of compulsory hospital insurance for all in formal employment or be wider in its range is still unclear, as is the form of collection and coverage.

Quality

Although much good healthcare is practiced in South Africa, concern is growing about the quality of care. Building a caring ethos and a greater respect for the dignity of patients and strengthening the work ethic are areas that will receive increased attention. Measures to offset perverse incentives and to increase the use of evidence-based medicine will also certainly grow. In addition, the government is increasingly committed to promoting consumer awareness as evidenced by its educational campaigns and the development of a patient's charter.

Notes

1. Although South Africa is now a nonracial democracy, the deeply rooted inequities in the society and its health status and health-care—born of colonialism and exacerbated under apartheid—live on. Hopefully these inequalities will also become part of South African history before too long. For the moment, it remains impossible to accurately reflect the South African reality without reflecting racial differences. In this chapter, the term "black" refers to all people of color discriminated against by apartheid; the term "Africans" refers to those of African origin (Nguni, Sotho, Tsonga, and Venda), "coloreds" (this is the term used in South Africa) to those of mixed descent, and "Indians" to those whose forebears hail from the Indian subcontinent. South Africa is truly a multicultural society and has 11 official languages.
2. Based on economically active people who did not work during the seven days before the interview who wanted to work and were available to work within a week.

REFERENCES

Boulle, A., Blecher, M., and Burn, A. 2001. "Hospital Restructuring." In *South African Health Review: 2000,* edited by A. Ntuli and N. Crisp, pp. 235–50. Durban: Health Systems Trust.

Bradshaw, D. 2001. Personal communication. August.

Burger, D. (ed.) 2000. *South African Yearbook, 2000.* Cape Town: Rustica Press.

Cancer Association of Southern Africa (CANSA). 2000. "Histologically

Diagnosed Cancers 1993–1995: Summary Statistics." Retrieved July 2000 from http://www.cansa.co.za.

Constitutional Assembly. 1996. *Constitution of the Republic of South Africa, 1996.* Act 108 of 1996.

Council for Medical Schemes. 2000. *Report of the Council of Medical Schemes 1999.* Pretoria: Council for Medical Schemes.

Crisp, N., and Ntuli, A. (eds.) 2000. *South African Health Review, 1999.* Durban: Health Systems Trust.

Department of Health. 1999. *Health Strategic Framework: 1999–2004.* Pretoria: Department of Health.

Hospital Association of South Africa. 2001. *Health Annals 2001.* Johannesburg: HASA.

National Department of Health. 2001. *National HIV Prevalence Survey 2000.* Pretoria: National Department of Health.

Ntuli, A., and Crisp, N. (eds.) 2001. *South African Health Review, 2000.* Durban: Health Systems Trust.

South African Medical Research Council and Macro-International. 1998. *South African Demographic and Health Survey: Preliminary Report.* Pretoria: Department of Health.

Statistics South Africa. 1998. *The People of South Africa Population Census: Census in Brief.* Pretoria: Statistics South Africa.

———. 2000. "2000 Statistics." Retrieved July 2000 from http://www.statssa. gov.za/releases/demograp/p0302.htm.

The Equity Gauge. 2000. "The Equity Gauge Project." Retrieved July 2000 from http://www.hst.org.za.

van Rensburg, D., and van Rensburg, N. 2000. "Distribution of Human Resources." In *South African Health Review: 1999,* edited by N. Crisp and A. Ntuli, pp. 201–32. Durban: Health Systems Trust.

Whelan, P. 2001. "A Review of Provincial Health Budgets 2001/02. IDASA Briefs." Retrieved July 2001 from http://www.idasa.org.za.

World Health Organization. 2000. *The World Health Report 2000. Health Systems: Improving Performance.* Geneva: World Health Organization.

BOTSWANA

Scott Stewart

Background Information

Botswana sits at the center of the southern African plateau bordered by South Africa, Zimbabwe, Namibia, and Zambia. It covers approximately 582,000 square kilometers, an area that is slightly smaller than the U.S. state of Texas and a little larger than France. The Kalahari Desert, which is characterized by arid and semi-arid savanna, spreads across nearly 80 percent of the country's land mass from the southwestern corner of the country (Granberg and Parkinson 1988). Annual rainfall averages range from approximately 250 to 650 millimeters (Main 1987). Botswana's only perennial interior riparian system is a portion of the Okavango Delta swamplands in the northeast. The north and northeast have some forest and farmland; the east comprises grasslands that are only marginally more fertile than the desert proper.

More than half of the country's population, estimated at nearly 1.6 million (Census Bureau 2000), live within 100 kilometers of the capital city of Gaborone; another 30 to 40 percent are concentrated along the major north-south transportation corridor running from the country's only other city, Francistown, in the northeast, through Gaborone to the border with South Africa (Campbell 1995). The rest of the population is distributed through the north and, more sparsely, throughout the Kalahari. Known collectively as Batswana, the people of this nation are employed in construction, trade, public and domestic service, and, primarily, subsistence farming and herding. Their per capita income was estimated at U.S.$3,310 in 1997 (World Bank 1999), which is high by African standards. However, such relative wealth has not always been the case, and it belies significant structural and medical challenges for the delivery of healthcare in this country. Additional demographic information is provided in Tables 23.1 and 23.2.

Brief History

Groups of Batswana have lived in present-day Botswana for hundreds of years. However, much of their expansion across the countryside was in flight from an intense conflict in the south known as the Difaqane, which began about 1820 and lasted nearly 20 years. As they migrated, emergent Batswana groups allied themselves with or subjugated the Bangologa and Khoe-San

TABLE 23.1
General Demographics

	1981	1991	2001	2025
Population in millions	0.9	1.3	1.6	1.2
Annual growth rate of preceding decade	4.7%	3.5%	1.9%	−1.2%
Infant mortality per 1,000 live births	71	45	62	54
Under-five mortality per 1,000 live births	109	56	98	
Life expectancy at birth (years)	56	65	39.3	33.2
Total fertility rate per woman	6.4	5.1	3.8	2.3
Percent urbanized	18	46	60	90

SOURCE: MFDP (1997); Census Bureau (2000); WHO (2000); UNDP (1998).

groups they encountered. Beginning around 1950, the principal leaders of the independent Batswana groups north of the Molopo and Limpopo rivers made a series of unsuccessful requests to the British for protection against the South African Boers, who settled the Transvaal beginning in the 1830s and began to seek control of the Batswana and their territory to the northwest. The British government finally established the Protectorate of Bechuanaland in 1885 to prevent expansion by the Boers from the southeast and by the Germans from the southwest. A major factor in the British decision was likely the protection of the major north-south route for transportation of trade goods and migrant labor (Tlou and Campbell 1984).

When it gained independence in 1966, Botswana was one of the poorest countries in the world; it had no direct access to the sea, and it

TABLE 23.2
Economic and Social Indicators

GNP per capita (U.S.$), 1997	3,310
GNP per capita (P.P.P.$), 1997	7,430
Human Development Index score, 1995	0.678
Percent of GNP spent on health	4.2
Public expenditure as percent of total health expenditure	61
ODA inflow as percent of GNP	1.6

NOTE: ODA = official development assistance.
SOURCE: UNDP (1998); World Bank (2001); World Health Organization (2000).

was surrounded by undemocratic, racist regimes. The Protectorate administration had done little to advance the social and economic development of the Batswana. Per capita income at the time has been estimated at 45 to 60 South African Rand (ZAR) (although exact worth in U.S. dollars is not available, ZARs are substantially less than U.S. dollar equivalents). At that time, Botswana had only 20 kilometers of paved road and severely limited communications and power networks (Hartland-Thunberg 1978). Its 175 schools have been credited more to missionaries and tribal authorities than the administration (Tlou and Campbell 1984). Of an estimated population of 520,000 (Mukamaambo 1994), only 40 had university degrees (Samatar 1999). The best source of wage-paying employment was in the mines of South Africa, which drew nearly one-third of Botswana's men between the ages of 20 and 40 years (Granberg and Parkinson 1988). Thus, the independent Republic of Botswana began with what appeared to be a meager chance of survival.

Current Situation

Since gaining its independence, however, Botswana has emerged as a notable success. Ten years after independence, Botswana had expanded its network of paved roads by a factor of 50, had established a telecommunications system, and was completing a power grid in the eastern part of the country. By 1996, Botswana had an estimated 4,343 kilometers of paved roads (CIA 2001), a national telephone system using microwave and optical fiber technology, and an autonomous national power grid. Gross national product per capita grew by 9.9 percent annually from 1965 until 1980 and 6.2 percent per year from 1980 to 1993 (Hope 1997).

Harvey and Lewis (1990) attribute Botswana's progress to three key factors: "luck, attention to key issues of economic management, and skill in negotiating with outsiders." The discovery and mining of significant mineral deposits, including diamonds, certainly have contributed to Botswana's success. However, fiscal prudence, a dynamic participatory planning process, and strong democratic traditions have allowed the Batswana to manage these resources effectively. Equally important has been the Batswana's ability to pursue their own objectives while maintaining peace with historically oppressive neighbors and to maintain control over the development process as recipients of assistance from friendly governments.

Governance

Botswana is a parliamentary republic with a functioning judiciary system that is based on Roman-Dutch and customary law. Suffrage is accorded to all citizens 18 years old and older. Elections have been held every five years since independence for Parliament and for district and town councils and land boards. Botswana's is a multiparty system, although the ruling party in Parliament has never changed.

Community Services

At the local level, a strong, indigenous tradition of civic participation persists in all realms, from interaction among the community and central and district level agencies to the Setswana equivalent of ordinary town meetings. Besides commerce, many functions remain under the control of the government of Botswana, either directly through a government ministry or via the district councils, which are largely funded by the central authorities. Therefore, education, social work, healthcare, and agricultural extension services do not originate from within communities, and community-level providers of these services (e.g., teachers, healthcare workers) are typically not from within the community. Rather, they will have been assigned to work in a particular community by a central personnel agency in coordination with the line agency for which they work, and they may rotate to a new assignment after two to five years.

Education

Botswana has the goal of universal access to basic education, although as many as 15 percent of children may not currently attend schools (Leburu-Sianga 1994). In 1991, nearly 20,000 children were enrolled in senior secondary school and 50,000 in junior secondary school, but 30 percent of children had never attended school at all. By 1996, an estimated 81 percent of primary-school-aged children and 45 percent of secondary-school-aged children were enrolled in school (World Bank 1999). Botswana has a national university, two teaching colleges for secondary school teachers, and several primary-teacher-training centers. Education is generally funded by the central government through grants to district authorities; teacher training is administered directly by the Ministry of Education. School health programs are common in Botswana, and they are supported by local authorities through staff from local health facilities. Table 23.3 provides details regarding net enrollments.

TABLE 23.3
Education
Indicators

	1995–96
Adult literacy rate, male	81
Adult literacy rate, female	60
Net primary school enrollment	81
Net secondary school enrollment	45

SOURCE: UNDP (1998).

Economic Activity

Botswana's economic growth, which averaged 10.7 percent annually from 1979 to 1989, was estimated at 4.7 percent ten years later. Key exports include diamonds, other minerals, and beef. Services account for more than half of the gross domestic product and employ roughly one-third of the labor force. Agriculture employs nearly half the labor force, but this is primarily for subsistence and accounts for less than 5 percent of the GDP. Meanwhile, total unemployment is estimated at 21.5 percent (World Bank 1999). Despite the relatively high per capita income, at least one-third of Botswana is thought to live in poverty (UNDP 1998).

Population Dynamics

Although it is slowing, Botswana's population growth has been rapid since independence. Annual growth rates were estimated at 4.7 percent in the 1970s and 3.5 percent in the 1980s; total fertility fell from 7.1 in 1981 to 5.4 in 1991. These figures are thought to have been significantly reduced in the last decade due to the positive effects of socioeconomic development and the severe impact of HIV/AIDS. Current estimates of population growth and total fertility are 1.9 percent and 3.8, respectively (Census Bureau 2000). In 1991, 47 percent of the population lived in urban areas. The growth rate of the urban population from 1981 to 1991 was nearly 14 percent, due both to migration and to the reclassification of settlements. The enumerated rural population remained stable during the same period (Mukamaambo 1994; van der Post 1994).

Context: Health Needs

HIV/AIDS is clearly the most pressing healthcare problem in Botswana today. Adult HIV seroprevalence is estimated at more than 30 percent nationally based on sentinel surveillance conducted at antenatal clinics (Census Bureau 2000). Outside of Gaborone and Francistown, little variation is seen between rural and urban HIV prevalence rates. Until recently, pharmacological treatments for AIDS commonly found in OECD countries have not been available in Botswana due to their cost. Currently, a nascent antiretroviral distribution program receives substantial support from international donors, private foundations, and pharmaceutical companies. However, the effectiveness and sustainability of that program remain unclear.

The HIV/AIDS epidemic is threatening the remarkable development gains described above. Infant mortality, having fallen from 100 deaths per 1,000 live births in 1971 to 45 per 1,000 20 years later, is currently estimated at 62 per 1,000 (Census Bureau 2000). One observer notes that 68 percent of all children's deaths are attributable to AIDS (Hilmers 2000).

Life expectancy, having increased from 55 to 65 years from 1971 to 1991, was recently estimated by the U.S. Census Bureau at only 39 years due to the impact of AIDS (Census Bureau 2000). The mortality rate for Batswana between the ages of 15 and 59 years is nearly 75 percent (WHO 2000).

Other healthcare needs exist, although none are as severe as HIV/AIDS. Generally, Botswana's socioeconomic progress is leading to a shift in disease patterns toward more chronic, noncommunicable conditions including cardiovascular disease and diabetes. However, infectious disease remains important, and the healthcare system must be capable of functioning effectively at both ends of the epidemiological spectrum. Additional information concerning health needs is located in Table 23.4.

Malaria is seasonally epidemic in the wetter, northern half of Botswana; its incidence is highly dependent on rainfall. Case fatality rates are between 0.2 and 0.5 percent. The prevalence of schistosomiasis among children has declined from 80 percent to about 8 percent during the past 20 years. Healthcare workers were treating 22 cases of leprosy in 1996, but the government expected to eliminate leprosy by 2000 (MFDP 1997). Tuberculosis case rates, having fallen to 202 per 100,000 people in 1989 from 506 per 100,000 in 1975, had increased again by more than 100 percent to 444 per 100,000 by 1996; this increase is attributed to the spread of HIV and HIV coinfection with tuberculosis (Kenyon et al. 1999).

National immunization coverage has declined since the late 1980s. Coverage ranged from 71 to 92 percent for individual vaccinations in 1994, although only 57 percent of children were fully immunized according to UNICEF standards (MFDP 1997). Prevalence of malnutrition among children under five years ranged from between 13 and 15 percent during the

TABLE 23.4

Morbidity and Mortality Measures)

Leading Causes of Inpatient Morbidity, 1994	Percent of Discharges	
Pneumonia	6.9	
Ill-defined intestinal infections	6.1	
Abortions	6.1	
Other ill-defined conditions	6	
Direct obstetric cause	5.7	
Pulmonary tuberculosis	5.2	
Estimated prevalence of HIV among adults	**Low-risk**	**High-risk**
Major urban areas (Gaborone/Francistown)	43.0%	60.4%
Outside major urban areas	32.7%	50.8%

SOURCE: MFDP (1997); Census Bureau (2001).

same period; severe malnutrition has fallen to less than one-half of one percent. Infant mortality had fallen to 45 per 1,000 live births by 1991 from 71 in 1971. Regional variations exist that should be considered. Furthermore, largely because of the impact of AIDS, infant mortality has increased since 1991 to a projected rate of 62 per 1,000 live births in 2001 (Census Bureau 2000). Additional information concerning access to health-enhancing factors can be found in Table 23.5.

Organization and Management of the Health System

Modern healthcare services were first organized under the auspices of various missions in the 1920s and 1930s and supplemented by a few hospitals built and administered by the colonial government. These, apparently, were fairly separate efforts with little central coordination. By the 1970s, the newly established Republic of Botswana had adopted a policy of universal access to healthcare (Maganu 1994) and begun a program of health-services extension that was heavily reliant on primary care (MFDP 1997).

Today, the public sector continues to play a pervasive role in Botswana's healthcare system; the fact that the majority of services are delivered through public healthcare facilities helps to preserve that role. Responsibility at the central level is shared by two ministries. The Ministry of Health (MOH) is responsible for planning, policy, technical oversight, and administration of most of the hospital system. The Ministry of Local Government, Lands, and Housing (MLGLH) maintains responsibility for the delivery of primary healthcare services, largely through local government authorities.

The Ministry of Health

Botswana's MOH defines its role as "policy maker, professional guide and supervisor of health care in its entirety in Botswana, irrespective of the provider or institution" (MFDP 1997). A private-sector system of health-

TABLE 23.5 Percent Access to Health-Enhancing Factors

Access to health services	89
Within 15 km of primary healthcare facility (rural/urban)	83/98
Within 8 km of primary healthcare facility (rural/urban)	75/94
Access to safe water	93
Access to sanitation	55
Immunization levels,* 1994	57

* Percent of children fully immunized according to WHO guidelines.
SOURCE: UNDP (1998); MFDP (1997).

care exists that is both compatible and cooperative with the public system, but it is comparatively quite small and based typically in urban areas.

Given the nation's tradition of participation in governance, policy formulation is typically an inclusive process. The MOH is the first voice of authority with regard to health policy at the parliamentary level; it facilitated the adoption of the National Policy on HIV/AIDS in 1994 and the National Health Policy in 1995. Departments within the MOH commonly sponsor local and national workshops to discuss healthcare issues and develop recommendations for policy formulation. The MOH sets standards of equipment for facilities as well as guidelines for care; it retains the power of licensure and controls the import of pharmaceuticals and medical equipment.

The MOH is a strong adherent to the principles of primary health set forth in the Alma-Ata declaration of 1978 (MFDP 1997). The Primary Health Care Department, which is made up of separate divisions for family, community, and dental health; rehabilitation services; and an independent AIDS/sexually transmitted diseases unit, has arguably the greatest influence of any MOH department on a citizen's life. Through its divisions and their constituent units, the Department of Primary Health Care sets standards for maternal and child health and nutrition and occupational and environmental health. The AIDS/sexually transmitted diseases unit is operated as a distinct entity within the department, and it is charged with planning and coordinating national AIDS prevention programs. The Primary Health Care Department supports primary prevention activities through its Health Education Unit and a unit devoted to the expanded program on immunization and diarrheal disease control. The Division of Primary Health Care Support implements programs designed to strengthen district-level management and support all levels of administration in the primary health system. The breadth of these activities extends the Department of Primary Health Care's influence across all levels of healthcare.

The Department of Hospital Services oversees the hospital system from primary through tertiary care and coordinates the planning of personnel, equipment, and capital development in response to demographic and epidemiologic trends. Hospital operations are under the direct control of the MOH through this department.

The MOH's Department of Technical Support Services coordinates policy with respect to a variety of issues that have an impact on quality of care. This department maintains final responsibility for equipment and commodities, including pharmaceuticals. It also oversees pharmacy, laboratory, and blood transfusion services throughout the healthcare system.

Finally, the Department of Manpower Services is responsible for human resources planning and development. It coordinates entry-level training for all cadres of healthcare providers, and it sets policy for licensure and practice, playing a role in determining the distribution of human resources, often in coordination with MLGLH. Human resources are discussed further below.

Ministry of Local Government, Lands, and Housing

The MLGLH is a vast ministry, with responsibilities for district administration and support to local government, town, and regional planning; land management and conservation; family and social welfare; and housing. Because a decentralization program begun in the mid-1980s has moved the majority of the primary healthcare system to the oversight of local authorities, the MLGLH has its greatest influence on the healthcare system through support to local governments.

The MLGLH's Department of Local Government and Development maintains a health office that provides support to local authorities for the administration of their healthcare programs. Such support includes assistance in planning, compliance with national policy, coordination of selected training initiatives, and oversight of human and other resource allocation among local authorities. This office is the official liaison between the MOH and departments of health in the town and district councils.

Local Authorities

Health departments within each town and district council oversee the delivery of primary healthcare. Within their respective jurisdictions, these health departments have increasing responsibility under decentralization for supervision and operations, allocation of resources, planning and implementation of discrete programs, and quality assurance. Technically, local authorities constitute governmental entities independent of the MLGLH. However, the MLGLH potentially has enormous influence on the functioning of district health departments given its role in oversight and coordination of district health plans and the attendant allocation of resources. Thus, district health departments, which typically lack resources, must navigate a difficult balance between ministerial and local influence.

Financing

A small proportion of the population pays out-of-pocket for private healthcare services. Employer-funded health insurance exists, but it is limited to that portion of the population fully employed by participating organizations. The vast majority of healthcare financing is provided through the public sector.

Generally Botswana's budget is broken down into recurrent and development expenditure. Recurrent expenditure is for salaries, supplies, maintenance and replacement of equipment, and other expenses of an ongoing nature, including a large portion invested in training costs. Development expenditure is for capital investment such as facilities, new equipment, pilot programs, one-time training, and research. Because a large proportion of recurrent expenditure for healthcare is channeled through local authorities as payment for salaries, vehicle maintenance, and utility payments, the exact amount of healthcare expenditure is difficult to ascertain.

Planning

In general, development planning in Botswana is led by the Ministry of Finance and Development Planning (MFDP), with substantial input from line ministries and local authorities; it is an evolving process that has active participation and integration with day-to-day decision making as its key goals. The typical plan period is seven years. The current National Development Plan is NDP 8, which covers the period from 1997 through 2003.

As the process begins, the MFDP identifies and disseminates a paper outlining key issues related to national economic performance to line ministries, local authorities, and other consultative bodies. Coordinated through planning units with close ties to the MFDP, line ministries respond with key-issues papers relevant to their sectors of responsibility, which are widely distributed for comment and discussion. In the midst of this dialog, the MFDP determines and distributes budget parameters for the line ministries to use in developing key strategies and, finally, in planning identifiable projects for concurrence by the MFDP and approval by Parliament in its adoption of the plan. Plan implementation is monitored jointly by the MFDP and specific implementing agencies (Samatar 1999).

Decentralization of the primary healthcare system adds some complexity to the planning process in the health sector. The MOH is responsible for health planning at the ministerial level, but it has neither direct control nor any real financial influence over the district health teams. The district health teams are funded within the overall plans of the relevant local authorities, which typically are financed through a combination of limited local revenue and substantial grants from the central government.

Although planning for vertically managed services such as hospital services and manpower training is completed at the central level, a more complex process is required to promote compatibility among the health plans of local authorities and the MOH. First, the MOH requests information from the district health teams regarding health status, service provision, and resource use. After this information is analyzed, guidelines are sent to districts and facilities to form the basis of subsequent discussion. These guidelines include information regarding recent experience, national programs and targets, and resource availability. Following consultation between local and central authorities, district health teams develop and submit their plans to the MLGLH within the overall district plans. Further technical consultation and negotiation then ensues among the MOH, the MLGLH, and local authorities to reconcile the now several discrete plans into a functional whole that is defensible before the MFDP and Parliament (Bloom et al. 1991). Obviously, this process relies heavily on good-faith consultation and cooperation among all parties involved.

Health Resources

Human resource constraints are a perennial problem in all of Botswana's development sectors. The country's small, sparsely distributed population and relatively sophisticated training requirements exacerbate the problem in the health sector. Training capacity exists domestically for registered nurses, midwives, nurse practitioners, anesthetic nurses, pharmacy technicians, x-ray assistants, and dental therapists. As of 1996, all other categories of service provider were required to train outside the country. To meet shortages, the MOH and the MLGLH regularly recruit from other countries in Africa and further abroad. Additional assistance, particularly with professional human resources, historically has been available through cooperation with various donor agencies. However, donor assistance has decreased in Botswana during the last decade.

In 1996, all but 20 of the physicians in the government's employ were expatriates; at least half of those 20 were in administrative positions. Given the shortage of physicians, nurses are the backbone of Botswana's primary healthcare system. Accordingly, they command considerable influence with regard to healthcare policy and planning. Nurse-matrons often supervise district health teams, and those with graduate training in public health have risen to head full ministerial departments. Tables 23.6 and 23.7 provide details regarding the available human resources in the health system.

	Number	Population per Facility
National referral hospital	2	747,500
District hospital	16	93,438
Primary hospital	14	106,786
Clinic with maternity ward	76	19,671
Clinic without maternity ward	133	11,241
Health post	314	4,761
Total fixed facilities	555	2,694
Mobile health stop	687	2,176

TABLE 23.6
Number and Type of Health Services Facilities and by Population

SOURCE: MFDP (1997).

TABLE 23.7
Human
Resources
per 1,000
Population
by Type

	Number (public and private)	Population per Healthcare Provider
Physicians	393	3,804
Dentists (public only)	10	149,500
Nurses	3678	406
Community health workers	714	2,094
Hospital administrators (public only)	25	59,800
Midwives (public only)	736	2,031
Family nurse practicioners	30	49,833

SOURCE: MFDP (1997).

Preservice nursing training takes place through six institutes of health sciences, which are attached to referral hospitals for practical work. These semi-autonomous institutes are overseen by the Department of Manpower Resources in the MOH.

Most public healthcare facilities are reasonably well equipped. In a 1996 situation analysis of the maternal and child health program, 93 percent of the sites visited had piped water, 84 percent had waiting rooms, and 84 percent had working toilets (Maribe et al. 1996). However, 40 percent had neither main nor solar electricity. Except for an examination lamp and a vaccine refrigerator, the equipment necessary to provide maternal and child health and family planning services was available at nearly all facilities. Diagnostic and screening facilities for sexually transmitted diseases and HIV/AIDS existed at nearly all hospitals, but they were rare at smaller facilities.

Pharmaceuticals and medical supplies are purchased by tender through the Central Medical Stores (CMS) in accordance with a registry of drugs and supplies approved for distribution in Botswana. The CMS falls under the MOH's Department of Technical Support Services. Requisitions for commodities are made by individual facilities directly to the CMS on the basis of simple inventory control procedures applied by facility personnel; the CMS then ships directly to the facility. District health teams are copied on paperwork. Shortages of commodities are not common, although they do occur. Problems of commodity management seem to lie primarily within the individual facility rather than across the distribution system and involve issues such as inadequate record keeping. The situation analysis mentioned above found that, although nearly all facilities had a stock book available, only about 70 percent maintained it adequately with regard to vaccines, drugs for sexually transmitted disease, or family planning commodities (Maribe et al. 1996).

Expensive, highly specialized equipment is more problematic. For example, computed tomography scanning services were routinely purchased from the private hospital by the national referral hospitals in the 1990s; the MOH plans to install the necessary equipment in referral hospitals by 2003. The expense associated with dental equipment has impeded the ability of oral health services to develop any sizable domestic capacity for the delivery of care, at least within the public sector. Reliance on South African resources for oral health services remains significant (MFDP 1997).

Service Delivery

The primary healthcare system operated by the local authorities is made up of a network of clinics, health posts, and mobile stops, with descending scopes of care. Services strongly emphasize education and prevention. Service delivery is integrated, meaning that within the normal scope of care, any given service should be available to the public on any given day. Thus, a mother should have access to care for her children (e.g., immunizations, growth monitoring) and herself (e.g., family planning, other services) in a single trip to a facility. This is considered an important factor in encouraging the use of services.

Mobile stops are operated from nearby clinics in areas with no fixed facility and provide limited primary healthcare services. Services may include the routine monitoring of child and prenatal health, the diagnosis of common illnesses, the dispensation of a limited range of medicines or family planning commodities, and health education. New enrollees and complex cases are referred to health posts or clinics for consultation.

Health posts have fixed facilities, usually limited to three rooms and outdoor plumbing facilities. Staffed by one nurse and a family welfare educator (community health worker), health posts deliver a broader range of services, including expanded maternal and child health, school and environmental health, and first aid. Health posts receive periodic visits from supervising clinics. Health education, case finding, and follow-up are important functions of the health post, particularly in communities without a resident clinic. The family welfare educator plays a key role in this regard.

Clinics generally are placed in villages with populations of 3,000 or more. They have several rooms, a covered waiting area, and at least one vehicle used for patient transportation, the operation of mobile stops, and visits to other facilities. Clinics may be staffed with several nurses but rarely have a physician, except for maternity clinics in larger urban areas. Clinics provide all of the primary care services available at their subsidiary facilities, and they are augmented with clinical and laboratory support. As such, clinics have a much greater role in providing curative care. Delivery services also are provided at maternity clinics. (See Table 23.6 for the number and type of facilities by population.)

As indicated, patients may access the healthcare system at mobile stops, health posts, or clinics. If a patient's primary facility does not offer needed services, the individual is referred to a higher-level facility for care, from health post to clinic and from mobile stop to clinic or health post. Clinics refer patients to primary hospitals as necessary. Primary hospitals have 20 to 70 beds for general, maternity, and tuberculosis care; they offer more complete laboratory services and outpatient services than clinics do, and they include x-ray and surgery facilities. Primary hospitals are distributed according to population and other factors related to physical accessibility.

In addition to receiving patients from their own community, district hospitals receive referrals from primary hospitals. With 71 to 250 beds, district hospitals offer special services for complex cases and a broader range of surgical and rehabilitative care. District hospitals are placed in major villages and towns. They refer clients to one of two national referral hospitals as required, as these two hospitals offer an extended range of specialty care in addition to the full range of care found at other points in the system. When needs are so specialized that national referral hospitals cannot meet them, referrals may be made to facilities in South Africa or, occasionally, to the private hospital in Gaborone.

Private and traditional healthcare delivery operates alongside and often in step with the public healthcare system. Private physicians are licensed by the government and generally practice in major villages and towns; they hold consultations and provide outpatient care from private offices. Privately operated laboratories exist, but they may rely on South African facilities for test results. Clients who require specialty care commonly are referred to private facilities outside the country or to a private hospital—the first in Botswana—in Gaborone. Referral of patients by private physicians to public facilities within Botswana would likely require enrollment in the public system as a new case, but work already completed by the referring physician may reduce the time required for diagnosis and treatment plans.

A major difference between the public and private healthcare systems is cost to the client. Public services charge a token fee, which is often waived in practice, amounting to about U.S.$1 for the first encounter annually and less thereafter. Clients of private providers typically pay cost plus a fee, and fees may vary from one provider to the next. Reasons for seeking care through private providers may include convenience (lines at public clinics can be long in urban areas and appointments are rare), increased privacy, or perceptions of differences in quality; that this situation could lead to some stratification of care-seeking behavior by income is readily apparent. However, with the possible exception of oral health services, indications of real differences in technical quality are unproven.

As is the case in many African societies, Batswana have many strongly held traditional explanations for physical and spiritual ailments. Traditional healthcare providers range from birth attendants to herbalists and faith healers. Individuals often seek care from a traditional healer for certain ailments and a modern healthcare provider for others without any thought of inconsistency. Additionally, some may seek palliative treatment at modern facilities while relying on traditional healers to cure the source of illness (Steen and Mazonde 1999). To a large extent, traditional healers are integrated into Botswana's primary healthcare system (Haram 1991; Chipfakacha 1999). Central-level and district authorities often host seminars designed to exchange views with traditional healers and, particularly, to recruit their assistance in case finding and referral. Traditional medicine in Botswana rests on a complex system of theory and practice that goes well beyond the scope of this chapter. Interested readers should look into the works cited here for additional references.

Botswana has no formal system of long-term care. Elders are generally active participants in extended households; the family provides their care. Rehabilitation of both mental and physical disabilities is typically based in the community. Training and other services are coordinated by private, not-for-profit institutions that receive some government funding and collaborate with public health or social welfare workers. Institutional mental health services are based in a single mental hospital.

Prospects for the Future

Botswana's most difficult challenge of the future is already upon it. The country's first case of AIDS was diagnosed in 1985, and aggressive preventive action was taken almost immediately. Steps were taken to protect the blood supply, public education campaigns increased in volume and directness, and productive partnerships were formed between the public and private sectors. Yet, as in so many other countries on the African continent, the HIV epidemic rages.

Now, with HIV prevalence at levels far above what previously was thought possible, AIDS threatens the important development gains that have led some to call Botswana "an African miracle." Local media report that nurses are leaving their posts en masse out of helplessness as well as fear of infection. Concern exists that the educational system will founder if teachers cannot be kept healthy or afford to stay at post. Given the perennial shortage of skilled human resources that this country faces and the level of mortality among the most economically active age groups, no sector of the economy can remain untouched.

Some point with hope to the experiences of Thailand and Uganda, where HIV prevalence has declined in recent years. However, it is not yet clear that such declines will be realized in southern Africa through anything more than the mortality of those already infected. Meanwhile, the substantial resources required to provide care for opportunistic infections related to the epidemic will detract from the nation's ability to complete its epidemiologic transition. Sadly, the future may well hold the past.

REFERENCES

Bloom, G. H., Lenneiye, N. M., Maganu, E. T., and Tselayakgosi, M. 1991. "Health Programme Planning for Consolidation and Quality." *World Health Forum* 12: 90–95.

Campbell, E. K. 1995. "Population Distribution and Urbanisation." Paper presented to the 1991 Population and Housing Census Dissemination Seminar in May 1995. Gaborone: Central Statistics Office, Ministry of Finance and Development Planning, Republic of Botswana.

Granberg, P., and Parkinson, J. R. 1988. *Botswana: Country Study and Norwegian Aid Review.* Bergen: Chr. Michelson Institute.

Haram, L. 1991. "Tswana Medicine in Interaction with Biomedicine." *Social Science Medicine* 33: 167–75.

Hartland-Thunberg, P. 1978. *Botswana: An African Growth Economy.* Boulder: Westview Press.

Harvey, C., and Lewis, S. R., Jr. 1990. *Policy Choice and Development Performance in Botswana.* New York: St. Martin's Press.

Hilmers, D. C. 2000. "A View from There." *Journal of the American Medical Association* 284 (1): 98.

Hope, K. R., Sr. 1997. *African Political Economy: Contemporary Issues in Development.* Armonk, NY: M. E. Sharpe.

Kenyon, T. A., Mwasekaga, M. J., Huebner, R., Rumisha, D., Binkin, N., and Maganu, E. 1999. "Low Levels of Drug Resistance amidst Rapidly Increasing Tuberculosis and Human Immunodeficiency Virus Co-Epidemics in Botswana." *International Journal of Tuberculosis and Lung Disease* 3 (1): 4–11.

Leburu-Sianga, F. M. 1995. "Review of Educational Achievements in Botswana Education 1971–1991." Paper presented to the 1991 Population and Housing Census Dissemination Seminar in May 1995. Gaborone: Central Statistics Office, Ministry of Finance and Development Planning, Republic of Botswana.

Maganu, E. 1994. "Health Prospects for Botswana into the Next Century: Interaction of Health Status and Socio-Economic Conditions." *Botswana in the 21st Century,* edited by S. Brothers, J. Hermans, and D. Nteta. Gaborone: The Botswana Society.

Main, M. 1987. *Kalahari: Life's Variety in Dune and Delta.* Republic of South Africa: Halfway House, Southern Book Publishers.

Maribe, L., Maggwa, B. N., Baakile, B., and Miller, R. A. 1996. "A Situation Analysis of the Maternal and Child Health/Family Planning Program in

Botswana." New York: The Population Council.

Ministry of Finance and Development Planning (MFDP), Republic of Botswana. 1997. *National Development Plan VIII*. Gaborone: Government Printer.

Mukamaambo, E. P. 1995. "Demographic and Socio-Economic Situation in Botswana." Paper presented to the 1991 Population and Housing Census Dissemination Seminar in May 1995. Gaborone: Central Statistics Office, Ministry of Finance and Development Planning, Republic of Botswana.

Samatar, A. I. 1999. *An African Miracle: State and Class Leadership and Colonial Legacy in Botswana Development*. Portsmouth: Heinemann.

Steen, T. W., and Mazonde, G. N. 1999. "Ngaka ya Setswana, Ngaka ya Sekgoa or Both? Health Seeking Behavior in Botswana with Pulmonary Tuberculosis." *Social Science and Medicine* 48: 163–72.

Tlou, T., and Campbell, A. 1984. *History of Botswana*. Gaborone: Macmillan Botswana Publishing.

United Nations Development Programme (UNDP). 1998. *Human Development Report 1998*. New York: Oxford University Press.

U.S. Census Bureau. 2000. International Data Base. Retrieved March 2002 from www.census.gov/cgi-bin/ipc.

———. 2001. HIV/AIDS Surveillance Database. Retrieved March 2002 from www.census.gov/ipc/www/hivaidsd.html.

U.S. Central Intelligence Agency (CIA). 2001. *The World Factbook 2001*. Washington, DC: CIA.

van der Post, C. 1995. "Internal Migration." Paper presented to the 1991 Population and Housing Census Dissemination Seminar in May 1995. Gaborone: Central Statistics Office, Ministry of Finance and Development Planning, Republic of Botswana.

World Bank. 2001. *World Development Report 2000/2001: Attacking Poverty*. New York: Oxford University Press.

World Health Organization (WHO). 2000. *The World Health Report 2000*. Geneva: World Health Organization.

BRAZIL

Rui Portugal and Alexandre V. Abrantes

> *Health is the right of everyone and the duty of the*
> *State, guaranteed via social and economic policies*
> *which aim for the reduction of the risk of disease and*
> *other injuries and universal access to activities and*
> *services for its promotion, protection and recovery.*
> —*Article 196, Brazilian Constitution*

Background Information

Brazil is geographically the fifth largest country in the world, with the sixth largest population. Brazil's land mass of 8,547,404 square kilometers covers nearly half of the continent of South America, stretching 4,320 kilometers from north to south and 4,328 kilometers from east to west, with a western land frontier of 15,719 kilometers and an Atlantic coastline of 7,408 kilometers (PAHO 1998; CIA 2000). That land mass supports a population of 166.1 million inhabitants according to 2000 estimates, yielding a population density of 18 people per square kilometer. However, that population is unequally distributed throughout the country. The north, the largest region, occupies 45 percent of the national territory but supports only 7 percent of the population; the southeast occupies 11 percent of the territory and has 43 percent of the population. Approximately 77.6 percent of the population is urban (PAHO 1998). In 1997, the Human Development Index score for Brazil was 0.793, giving it a general ranking of 79 (UNDP 2000). Approximately 30 percent of the population lived in poverty in that year, with significantly higher percentages in the northeast and northern regions and in rural areas (39 percent), whereas poverty in the more industrialized states (chiefly in the southeastern region) is described as increasingly urban. The nine states in the northeast have the lowest socioeconomic indicators in the country. The Brazilian fertility rate has decreased rapidly in recent decades, from 2.57 children per woman in 1991 to 2.4 in 1997 (PAHO 1998; World Bank 2000). Life expectancy at birth increased by 3.9 years (6.3 percent) between 1980 and 1990 (PAHO 1998). Additional demographic data are provided in Table 24.1.

The Brazilian population is derived from four ethnic sources: the indigenous Indians, the colonizing Portuguese, the enslaved African blacks,

TABLE 24.1
General
Demographics

Population in millions	167.9
Infant mortality per 1,000 live births	30.1
Under-five mortality per 1,000 live births	44.2
Life expectancy at birth (years)	67.8
Fertility rate	2.4
Percent urbanized	77.6

SOURCE: WHO (1999); DATASUS (1997, 1998); PAHO (1998).

and various immigrant groups from Europe and Asia. Currently the majority of the population claims a mixed lineage. Ethnic disparities are evident in the lower wages received by blacks and those of mixed race (including other dark-skinned groups), who make up 44 percent of the total population and who, in 1990, earned on average only 68 percent of the amount earned by Caucasians (PAHO 1998; World Bank 2000).

Brazil is a federal republic consisting of 26 states, the Federal District, and 5,507 municipalities, the political, fiscal, and administrative autonomy of which are guaranteed in the Brazilian Constitution of 1988. The Brazilian economy is the largest in Latin America and the tenth largest in the world. Still, the nation remains largely agricultural; processed and unprocessed agricultural products account for about one-third of exports, and agriculture, forestry, and fishing account for 14 percent of the gross national product. The country is richly endowed with metals and other minerals and claims almost one-third of the world's iron reserves. Industrial production accounts for 36 percent of the GNP, and sales of mechanical equipment, cars, chemicals, textiles, and other manufactured goods account for the majority of exports. Service industries account for 50 percent of the economy (PAHO 1998; World Bank 2000).

In 1994, the Real Plan (named for the country's new currency unit, the real) was launched in an effort to foster growth in per capita income and spur a redistribution of wealth. As a result, the poorest half of the population saw its share of national revenues increase by 1.2 percent, whereas that of the richest 20 percent decreased by 2.3 percent. The per capita gross domestic product grew from U.S.$4,305 in 1994 to U.S.$4,630 in 1999. In 1999, the annual inflation rate was 6 percent as compared with rates of as much as 45 percent per month just a decade earlier. See Table 24.2 for additional economic data (CIA 2000; World Bank 2000).

Although the unemployment rate is relatively low, the quality of jobs has deteriorated. The proportion of workers employed in the formal sector has fallen from 60 to 50 percent, whereas the proportion of self-employed workers, who are excluded from the benefits and protection of labor leg-

GNP per capita (U.S.$)	4,630
Real GDP per capita (P.P.P.$), 1998	6,100
Human Development Index score	0.739
Percent of GNP to health	6.52
Percent of health budget in public sector	9.39
Unemployment rate (percent)	7
Poverty rate (percent)	30

FIGURE 24.2
Economic and
Social
Indicators

SOURCE: World Bank (2000); CIA (2000); UNDP (2000); WHO (1999); DATASUS (1997).

islation, has increased (CIA 2000; World Bank 2000).

Job security has decreased even in the face of improved economic indicators, but educational levels have improved significantly in recent decades, with a reduction in illiteracy, an increase in school enrollment, and a rise in the average number of years of schooling. Nevertheless, the illiteracy rate remained as high as 15 percent in 1998. Additional information about the education of the Brazilian population is provided in Table 24.3.

Context: Health Needs

Mortality levels in the Brazilian population have declined significantly in recent decades, even after controlling for underreporting of 20 percent according to estimates by the Brazilian Geography and Statistics Institute; this reduction primarily reflects the decline in mortality in children younger than five years old. In 1998, the mortality of this age group was 44 per 1,000, and infant mortality was 30.1 per 1,000. This represents a significant decrease from the early 1990s, when rates stood at 58 per 1,000 for children under five years and at 40 per 1,000 for infants. Half of all infant deaths occur in the northeast, which is the poorest region of the country (PAHO 1998; World Bank 2000).

	Male	Female
Adult literacy rate (percent)	85.4	84
Primary school enrollment (percent)	97	97
Secondary school enrollment (percent)	66	66

TABLE 24.3
Education
Indicators

SOURCE: World Bank (2000).

The maternal mortality rate also dropped significantly from 1982 through 1997 from 156 to 59.1 per 100,000 live births, largely because of improvements in access to prenatal and postnatal maternal care. Data from a national study conducted in 1997 show that 96.9 percent of births in urban areas took place in healthcare institutions (78 percent in rural areas) and that 86 percent of the mothers had received prenatal care (World Bank 2000).

Although access to health-enhancing factors such as clean water and immunizations remains a source of concern, the situation is improving. As indicated in Table 24.4, the majority of the Brazilian population is now connected to a clean water supply and sewer system or septic tank. However, of the total amount of wastewater collected, only 20 percent is treated at a water purification plant.

The National Immunization Program has reported high routine coverage of infants that are less than one year old (Table 24.4). However, coverage is still very low for hepatitis B because the vaccine is not offered free of charge (PAHO 1998). The immunization program still uses various campaigns to inform and increase access for the population.

Analysis of 1997 deaths by cause shows that noncommunicable diseases account for the majority of deaths. During the period from 1990 to 1994, 33.9 percent of reported deaths were attributed to cardiovascular diseases, which are the leading causes of death in all regions of the country. Injury and poisoning (external causes) account for close to 15 percent of all deaths from defined causes. Notably, between 1977 and 1994, the death rate due to homicide increased 160 percent nationwide. Among external causes of death, one of the most prevalent in Brazil is traffic accidents, which increased rapidly until the mid-1980s and then began to decrease slightly in 1990. Many automobile-related deaths involve pedes-

TABLE 24.4

Access to Health-Enhancing Factors (percent)

Access to health services	95
Access to safe water	76
Access to sanitation	60
Immunization levels	
Polio	89.5
Tuberculosis	117.4
Hepatitis B	5.6
Measles	108.5
Diphtheria	78.7
Use of contraception	55.4

SOURCE: DATASUS (1995, 1997).

trians (PAHO 1998; DATASUS 2000). Detailed information about the most common causes of hospitalization can be found in Table 24.5.

Tropical communicable diseases are common throughout Brazil, although they may be particularly prevalent in specific areas. For example, more than 99 percent of the 463,993 cases of malaria reported in 1997 occurred in the Amazon region. As for most developing nations, AIDS is a major health threat. As of February 1997, the cumulative number of AIDS cases in Brazil was 103,262 (20,026 in 1997 and 18,774 in 1998); 74 percent of these cases were in the southeast region. Between 1997 and 1998, the mean cumulative incidence for the country as a whole was 74 cases per 100,000 inhabitants. The mortality rate of AIDS is slowing as a result of access to new medications and a reduction of the infection rate, which undoubtedly has been facilitated by increased health promotion and health education programs. The incidence of tuberculosis, which occurs as an opportunistic infection in 15 percent of AIDS cases, remains high at 52.19 per 100,000 inhabitants (PAHO 1998; World Bank 2000; WHO 2000).

Malnutrition has been a constant health threat in Brazil, especially among children. During the past two decades, a steady decline has been reported in malnutrition among children five years old and younger, with a reduction of 60 percent between 1975 and 1989 and of 20 percent between 1989 and 1996. (Malnutrition is defined as weight-for-age two standard deviations or more below the expected mean value.) Still, although great strides are being made, malnutrition remains a serious problem (World Bank 2000).

The most recent data on the distribution of mental disorders in the Brazilian population come from a study conducted in 1990 and 1991 in three metropolitan regions. Neurotic disorders, especially anxiety and phobia disorders, were found to be most prevalent, with rates ranging from 7.6 percent in São Paulo to 17.6 percent in Brasilia. Mental health care is included by legislation in the public healthcare system as an important component of the health of the population (Ministério de Saúde 2000). However, most mental health care is still provided in mental health hos-

TABLE 24.5
Leading Causes of Hospitalization

Causes	Percent
Obstetrics	26
Cardiac and circulatory disease	9
Respiratory infections	17
Infectious diseases	8
Cancer	3

SOURCE: DATASUS (2000).

pitals. Mental health community services are not well distributed in the country.

Drug use is also a growing problem in Brazil, especially among young people. Surveys conducted in 1987, 1989, and 1993 in primary and secondary schools in ten cities showed that the six most frequently used drugs were alcohol, tobacco, solvents, tranquilizers, amphetamines, and marijuana. Alcoholism and drug use together account for close to 20 percent of all hospitalizations for mental disorders. An estimated 30 million Brazilians smoke cigarettes, and 80,000 deaths each year are related to tobacco use (DATASUS 2000).

Organization and Management of the Health System

The Brazilian health system is in transition, and this is undeniably affected by the broad socioeconomic changes in the country in recent decades. Healthcare reform was written into the Federal Constitution of 1988, but practical implementation of the Unified Health System (Sistema Único de Saúde [SUS]) was not undertaken until 1990, when the National Social Insurance Institute for Medical Care was transferred to the Ministry of Health and Laws 8080 and 8142/90, known as the Organic Health Laws, were enacted (Buss and Gadelha 1996).

The SUS integrated all public healthcare services, including those supplemented by private facilities, in a decentralized and hierarchical network with a single command center at each level of government (federal, state, and municipal). This arrangement allows citizens some control over state actions regarding health and healthcare. These principles of decentralization and public involvement were extended to state and municipal legislation (Araújo-Júnior 1997; Atkinson et al. 2000). Healthcare delivery institutions remain predominantly private but with predominantly public financing (Fielder 1996).

Other systemic changes since the late 1980s include the following:

- Access to specialty care is no longer limited to Social Security beneficiaries.
- Decisions about priorities and health service delivery have been transferred to managers with greater patient contact.
- Public participation has increased through both health conferences and the health councils, which now include the organized representation of professionals and consumers.
- Substantial improvements have been seen in many health areas. For example, prenatal care coverage increased from 74 to 85 percent, and deliveries in health facilities grew from 80 to 91 percent, contributing to a 41 percent drop in infant mortality and a 30 percent drop in maternal mortality (Almeida 2000).

Brazilian health sector reform, as conceived and implemented at the end of the 1980s, was one of the last expansionist reforms of the decade (PAHO 1998). It was based on the ideas that have generally shaped health system organization in the postwar world and strongly influenced by the philosophy of the state as service provider. Health sector reforms have focused on strengthening the public sector; increasing and diversifying financial resources; decentralizing the system; rationalizing the supply and delivery of services; and reorganizing sectorial interests, with a new definition of the public/ private relationship. In the long term, the SUS managerial model aims for accessibility and equity along three principal vectors of reform:

1. consolidating a comprehensive, decentralized system by harmonizing functions across levels of government and integrating services of varying scope and complexity
2. investing authoritative bodies with the power to make decisions about the health system and to conclude agreements between the parties involved in the management of services, with a focus on creating and maintaining partnerships
3. assigning local authorities the responsibilities for effectiveness and equity of care provided to the population in each territorial unit, especially at the municipal level (Almeida 2000)

The development of the system, however, has been fraught with contradictions and conflicts because of both domestic and international political and economic conditions as well as constraints of the reform process itself (Buss and Gadelha 1996). Since the implementation of reforms, Brazil has struggled with a series of conflicts of interest. Outstanding among them is the conflict between states and the federal principles underlying SUS, compounded by a strong upsurge in neoliberal, free-market thinking. For users, an immense gap still remains between constitutionally guaranteed rights to healthcare, which is the normative rationale of the system, and its actual implementation. Substantial socioeconomic inequities in access and care persist, along with pervasive user dissatisfaction with the quality and availability of services.

The SUS administration is not staffed by permanent professionals. Rather, administrators change with each change of local or national government; these personnel shifts are usually based on political criteria and do not take technical competence into account. This has been a major obstacle to the continuation of the various programs. Notwithstanding this fluidity, the main conceptual and operational principles of the SUS have endured because of the activism of public health professionals and various social movements (Buss and Gadelha 1996; Almeida 2000).

The Brazilian health system is a complex network of service providers and service purchasers that are simultaneously interrelated, complementary, and competitive, thereby forming a complicated public/private mix funded primarily by public resources. The system is composed of three main subsectors (Buss and Gadelha 1996; Ameida 2000):

1. the public sector, which is made up of publicly financed health services at the federal, state, and municipal levels and the armed forces, which have their own separate healthcare services
2. the private sector (both for-profit and not-for-profit), which is contracted by the public sector and paid through reimbursement systems and is made up of publicly financed and privately provided services
3. the free choice private sector, which is financed with out-of-pocket payments or by corporate health insurance and is made up of privately financed services with different levels of insurance premiums and tax subsidies

Unlike the situation found in most healthcare systems, general practitioners do not play a dominant role in the Brazilian system, which is primarily focused on specialized and curative care. The system is hospital-centered, largely as a result of the design of Social Security benefits at the inception of the system in the 1960s. The most significant innovation in recent reforms is the priority given to basic care, which is understood as a "package" of procedures to be provided locally according to certain parameters and financed through the Basic Operational Guidelines (Piso Assistencial Básico) distributed per capita to municipalities. At the same time, financial incentives are being put in place to encourage the introduction of two programs, the Family Health Program and the Community Health Agents. These two programs are intended to improve the primary healthcare balance in contrast with the current curative medical focus (PAHO 1998). Public health services and private services that work under contract to the government within the framework of the SUS cover 75 percent of the population. Most inpatient hospital services are provided under a system of public reimbursement for services provided by private entities. Eighty percent of hospitals that provide services within the SUS are private. In contrast, public establishments provide 75 percent of outpatient care within the SUS.

The federal tier of the system is legally responsible for formulating and implementing national health policy. It is also in charge of system planning, assessment, control, and funding distribution. The decision-making process at that level involves three agencies. The National Health Council, which includes representatives of government agencies, service providers, healthcare professionals, and consumers, approves strategic planning and monitors implementation of the nation's healthcare policy. The Tripartite Intermanagerial Committee, whose members include representatives from the Ministry of Health, the National Council of State Health Secretaries, and the National Council of Municipal Health Secretaries, is designed to approve the rules for operating the system. The Ministry of Health manages the federal allocation of funds under the supervision and approval of the National Council of Health and proposes the operating rules to be approved by the Tripartite Intermanagerial Committee. This management structure is mirrored at the state level (State Health Secretariat, Bipartite Intermanagerial Committee, and State Health Council) and municipal level (Municipal Health Secretariat and Municipal Health Council) and coordinated by the respective health secretaries. Functions at the state level involve service coordination, distribution of financial resources, and decisions related to complex specialized technological interventions. These state-level functions are still evolving, as the decentralization process has until recently focused on the municipal level. The municipalities are responsible for handling the delivery of goods and services for health promotion, preventive care, healthcare, and rehabilitation (Buss and Gadelha 1996; Almeida 2000; Araújo-Júnior 1997).

Thus, despite differences in the organization of the system in the different states, the municipalities are generally responsible for managing the facilities operating at the primary and secondary levels, whereas the state manages those for tertiary referral and coordinates the regional referral and back-referral networks. In addition to operating under contract with state and municipal health secretariats to provide public health services, commercial and not-for-profit private facilities may also be paid directly by patients or as participants in some form of supplemental medical care; these services are heavily concentrated in the southeastern region.

The reform process has required deep changes at the technical-operational level, demanding a capacity-building effort as well as a revision of values, habits, and procedures. A number of recent studies have revealed at least two important problems: (1) radical devolution of power to the municipal level has led to greater fragmentation of the system, divesting the states of authority; and (2) the very composition of the various intermanagerial committees reproduces existing power relations, thereby maintaining historical inequities in the distribution of resources. Nevertheless, several innovative experiments are underway at the local level throughout the country (Atkinson et al. 2000; Araújo-Junior 1997).

The private medical care system operates under one of five primary arrangements (Buss and Gadelha 1996; Lewis 1995):

1. Group medicine, consisting of medical enterprises that administer health plans for individuals, families, and enterprises, have a care structure that includes their own and accredited facilities.
2. Medical cooperatives, which are organized by cooperating physicians and accredited hospitals and services, also offer health plans for individuals, families, and enterprises.
3. Health insurance administered by insurance companies gives the insured a choice of physicians and hospitals while reimbursing expenditures.

4. Self-management, which is the arrangement used by large enter-
    prises that finance and administer their own services, offers med-
    ical and hospital care exclusively to enterprise staff and their
    dependents.
5. Administration plans resemble self-management except that they are
    administered by enterprises hired to mediate service delivery.

Although the SUS is supervised by the National Health Quality
Control Institute (which serves as a national reference and quality-control
laboratory for an integrated network of state and university institutions),
private insurance plans, which cover approximately 25 percent of the population, are not strictly regulated.

Health Resources

In April 2000, Brazil had 487,338 available hospital beds, which was a total
of 3.6 per 1,000 inhabitants; 25 percent of these were in the public sector
and 75 percent were in the private sector. The vast majority of psychiatric
hospital beds (100,749, of which 30 percent are in public-sector facilities)
are concentrated in the southeast (63 percent) as compared with the north
(less than 1 percent) and the northeast (18 percent). The southeast and southern regions of the country possessed about 60 percent of the total installed
capacity in terms of establishments and available beds. In short, distribution
of hospital resources in Brazil is grossly inequitable. More than one-third of
Brazil's municipal districts (generally those with less than 5,000 inhabitants)
have no hospitals and lack even simple clinics (Buss and Gadelha 1996;

TABLE 24.6

Number and
Types of
Health
Services
Facilities and
per 1,000
Population

	Number	Per 1,000 Population
Hospitals	6,449	0.04
Public	2,224	0.014
Private	4,069	0.025
Hospital beds	487,338	3.6
Public		0.9
Private		2.7
Health centers	33,319	0.2
General clinics	1,745	0.011
Specialty clinics	4,577	0.028

SOURCE: DATASUS (2000).

DATASUS 2000). See Table 24.6 for additional information on health facilities.

Although specialized care and hospital care are concentrated in the private network, the basic public health services network is composed mainly of primary health service facilities, including health units, health centers, and emergency services. The system underwent a marked expansion from 1980 to 1986, largely in health centers (9 percent per year). Their numbers have increased nearly five-fold in recent decades as a result of rationing measures aimed at cost containment, which restricted hospital admissions and encouraged outpatient care. Since implementation of the SUS, the decentralization process has been intensified, accompanied by further growth in the number of health units and outpatient clinics (6 to 7 percent per year), despite the reduction of federal investments from 1990 to 1992. This has varied across the regions, with higher growth rates in the north and south (Almeida 2000; DATASUS 2000).

At the secondary level of care, public facilities serve an estimated 70 percent of the population. Regional disparities are striking here, too. Southeast Brazil has twice as many hospital beds at 4.3 per 1,000 population as the north with 2.1 per 1,000 population. The disparity persists in overall hospitalization rates as well as hospitalization under the SUS (Almeida 2000).

Brazil has more than half a million health professionals, and 50 percent are physicians (Table 24.7). Although a shortage of qualified nursing personnel persists, historical series constructed by professional councils show a real increase in the numbers of nurses and dentists and a stable supply of physicians relative to the total population. Women are entering the medical profession in increasing numbers; in 1996, 31.9 percent of all practicing physicians in the country were women. The distribution of health services and health professionals in the country is characterized by a heavy concentration of human resources in the most developed regions and in the state capitals.

The health sector accounts for about 8 percent of all jobs in the formal economy of Brazil. One-third of all health sector jobs are in the public administration sector at one of the three levels of government. Health

Physicians	1.34	**TABLE 24.7** Human Resources per 1,000 Population by Type
Nurses	.45	
Auxiliary nurses	2.22	
Dentists	.64	
Pharmacists	.35	

SOURCE: DATASUS (2000).

professionals commonly maintain more than one job, either within the public sector, the private sector, or both (World Bank 2000).

Brazil is among the world's ten largest consumer markets for drugs, with a 1.5 percent share of the world market. The pharmaceutical industry directly generated 47,100 jobs in 1996, with overall investments of U.S.$200 million that year. The sector comprises some 500 companies, including drug producers, chemical-pharmaceutical industries, and importers; 5,200 pharmaceutical products are available to Brazilians in 9,200 different forms. In 1996, the national immunization program used 196 million doses of 26 different types of vaccines and sera worth approximately U.S.$84 million. Of this amount, close to 76 million doses were manufactured in the country, which was sufficient to meet the total demand for bacillus Calmette-Guérin (BCG, a type of tuberculosis), tetanus toxoid, double antigen, yellow fever, and human and canine rabies vaccines as well as antivenin, antitetanic, antipertussis, and antirabies sera (World Bank 2000).

The National List of Essential Drugs was instituted in 1975 to serve as a guide for the selection of drugs in public health services. It has been updated periodically, with the last revision in 1998. The new list contains 315 active principles in 475 dosage media designed for the prevailing pathologies in Brazil. Under the Basic Drug Program, the Ministry of Health transfers about 1.30 Reals per capita each year to states and municipalities for the decentralized procurement of many of these drugs, which are intended for use in primary care. The Ministry of Health retains purchasing and distribution responsibility for those drugs required by standard treatment protocols for HIV/AIDS (an extraordinary achievement); Hansen's disease, tuberculosis, malaria, leishmaniasis, schistosomiasis, and other endemic diseases, as well as for insulin and a variety of immunobiologicals and blood products for which economies of scale justify continued centralized procurement. Expensive drugs (e.g., growth hormone, posttransplant immunosuppressants) and other drugs for ongoing use are listed in the tables of outpatient and hospital procedures. The Ministry of Health reimburses state and local health secretariats for these drugs on a monthly basis on presentation of vouchers verifying quantity dispensed (World Bank 2000).

Consumption of medical and hospital equipment and materials in Brazil in 1995 totaled close to U.S.$2 million, which represented 1.7 percent of the world market for these products. Domestic industries met about 60 percent of internal demand, with equal participation by the public and private sectors.

The national capacity for research and training in public health is powerful, with 17 reputable specialized institutions offering master's programs (8 of them doctoral programs as well), 10 technical training schools for services planning/management and epidemiology, and more than 100 public health departments in the faculties of medicine and nursing.

Service Delivery

Access to healthcare services in Brazil varies by family income, regardless of region. Nonetheless, across-the-board expenditures for outpatient and home services have increased since the 1990s relative to those for hospitalization. Innovations contributing to increased use of outpatient services include the following (Almeida 2000):

- strategies to modify the basic model of care, including the formation of family health teams, training of community health workers, and replacement of fee for service with direct transfers of fixed per capita sums to the municipal health funds
- adoption of new care technologies as a substitute for hospitalization
- innovative trials of a tiered hospital system in different municipalities
- the establishment of intermunicipal consortia and interstate clearinghouses for guaranteed referral to services of intermediate and high complexity
- better monitoring of the invoicing procedures of service providers and intensive fraud prevention

In addition, since 1995, the progressive adoption of integrated programming and resource allocation has made a gradual reorientation of healthcare priorities possible.

Since 1994, the Ministry of Health has adopted a family health program as a framework for reorganizing primary healthcare. The program seeks to incorporate health promotion into traditional medical care through reorganized health units that focus on families and their social relations within a given area. Several national programs are also aimed at ensuring comprehensive care for the health of women, children, and adolescents. For example, since 1995, a project aimed at reducing infant mortality has been coordinating specific maternal and child health and basic sanitation activities in the 913 municipalities with the highest levels of poverty since 1995.

Public health services are delivered primarily by municipalities. The municipality—or, if it cannot, the state—is responsible for monitoring delivery of the various public health services under its jurisdiction. The vast majority of these services are provided by public facilities and vary with the local epidemiological profile. States and municipalities provide for the promotion, prevention, and control of Hansen's disease, tuberculosis, vaccine-preventable diseases, cholera, zoonoses, as well as the treatment of bites or poisoning from venomous species in the manner prescribed by the federal level. In addition, the state and sometimes even the municipal health secretariats maintain programmed lines of action (for which they provide the standards) for monitoring and control of disorders not covered by the

Ministry of Health but that they consider important in the morbidity and mortality profile of their populations. Thus, many local health agencies have begun to monitor hypertension, diabetes, external causes, and cancer in their populations.

The treatment and prevention of communicable diseases is gradually being taken over by the general public facilities system, although some parallel facilities of the National Health Foundation (Fundação Nacional de Saúde) still fight vector-borne diseases (e.g., malaria, leishmaniasis, Chagas' disease, schistosomiasis) and provide patient care and required environmental control measures. All three spheres of government conduct health-promotion campaigns with intensive media support as well as campaigns for the early detection of diseases such as breast and cervical cancer.

Prospects for the Future

Full implementation of the constitutional and legal guidelines underlying Brazil's SUS will depend on a large number of factors. Success will require the effective integration of healthcare policy with other social policies and must take into account the requirements for local strategies to tackle the marked inequalities observed in the Brazilian healthcare system. It will require the transformation of a welfare model based on medical and hospital treatment into a fully integrated healthcare model that stresses health promotion and health protection and prioritizes primary healthcare for both the individual and the community. This must be accomplished through a continuing process of decentralization to the states and municipalities accompanied by greater public participation and control mechanisms.

The main obstacle to consolidation and reform is the inability to contain the fiscal deficits at all three levels of government. By preventing the expansion and replacement of technical staff and decreasing remuneration in the public sector, these continued deficits complicate team building and delay the introduction of management and information technologies capable of supporting the full exercise of strategic government functions.

Some particular goals should take priority in future reform efforts:

1. Expenditures for outpatient and home services should increase relative to those for hospitalization, reflecting an increased focus on primary and preventive care.
2. Social participation in the management of health systems should increase. Many public hospitals are already setting up councils or other advisory bodies directly linked to their management and including significant consumer representation.
3. Hospital accreditation and the technological and economic assessment of procedures should become a focus of improving quality.

Although quality improvement methodologies are becoming more common, they are not yet part of the culture and are not requirements for service providers or for the inclusion of new procedures in the remuneration schedules of the SUS.

4. Inequities of access and quality among different regions and population groups must be diminished.

5. Continued improvement should be sought in such health indicators as infant mortality and disease prevention.

REFERENCES

Almeida, C., Travassos, C., Porto, S., and Labra, M. E. 2000. "Health Sector Reform in Brazil: A Case Study of Inequality." *International Journal of Health Services* 30 (1): 129–69.

Araújo-Júnior, J. L. 1997. "Attempts to Decentralise in Recent Brazilian Health Policy: Issues and Problems, 1988–1994." *International Journal of Health Services* 27 (1): 109–24.

Atkinson, S., Medeiros, R. L. R., Oliveira, P. H. L., and de Almeida, R. D. 2000. "Going Down to the Local: Incorporating Social Organisation and Political Culture into Assessments of Decentralized Health Care." *Social Science and Medicine* 51: 619–36.

Buss, P., and Gadelha, P. 1996. "Health Care Systems in Transition: Brazil Part I: An Outline of Brazil's Health Care System Reforms." *Journal of Public Health Medicine* 18 (3): 289–95.

DATASUS—Rede Intergencial de Informações. 2000. "Informação de Saúde." Retrieved 20 June 2000 from www.datasus.gov.br.

Fielder, J. 1996. "The Privatisation of Health Care in Three Latin American Social Security Systems." *Health Policy and Planning* 11: 406–17.

Lewis, M. A., and Medici, A. C. 1995. "Private Payers of Health Care in Brazil: Characteristics, Costs and Coverage." *Health Policy and Planning* 10: 362–75.

Ministério da Saúde do Governo Brasileiro. 2000. "Legislação de Saúde." Retrieved 20 June 2000 from www.msaude.gov.br.

Pan–American Health Organization (PAHO). 1998. "Brazil. Profile of the Health Services System." Retrieved 20 June 2000 from www.opas.br.

United Nations Development Programme (UNDP). 2000. "Human Development Report 1999." Retrieved 20 June 2000 from www.undp.org.

U.S. Central Intelligence Agency (CIA). 2000. *The World Factbook 1999.* Retrieved 21 June 2000 from www.civ.gov.

World Bank. 2000. "Brazil." Retrieved 20 June 2000 from www.worldbank. org/data.

World Health Organization (WHO). 1999. "The World Health Report. Making a Difference." Retrieved 28 June 2000 from www.who.int.

———. 2000. "The World Health Report." Retrieved 28 June 2000 from www.who.int.

MEXICO

Anna Johnson, Ana María Carrillo, and Juan Jose García

Background Information

Before the end of the nineteenth century, Mexico's health system was a loose conglomerate of "rural, traditional societies, closed to changes, illiterate and with authoritarian government schemes" (Sepúlveda and Gómez 1997). Since then, even isolated rural communities have replaced the traditional health practices with at least some degree of evidence-based medical philosophy and technology. Rapid industrialization and urbanization resulted in Mexico City becoming one of the largest cities in the world, with approximately 17.8 million residents (INEGI 2000). In contrast with the dense urbanization of Mexico City, however, are approximately 170,000 rural towns of fewer than 500 inhabitants each. Mexico's epidemiological profile is a result of conflicting trends: on the one hand are industrialization, urbanization, and new lifestyles, and on the other are continuing poverty and indigence (Morelos 1999).

Increased industrialization brings increased pollution, which has become a great concern for major Mexican cities. According to the Mexican National Environmentalist Groups, in 1990, approximately 100,000 children in Mexico City died as a result of air pollution; 250,000 children and adults suffered from eye diseases; up to 10 percent of children under the age of 16 suffered from pollution-induced asthma; and 5 million people within the city suffered from respiratory diseases (Saad Sotomayor 1990). Increased urbanization has also led to overcrowding and the reemergence of infectious diseases. For example, a June 1998 study revealed a prevalence of approximately 25,000 cases of rubella in Mexico (CDC 2000).

The recent move to cities has also been cited as one of the reasons for the increase in disease risk factors such as smoking and alcohol abuse, poor diet, and a sedentary lifestyle. Indeed, data collected in the Federal District in 1993 show that almost three-fourths of children between the ages of 12 and 18 years had consumed alcohol at some time, and alcohol consumption among teenagers has increased. A similar study showed that more than one-fourth of Mexicans between the ages of 12 and 65 years reported being current smokers, and one-fifth reported being former smokers. According to this report, approximately half of the current smokers are between 16 and 20 years old; the highest prevalence of smoking has been reported within Mexico City (PAHO 1999). According to 2000 census data, 118 Mexicans die each day from smoking-related illnesses. In addition, although national law prohibits the sale of tobacco products to people less than 18 years old, the prevalence of smokers between the ages of 12 and 17 increased from 7.7 percent in 1988 to 11.7 percent in 1998 (SSA 1998).

Risk factors including smoking and alcohol consumption are implicated in diseases such as cancer, diabetes mellitus, cardiovascular diseases, accidents, suicide, and violence (Medina 2000). These risk factors have also been shown to be correlated with promiscuity, which exposes the population to an increased incidence of sexually transmitted diseases including HIV/AIDS and hepatitis B (PAHO 1999). Although Mexico ranked sixty-ninth globally in the accumulated number of HIV cases reported in 1997, it ranked only thirteenth in the total number of cases reported. Although its incidence rate as of 1997 was low as compared with other countries in the Americas (eleventh in accumulated cases), controlling the spread of HIV/AIDS is still of grave concern in Mexico, which had an annual average of more than 4,000 new cases in 1997 (PAHO 1997). One year later, in 1998, the prevalence of HIV in Mexico was estimated to be between 116,000 and 174,000 (Magis-Rodríguez et al. 1998). An additional 4,745 new AIDS cases were reported that year, with a rate of 4.93 new cases per 100,000 inhabitants, as well as 2,373 new seropositive cases, which resulted in a rate of 2.47 new such cases per 100,000 inhabitants (SSA 1999).

Although some of the most pressing health issues for Mexico today are quite different from those that plagued the nation only a few decades ago, other, more long-standing issues remain. Although chronic, degenerative diseases and accidents are quickly becoming leading causes of mortality, pneumonia and influenza, nutritional deficiencies, and infectious intestinal disease are still among the nation's top 20 causes of death. In addition, a recent resurgence of diseases such as cholera, malaria, and tuberculosis has occurred. The poorest segments of the population show significantly higher rates of infectious diseases and nutritional deficiencies (Frenk, Bobadilla, and Sepúlveda 1988), indicating an apparent epidemiological polarization of mortality and morbidity rates; similar polarization occurs between rural and urban populations (Calva 2000). The combined mortality rate of the five poorest states is twice that of the five richest ones, and according to the latest available data, 24.5 percent of deaths in Mexico occurred in localities with fewer than 2,500 inhabitants as compared with only 10 percent in those with one million inhabitants or more (Frenk 1997; SSA 2000).

The Economy

Industry in Mexico has continually diversified since the end of the nineteenth century. Currently, most major businesses are based in the region in and surrounding Mexico City, Monterrey, and Guadalajara. The economy has experienced strong growth since colonial times, particularly between 1940 and 1980. However, between 1970 and 1980, when Mexico seriously overborrowed from other countries, trade deficits grew and inflation soared to the point that significant foreign intervention was necessary. Since 1990, when more open-market and free-trade policies were introduced (particularly during the period 1998 to 2002), great improvement has been seen at the macroeconomic level.

However, these policies have benefited only a minority of the population. The Mexican Economic Analysis and Projection Center (CAPEM) estimates that the real minimum wage in Mexico has dropped by 67 percent since 1980. In other words, minimum wage today buys only one-third of the goods that it bought 20 years ago (World Paper 1999). Current economic reform proposals emphasize reducing the country's dependence on oil for revenues and strengthening the capital adequacy of the nation's banks (World Bank Group 1998). The problem of public debt, however, is the debt accumulated by private companies. The Institute for the Protection of Bank Savings (Instituto para la Proteccion del Ahorro Bancario) was created to shift the private debt of a group of bankers and businessmen into additional public debt, which all Mexicans must pay. This debt of about 850 million Mexican pesos is higher than either the external or the internal public national debt (López-Obrador 1999).

Mexico's gross domestic product of U.S.$410 billion in 1998 makes it the world's thirteenth-largest economy (World Bank Group 2000). Presently, Mexico has a per capita GDP of U.S.$8,300 and a per capita gross national product of U.S.$3,970. Its total external debt was U.S.$160.3 billion (1.25 percent of its GDP) in 1998, and its GDP growth rate was 4.8 percent in 1995 (World Bank Group 1998a). Still, Mexico's inflation rate (17.4 percent in 1998) continues to be high (CEPAL 2000). The unemployment rate of 3.9 percent in 1998 is deceptively low, as considerable underemployment exists, particularly in rural areas. In total, 35.8 million people make up the working class in Mexico. However, income across the nation is not equally distributed; the top 20 percent of workers account for 55 percent of income (CIA 2000). Indeed, poverty levels are very high in Mexico, with 36 percent of the population classified as poor between 1994 and 1997 (WHOSIS 2000). Table 25.1 provides details about selected economic measures for the country.

According to 1997 estimates, national health expenditures account for approximately 4.8 percent of Mexico's GDP. Of these funds, approximately one-third come from the public health sector, including national, regional, and local health entities. Per capita health expenditures in 1995 averaged U.S.$160. Although healthcare facilities and professionals are generally in adequate supply in urban areas, rural areas are typically understaffed and managed by medical students (Library of Congress 1996).

Although Mexico is historically characterized as an undemocratic country, during the governments of Carlos Salinas de Gortari (1988–94)

TABLE 25.1

Selected Employment and Economic Indicators, Mexico, 1997

Total labor force in millions	35.8
Labor force participation rate, percent	61
Unemployment rate	
Percent of total labor force	3.9
Percent of urban population, male	5.1
Percent of urban population, female	3.6
Percent of population living in poverty	36
GDP	
Total in billions of U.S.$, 1990	338.1
Per capita in billions of U.S.$, 1990	3.5
Per capita in U.S.$ using P.P.P.$	363
Average annual growth rate, 1989–98	3.3
Per capita average annual growth rate, 1989–98	5
Debt to GDP ratio	37.3
Consumer prices, average annual growth rate, 1999	16.6
Inflation, annual rate, 1998	17.4
Health spending	
Percent of total GDP	5.6
Public expenditure as percent of total health expenditure	41
Private expenditure as percent of total health expenditure	59.1
Out-of-pocket expenditure as percent of total health expenditure	52.9

SOURCE: CEPAL (2000); IADB (2000); OECD (2000); WHOSIS (1999); World Bank Group (2000); PAHO (1999).

and Ernesto Zedillo Ponce de Leon (1994–2000), the federal republic of Mexico moved toward democracy. This move occurred in large part as a result of the activities of opposition political parties and social organizations as well as international pressures. In the most recent presidential election, Vicente Fox of the National Action Party (Partido Accion Nacional) was elected president, ending the 71-year reign of the Institutional Revolutionary Party (Partido Revolucionario Institucional). Many people consider this the beginning of a new democratic era. Nevertheless, state elections are still conducted in a less-than-democratic manner (Sullivan and Jordan 2000).

General Demographics and Education

Spanning 1,972,547 square kilometers, Mexico is the third-largest country in Latin America (Library of Congress 1996). Its population grew from 13.6 million inhabitants at the beginning of the twentieth century to 25.8 million in 1950. According to the 2000 census, 97,361,711 people were living in the Mexican Republic as of February 14, with a ratio of 100 women for every 95 men, making Mexico the eleventh most populated nation in the world. Its population multiplied by a factor of 7.2 between 1990 and 2000 as compared with a population multiplication factor of only 3.7 worldwide and 2.2 for developed nations (INEGI 2000). With an annual growth rate of 1.73 percent in 2000, the national birth rate was estimated at almost 5 percent and the death rate at approximately 4.6 percent. Births per woman decreased from 7 in 1970 to 2.85 in 2000 (United Nations Population Fund 2002; CIA 2000).

Both infant and maternal mortality rates are high at 15.8 deaths per 1,000 live births as compared with an average of 5.3 deaths per 1,000 live births for more-developed countries (SSA 2000). The average mortality rate for children under five years old is 37 deaths per 1,000 live births. In 1900, life expectancy after birth was 25.4 years; by 1998 it had risen to 74.7 years, with women living longer than men on average. Almost three-fourths of the Mexican population lives in an urban setting, and almost 40 percent of the population lives below the poverty line (WHOSIS 2000). Poverty is more common in rural settings and among indigenous populations (Sepúlveda 1993).

The official language of Mexico is Spanish, although approximately 10 percent of the population belongs to one of the 56 indigenous groups of Mexico and speaks one of the 90 indigenous languages. Knowledge of English is increasing rapidly throughout the country, particularly among its younger citizens. The Mexican population is approximately 80 percent mestizo, 10 percent indigenous, 9 percent European, and 1 percent from another background. The dominant religion in Mexico is Roman Catholicism; 1990 census data report that approximately 90 percent of the population is Roman Catholic (Library of Congress 1996).

The Ministry of Public Education heads the education system at elementary and secondary school levels, and the Autonomous National University of Mexico does the same at preparatory school and university levels. Education is compulsory until age 14 and public education is free; private schools are available at all levels of education. Overall literacy rate in 1999 was approximately 90 percent, with male literacy estimated at 92 percent and female literacy at 87 percent. More than 14.5 million children were enrolled in primary school between 1997 and 1998, and nearly five million attended secondary school (PAHO 1999). Additional demographic and education data are provided in Table 25.2.

TABLE 25.2

Selected
Demographic
and Education
Data, Mexico,
1997

Total area (thousand square kilometers)	1,972.5
Population in millions	97.4
Population per square kilometer	47.8
Population growth rate, percent of total population	
Total, 1989–98	25.8
Urban, 1990–97	2
Percent urbanized	74.9
Age structure of population by percent of total population	
Less than 15 years	34.9
15 to 64 years	60.2
65 years and older	4.9
Median age in years	22
Males, percent of total population	48.7
Life expectancy at birth in years	74.7
Female	77
Male	72.4
Mortality rates	
Infants, deaths per 1,000 live births	15.8
Under five years, deaths per 1,000 live births	37
Maternal, deaths per 1,000 live births	53
Ages 15 to 64, deaths per 1,000 individuals	2.8
Total fertility rate (number of children per woman)	2.85
Percent of births delivered by trained personnel	84
Percent of low birthweight newborns (less than 2,500 grams)	7.0
Registered births in millions	2.7
Registered deaths in millions	0.44
Education	
Percent of population reaching grade 5	84
Expenditure on education as percent of central government expenditure, pre-primary through secondary schooling	24.5
Average years of schooling of the population over 25 years old	5.3
Illiteracy rate, percent of total population	10.0

SOURCE: IADB (2000); INEGI (1998); PAHO (1999); SSA (1998); UNICEF (2000); UNESCO (1999); WHOSIS (2000); World Bank Group (2000); CIA (2000).

Context: Health Needs

During the past century, Mexico has experienced a significant decrease in mortality rates. General mortality decreased almost tenfold between 1900 and 1998, from 35 to 4.6 deaths per 1,000 inhabitants (Bronfman and López 1999). At the same time, life expectancy has increased notably; for women it has increased from 42.5 years in 1940 to 77 years in 1998, and for men it has increased from 40.4 to 72.4 years during the same period (SSA 1998b). Still, one of the national health priorities is improving the treatment of common diseases. According to a study conducted by the Mexican Institute of Social Security, "errors in treating common diseases occur very frequently in primary healthcare practice" (Guiscafre et al. 1995). Although the quality of services provided to patients in urban settings is generally much higher than that offered in rural settings, both require significant improvement (Guiscafre et al. 1995).

Table 25.3 summarizes death rates for Mexico. In 1980, the three most common causes of death nationally were accidents, heart disease, and respiratory disease (INEGI 1984). By 1999, these had been replaced by heart disease, malignant neoplasms, and diabetes mellitus (INEGI 1999). According to the Mexican Committee for Basic Health Research in Mexico City, biomedical research priorities include chronic degenerative diseases, accidents, and cancers (Morissette 1997).

Pediatric Health

Children's health has improved greatly in Mexico during the twentieth century. Most notably, the average infant mortality rate has decreased from 288.6 of 1,000 live births in 1900 to 15.8 in 1998. In other words, today only one infant dies for every 18.3 who died a century ago. In 1991, polio was considered eradicated from the population. The incidence of other once-common pediatric diseases such as measles, whooping cough, diphtheria, neonatal tetanus, and diarrheal and respiratory diseases has been drastically reduced in recent years. Infant immunization rates in 1997 were 93 percent for diphtheria, tetanus, and pertussis; 94 percent for oral poliomyelitis vaccine; 99 percent for tuberculosis; and 84 percent for measles. Mortality from acute diarrheal diseases dropped significantly from 25.5 percent in the period from 1980 to 1985 to 7.6 in the period from 1990 to 1995. Similarly, mortality from acute respiratory infections dropped from 21.6 percent between 1980 and 1985 to 14.5 between 1990 and 1995. The overall rate of low birth weight is also relatively low, with only 8.1 percent of newborns weighing less than 2,500 grams in 1995 (PAHO 1999). Improvements in Mexico's health system and vaccination programs, as well as other factors, are credited for these positive developments (PAHO 1999).

Despite such improvements, inequities in children's health are prevalent. A recent evaluation of access to health services and the quality of pediatric healthcare services found that access to health services in rural com-

TABLE 25.3

Leading
Causes of
Mortality,
Mexico, 1998

	Deaths per 100,000 Persons
Cardiovascular disease	71.1
Malignant neoplasms	54.5
Diabetes mellitus	43.3
Accidents	36.8
Cirrhosis and other liver disease	28.2
Cerebrovascular disease	25.9
Perinatal disease	10.6
Pneumonia and influenza	15.6
Homicide and injuries	14.1
Malnutrition and other nutritional deficiencies	10.9
Pulmonary disease	10.7
Congenital anomalies	10.5
Renal failure	8.2
Bronchitis, emphysema, and asthma	7.6
Infectious and parasitic disease	6.9
AIDS	4.2
Anemia	4.0
Pulmonary tuberculosis	3.7
Suicide	3.5
Septicemia	3.3

SOURCE: INEGI (2000); SSA (2000).

munities is still a significant problem for adults and children. Other studies have shown that the quality of care delivered to Mexicans in rural communities is inferior to that provided in urban areas (Reyes et al. 1998). Regional variations in pediatric health are also prevalent. Although the central region of Mexico had an infant mortality rate of 22.3 deaths per 1,000 live births in 1995, the northern and southern regions had infant mortality rates of only 12.2 and 12.8, respectively. Under-five mortality rates follow this trend, with the central region showing a mortality rate of 21.5 deaths per 1,000 live births in 1995 and the northern and southern regions having rates of 14.6 and 17.3, respectively (PAHO 1999).

The primary causes of death in children have remained relatively stable during the past decade. According to 1998 public hospital records, the most common causes of mortality for children under one year were peri-natal disease (745 per 100,000), congenital anomalies (285.3 per 100,000), pneumonia and influenza (133.8 per 100,000), infectious and parasitic disease (85.1 per 100,000), accidents (54.5 per 100,000), and malnutrition and other nutritional deficiencies (47.9 per 100,000). The most common causes of death in children between one and four years during this same year were accidents (19.9 per 100,000), congenital anomalies (11.3 per 100,000), infectious and parasitic disease (10.5 per 100,000), pneumonia and influenza (9.6 per 100,000), and malignant neoplasms (4.7 per 100,000). Mortality in children between the ages of 5 and 18 years in 1998 was most commonly caused by accidents (11.8 per 100,000), malignant neoplasms (4.9 per 100,000), congenital anomalies (2 per 100,000), homicides (1.6 per 100,000), cerebral paralysis (1.2 per 100,000), and malnutrition and other nutritional deficiencies (1 per 100,000) (SSA 1998b).

Adult Health

In 1998, the main causes of mortality for people between the ages of 15 and 65 years were malignant neoplasms (40.2 per 100,000), accidents (39.7 per 100,000), cirrhosis and other liver disease (31.3 per 100,000), heart disease (29.9 per 100,000), diabetes mellitus (29.5 per 100,000), homicide (20.5 per 100,000), cerebrovascular disease (10.5 per 100,000), AIDS (6.7 per 100,000), renal failure (5 per 100,000), and suicide (5 per 100,000) (SSA 1998b). These illnesses are directly related to productive activities, unemployment, addictions, and urban living.

Women's Health

The majority of information currently available on women's health in Mexico is related to reproductive issues. Across the country in 1998, there were 1,430 maternal deaths, 89.4 percent of which were directly linked to childbirth. More recent data show that maternal mortality has increased to 5.3 deaths per 1,000 live births. Maternal mortality rates vary widely across different regions of the country; whereas the northern and northwestern regions have low to medium rates of maternal mortality, rates are high to very high in the south and southeastern regions. The underlying factors affecting maternal mortality vary across these regions as well. Whereas regions with lower maternal mortality rates credit the quality of healthcare, those with high rates blame lack or difficulty of access to care. Consequently, policymakers argue that programs to lower the overall national maternal mortality rates should differ in different regions according to their needs (Reyes et al. 1998). The National Midwives Program estimated in 1990 that widening the availability of training in handling high-risk pregnancies, currently offered only to midwives, could cut the current rate of maternal mortality in half by the year 2000. However, other determinants of maternal mortality, such as nutrition and living conditions, must also be considered (Carrillo, in press).

Use of prenatal care services among women covered by the Mexican Institute of Social Security is low as compared with other countries. Although 75 percent of women covered by the Institute start antenatal care during the first trimester, only 23.8 percent of these women make nine or more antenatal care visits, which is considered the threshold for adequate utilization of prenatal care services (Martínez-González, Reyes-Frausto, and García-Peña 1996). Between 1987 and 1996, the number of women covered by the national family planning program increased from 52.7 to 66.5 percent. The overall number of women who sought prenatal care from health workers has also increased during the past 20 years as indicated by a more than 50 percent increase in pregnancies supervised by medical personnel between 1978 and 1998. As of 1995, almost two-thirds of births were attended in public hospitals (PAHO 1999).

In terms of other related health issues, the main public health concerns for women in Mexico are cervical and breast cancer. In 1998, mortality from cervical cancer was 14 deaths per 100,000 women 15 years old and older; these 4,545 cases made up 8.6 percent of all malignant neoplasms. Mortality from breast cancer was 10.5 deaths per 100,000 women 15 years old and older, which accounted for 6.5 percent (3,380 deaths) from all malignant neoplasms that year (SSA 1998b). Cancer of the uterus is a primary cause of mortality among women in lower-income groups as a result of infrequent visits to the doctor; during 1995, approximately two-thirds of women in urban areas had pap tests performed as compared with only 30 percent in rural areas (PAHO 1999).

Health of the Elderly

The proportion of elderly in the population has increased rapidly in Mexico during the past century. In 1900, deaths of Mexicans 65 years old and older made up 8.3 percent of all deaths in the country. In 1980, this percentage had reached 31.3, and by 1998 it had reached 48.4 percent (García 2000). In 1950, people 60 years old and older made up approximately 5.6 percent of the population as compared with 6.2 percent in 1990 and a projected 12.6 percent in 2030. This change in age structure is attributed both to a decrease in fertility and to an increase in average life expectancy (Ham Chande 1993). Women predominate in this age group; whereas the ratio of men to women in the total population was 0.97 in 1999, the ratio of men to women in the over-65 age group was 0.81 (CIA 2000). The elderly are also more likely than those in younger age groups to live in rural areas.

The main causes of death for this group fall into the broad category of chronic-degenerative disease. In 1998, the main causes of mortality in the elderly population in Mexico were heart disease (1,132.6 per 100,000), malignant neoplasms (617 per 100,000), diabetes mellitus (549.4 per 100,000), cerebrovascular disease (418.7 per 100,000), respiratory disease (202.9 per 100,000), cirrhosis and other liver disease (188.5 per 100,000), pneumonia and influenza (177.8 per 100,000), and nutritional deficiencies (154.2 per 100,000) (PAHO 1999).

With regard to morbidity, the elderly population covered by the Mexican Institute of Social Security tends to live with both infectious and chronic disease simultaneously. In 1995, the most common causes of hospitalization in the elderly population were circulatory disease (17.8 percent of all discharges), genitourinary disease (16 percent), digestive disease (13.8 percent), and respiratory disease (9.5 percent) (PAHO 1999). In 1993, a national survey about chronic diseases in urban localities found that the prevalence of chronic diseases was higher than average among the elderly (García 2000); this trend poses a challenge for healthcare policymakers as the elderly population increasingly competes with other groups for healthcare services (Lara-Rodríguez et al. 1996).

Organization and Management of the Health System

Like many countries in Latin America, Mexico has developed a broad-based health system that comprises complex institutional structures. Although this system was developed to serve the health needs of the majority of the population, it excludes major groups from access to healthcare coverage. As in much of Latin America, the healthcare delivery system in Mexico is fraught with social inequity. Despite the protection of citizens' rights to access the healthcare system guaranteed by Article 4 of Mexico's Constitution, access to this system is in large part dependent on the user's place in the work force. Since the end of the nineteenth century, attempts were made to guarantee healthcare to railroad employees and miners (Carrillo 2000). In the 1940s, social security was established for employees of private companies, and in the 1960s, states guaranteed medical care for their government employees. Those connected to the formal employment sector are thus insured through their employers, whereas those outside of this system are either uninsured or insured through the private system (Fleury et al. 1998).

Such a system has resulted in a segmented delivery structure with three separate components: a social security system that covers workers in the formal sector, a public services system that provides services to a portion of the lower and middle classes, and a diverse private sector that covers Mexican citizens from various economic backgrounds (Fleury 2000). As of 1996, approximately half of the population was covered by the national social security system. Those covered include formally employed workers, members of production cooperatives, and small landowners and agricultural laborers (SSA 2000).

The social security system includes five distinct coverage systems, the largest of which is the Mexican Institute for Social Security. The Institute covers mainly private-sector employees and the self-employed and is funded primarily through federal monies, with some contributions from employers and beneficiaries. The Institute of Social Security and Services for State Employees (Instituto Mexicano de Seguridad y Servicios Sociales para los Trabajadores del Estado) covers federal employees and is funded in a similar manner. State government employees have a separate health insurance system that is funded jointly by the state and federal government. The federal government also funds the entire coverage system for Mexico's armed forces, known as the Secretaría de la Defensa Nacional (SEDENA) or Ministry of National Defense. Finally, PEMEX provides services to Petróleos Mexicanos employees and their families and is funded by federal, employer, and beneficiary monies.

Those not covered by the social security system may be covered by public services or the private sector. People from all income groups may be insured under the public service system, which is divided into three coverage systems. The largest of these is the Ministry of Health, the federally funded health insurance system. The Mexican Institute for Social Security–Solidarity system is also available for voluntary enrollment under the public service system, although the high cost and extensive requirements of participation in this system has made it an unpopular option. The National Institute for Indigenous Peoples (Instituto Nacional Indigenista) is the third coverage option available under public services. People not covered by either the social security or the public services systems may be covered by the private sector.

Because the three health insurance segments operate independently, historically little coordination of care has been seen among providers. Each segment has its own network of primary care divisions and its own secondary- and tertiary-level delivery systems. Within the private insurance segment, care is available only at the primary and secondary levels, and each facility operates independently. Throughout the health delivery system, services are based on the primary care model, where secondary and tertiary care is available only by referral from the primary care level (PAHO 1999).

Changes in the epidemiology, demography, and political atmosphere of Mexico and the world in recent years have led to a call for reform of the Mexican health system. The country is finally recognizing the need to improve equity and quality in the nation's healthcare delivery system. The most recent round of health reform began in the early 1980s. Prior attempts, which were hampered by economic difficulties and political disagreements, had only limited success. These reforms had a dual focus: first to unify the social security and public healthcare systems and second to extend coverage to more of the population (Fleury et al. 1998).

The reforms that produced the current healthcare system are thought to have resulted from two significant developments in Mexican history. First, in 1983, proposals were brought before the government for amendments to Article 4 of the Mexican Constitution to make healthcare a right for all. Second, in 1981, the president created the Health Care Services Coordination (Coordinación de los Servicios de Salud) to reduce expenditures and improve the efficiency and quality of healthcare by streamlining the national healthcare system. The focus of the reform was to modify Article 4 to allow for large "structural change" (Tamez and Molina 2000a).

The product of this effort was the National Healthcare System. Decentralization, modernization, and community participation were used to overhaul the system. Decentralization was the main focus of the reform effort, as multiple health systems were functioning at both state and national levels. The Health Care Services Coordination attacked the problem of centralization in two stages. Between 1983 and 1984, it focused on coordinating individual programs; in the following years, it concentrated on the goal of integrating the various organizations. Significant refinancing followed this period of restructuring. The modernization of programs and sectors as well as health promotion and education services necessary to improve community participation fell under the direction of the Ministry of Health and the Health Care Services Coordination. These reforms led to a change in the role and power of the Ministry of Health, as it had not before been involved in the planning or budgeting process.

By the mid-1990s, healthcare system reforms again became a national priority. Between 1980 and 1988, the public service system actually weakened, and attempts at reform were dropped until a second attempt was made (Fleury et al. 1998). In 1995, the Social Security Law was passed, which significantly changed the financial structure of the Mexican Institute for Social Security to increase its service capacity. With a new political regime, this second attempt at reform was more successful than the first. More political interest groups backed the government's attempts to decentralize the national system of social security and to decrease the number of uninsured by way of an improved public health delivery system. However, more reform is needed in financing and allocation mechanisms to continue this expansion of coverage and encourage more hospitals and clinics to participate in its network.

The effects of such reforms are numerous. First, they improved the organization of Mexico's public health system. One of the main objectives of the 1995–2000 Health Sector Reform Program was to improve the services available for the treatment of the most widespread epidemiological and demographic health issues. Under this newly organized system, the Ministry of Health manages the nation's health promotion initiatives by designing strategies for disease prevention and control and health education. The Ministry administers these duties through six departments: family health, comprehensive health of schoolchildren, comprehensive health of adolescents, healthy *municipios,* healthcare exercises, and development of educational content. The Ministry is also responsible for monitoring and testing the quality, safety, and efficacy of drugs produced and sold in the country and for regulating the marketing of these drugs. In addition, the Ministry is in charge of monitoring air quality and has recently focused efforts on reducing air pollutants from motor vehicle emissions, industries, and gas stations. In 1996, the Ministry made efforts to modernize its system of ensuring food safety in production, distribution, and consumption. Authorization for the use of chemicals is controlled under the Ministry's General Environmental Health Directorate. The Ministry of Health, along with the National Water Commission, manages the sanitation of Mexico's drinking water (PAHO 1999). Figure 25.1 provides a graphic representation of the major components of the Mexican Health System.

Financing

The Mexican National Health System (Sistema Nacional de Salud) has changed significantly since the 1980s, in large part because of economic forces. When oil prices plummeted in 1981, Mexico's interest payments rose along with its national debt, resulting in a near-collapse of the economy. Since 1995, the economy has experienced some improvement at a macroeconomic level, with increased foreign investment, growth of the GDP, and a decrease in inflation. Still, Mexico lives with a significant amount of debt. In an effort to reduce spending and free funds to make interest payments and pay down the debt, expenditures on public programs decreased from 10.1 percent in 1980 to 4.3 percent in 1989 (Valenzuela 1992). Education and health programs were most severely affected by the funding cut; health expenditures dropped from 2.5 percent of the gross national product in 1982 to 1.3 percent in 1988, and public health expenditures declined from 6.2 percent of total public expenditures to only 2.5 percent (López and Blanco 1993). Despite such drastic cuts in health expenditures, the early 1980s saw several attempts to increase health coverage. However, these attempts met with little success, as international creditors increased pressure on Mexico to repay old debt (Tamez and Molina 2000a).

Sixty-eight percent of Mexico's total health budget in 1997 was allocated to curative care (including hospitalizations), whereas 15 percent was directed toward administrative costs, 7 percent to preventive care, 6 percent to infrastructure, and 4 percent to other costs. Budget structures among the three main health sectors (social security, public services, and the private sector) differ widely, however. Whereas the Mexican Institute for Social Security and the Ministry of Health spend almost half of their budgets on salaries, the Institute of Social Security and Services for State Employees spends only 21 percent of its budget on salaries. Conversely, while the Institute of Social Security and Services for State Employees spends over half of its funds on operating expenditures, the Mexican Institute for Social Security spends 35 percent and the Ministry of Health spends 3 percent of its total budget on operating expenses. Private sector spending

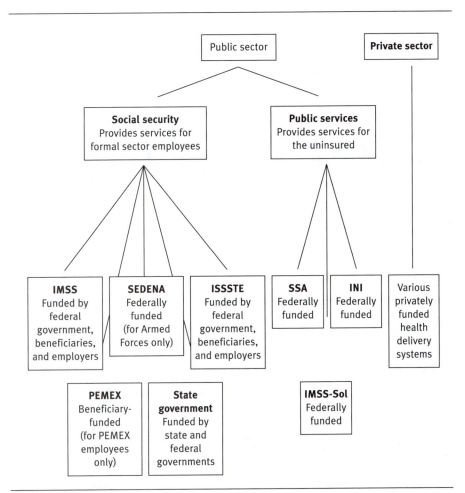

FIGURE 25.1

Flow Chart
Showing the
Major
Components
of the Mexican
Health System

is also different. Whereas the majority of private sector spending goes to curative care, fees account for 35 percent as compared with 27 percent for drug purchases and 20 percent for hospitalizations.

The largest health expenditures—66 percent of all national health expenditures in 1998 (World Bank Group 1998)—are made by the federally financed social security system, which serves approximately 52 percent of the population according to April 2000 estimates (World Bank Group 2000). Second in terms of expenditures is the private healthcare industry, which accounts for nearly half of all healthcare expenditures but serves only 2 percent of the population. Services for this sector are provided at various hospitals, private physicians' offices, health maintenance organizations, pharmacies, and ambulatory clinics across the country. Last in terms of expenditures is the Ministry of Health, which serves approximately 46 percent of the population. However, it has received increased funding from the government in recent years, as it serves sectors of the population that might otherwise be uninsured (SSA 2000). Most significantly, when the Social Security Law was passed in 1995, the financial structure of the

Mexican Institute for Social Security was changed so that the financial burden was shifted from payroll taxes to public financing through general revenues. This shift allowed for increased coverage—especially for those in the self-employed and informal sectors—and improved choice of providers (World Bank Group 1998).

According to 1994 figures, almost half of all health expenditures were financed by individual households; 28 percent of expenditures were covered by employers, 20 percent were covered by the federal government, and 3 percent were covered by state governments (PAHO 1999). Indeed, one of the major problems with the financing of the public health system originates from problems with the country's tax system. According to OECD (2000), "Mexico has by far the lowest level of tax revenues in relation to GDP among the OECD countries . . . [and] the low capacity for raising tax revenue severely limits the scope for public spending, including in areas where potential social returns are high."

The primary source of spending on health insurance is households, which accounted for 49 percent of the funding from 1992 to 1996. During the same period, employer contributions made up 29 percent and federal contributions made up 22 percent of health insurance financing. Since the enactment of the Social Security Act in 1997, state contributions to the health budget increased eightfold from 4.5 percent in 1996 to 28.5 percent in 1997; these funds were designed to replace much of the employer and beneficiary spending that had been steadily increasing (PAHO 1999).

In the private sector, out-of-pocket spending is increasing in proportion with other sources of funding. Private expenditures in urban areas are approximately 10 times higher for households in the highest income group than for those in the lowest income group. In rural areas, expenditures are 20 times higher among the wealthiest households (PAHO 1999). In addition, the cost of healthcare in rural areas has been found to be significantly higher than the cost of the same services in metropolitan areas (Villarreal-Ríos et al. 1996).

Social security reform implies a profound change in the guiding principles of healthcare organization and management. In Mexico, this has meant a shift away from a public model of social security and toward a model based on private administration. The steady decline of the minimum wage since 1982 has directly affected social security funding because premiums are a fixed percentage of workers' wages. Calculated with official data, the income loss suffered by the Mexican Institute for Social Security because of wage reduction from 1983 to 1994 was approximately 215 billion Mexican pesos. At the same time, government subsidies to social security were diminished. As a result, in the past 15 years, the fairly well functioning social security institutes have deteriorated because of salary cuts, gradual wear of equipment and installations, and lack of supplies (Laurell 1999); this decline in quality has been used by the government to justify the possible privatization of the social security system. Many political and health analysts fear that privatization will lead to an increase in the already large gap in access to quality healthcare services. Data on insurance coverage of the population in Mexico are provided in Table 25.4.

Health Resources

Health resources have grown steadily during the past few decades, and this trend is expected to continue. The largest number of physicians and nurses work within the public services' Institute of Social Security, followed by the public services' Ministry of Health. In 1995, the private sector was responsible for approximately half of all health expenditures and approximately one-third of the bed counts, physicians, and medical consultations. The influence of the private sector on health insurance is limited; it covered only 2 percent of the population in 1996. In all insurance segments, the concentration of medical staff is greater in urban areas than in rural areas (PAHO 1999).

　　The three health insurance segments operate independently, and each segment's facilities operate relatively independently of other health facilities. Under the Ministry of Health in 1997, a total of 372 hospitals and 14,978 outpatient clinics were available to its beneficiaries. During the same year, the Institute for Social Security offered its beneficiaries 438 hospitals and 3,208 outpatient clinics. Tertiary care is provided to beneficiaries from all segments and throughout the country through the Ministry of

Total number of insured people in millions	54.26	**TABLE 25.4** Insurance Coverage, Mexico, 1998
Social security		
Number insured in millions	50	
Percent of total population	50	
Percent of national health expenditure	43	
Public services		
Number insured in millions	N/A	
Percent of total population	N/A	
Percent of national health expenditure	13	
Private insurance		
Number insured in millions	1.92	
Percent of total population	2.0	
Percent of national health expenditure	45	

SOURCE: World Bank Group (2000); PAHO (1999); INEGI (2000).

Health's 11 national institutes of health. Nationally, there are little more than 2,000 private units have hospitalization services, where almost 25,000 physicians work. In addition, approximately 33,530 physicians offer health services independently (Lezana 2000). The Mexican health system fosters a variety of approaches to medical therapy; in addition to institutional medicine, homeopathic and chiropractic medical practices are prevalent. Chinese acupuncture, self-help health groups (e.g., Alcoholics Anonymous), popular/religious medical practices (e.g., Marian Trinitarian Spiritualism), home health, and other "traditional" medical treatment methods are also practiced throughout the country. Occidental medicine has reached the farthest corners of the country, but rural and indigenous populations still often prefer traditional systems of medical attention. Mexico has registered approximately 25,000 midwives in urban and well-communicated rural areas, and indigenous traditional medicine still plays a key role in the delivery of health services (PAHO 1997).

In terms of professional health resources, in 1996, 110,804 people worked in private medicine (51.4 percent of physicians and 24 percent of nurses). Of the 178,520 physicians employed by the private sector in 1996, 2.8 percent were general practitioners, 47.9 percent were specialists, and 5 percent were dentists; the rest were residents, interns, and other practitioners. That same year also saw 190 million medical consultations, 3.8 million hospitalizations, and 137 million auxiliary diagnostic services. Although no data are available, the use of traditional healing methods is known to be widespread, particularly in sections of the country with high concentrations of indigenous peoples. Data on health resources and utilization are provided in Table 25.5. Human resources distribution data are provided in Table 25.6.

Service Delivery

The main objective of the 1995–2000 Health Sector Reform Program is to reorganize the delivery system so that coverage may be expanded to more of the population. The program has made changes in the health delivery system to achieve this goal (PAHO 1999):

1. It established a system of insurance coverage for families under the Mexican Institute for Social Security.
2. It allowed social security beneficiaries to choose their own primary care physicians.
3. It developed a system that allowed individuals to buy into the social security system.
4. It made strides toward decentralizing health services for the uninsured population by transferring responsibility for their care to the states.

TABLE 25.5

Inpatient care	
Public hospitals (SSA and social security only)	810
Beds per 100,000 population	80.5
Population per hospital bed	827
Average length of stay in days	4.0
Physicians	
Total	129,000
Per 10,000 population	13.6
Nurses	
Total	172,000
Per 100,000 of population	181.1
Dentists	
Per 10,000 of population	1
Paramedics	
Total	190,877
Public health workers	
Total	463,611

TABLE 25.5 Health Resources and Use, Mexico, 1997

SOURCE: INEGI (1998); World Bank Group (2000); PAHO (1999).

5. It improved local participation in health delivery through the healthy *municipios* program, a program designed to strengthen local community leadership and its ability to define and implement local priorities and health promotion programs.

One of the program's greatest achievements has been the implementation of a plan to expand coverage to rural populations. By 1997, six million Mexicans in 18 states were covered under this new plan. The program also reorganized the health delivery system to give the Ministry of Health more regulatory control and to improve the coordination of health services for the uninsured. Furthermore, it separated the functions of financing and service delivery within the Institute for Social Security, in part by introducing more competition among service providers (PAHO 1999).

Through the Program, 121,000 jobs have been transferred to the states, along with 7,370 pieces of real estate and U.S.$1.1 billion. State and local agencies now share responsibilities for "the organization, operation, and monitoring of public and private health services, sanitary control of services to the population, and the fulfillment of health promotion and

TABLE 25.6
Distribution
of Human
Resources,
1996

	Public Services			Social Security		Private (1997)
	SSA	IMSS-Sol	IMSS	ISSSTE	PEMEX	
Physicians	37,620	5,434	47,813	15,945	2,393	17,649
Nurses	21,898	855	43,355	10,703	1,521	22,902
Administrative staff	27,955	2,187	22,126	10,858	1,549	N/A
Other staff	35,398	2,617	65,579	17,571	4,244	N/A

	National Health Service	
	Beneficiaries	Public Sector
Physicians per 100,000 population	113.4	110.9
Physician offices per 100,000 population	43.0	54.7
Census beds per 100,000 population	80.2	75.4
Daily consultations per physician	11.0	6.0
Hospital occupancy, percent of total beds	78.4	59.1
Surgical procedures per 1,000 population	33.4	18.7
Contraception use per 1,000 reproductive-age women	595.9	318.9

SOURCE: PAHO (1999); INEGI (2000).

orientation tasks" (PAHO 1999). Still, the Mexican federal government retains the authority to set health standards, control professional certification, accredit health delivery centers, regulate sanitary guidelines, generate national statistics, and decentralize services to the states (PAHO 1999).

Through such initiatives, the percentage of the population with access to health services has grown significantly. According to 1995 figures, 89 percent of the total population was covered by some form of health insurance (PAHO 1997). According to 1997 data, 51.4 million of these people were covered by the National Health Service (INEGI 1999). Still, with 11 percent of the population uninsured, more than 10 million Mexicans do not have access to institutional healthcare. According to national figures, of the 444,665 deaths that occurred in 1998, 48.3 percent (214,961 deaths) occurred in people with no access to social security. However, because of underreporting, the actual percentage is probably higher (SSA 2000). Clearly, further reform is essential.

Prospects for the Future

The hallmark of recent reform efforts continues to be a focus on expanding coverage to the uninsured, decentralizing the nation's health financing and delivery systems, and increasing the use of the private sector insurance market. Already the country has witnessed improvement in all three of these priority areas. Still, high costs and limited quality remain due to stratification in these systems that, although improved, remain inefficient. Inequities in access, cost, and quality among different employment and income groups remain significant problems for the Mexican healthcare system today. Although significant changes in the framework of health regulation have occurred during the past decade, still more change is needed (Tamez and Molina 2000).

Both in terms of access and quality of services rendered, the gap between the rich and the poor is wide and still growing. Those with access to institutional healthcare services are generally urban workers and their families in the middle to upper classes. Those without access to healthcare services are found most frequently within the unemployed or informally employed sectors of the nation (Londoño and Frenk 1997).

In conclusion, each of the three healthcare sectors—social security, the public sector, and the private sector—function differently and independently. Problems associated with this segregation of markets include waste of resources, duplication of services, monopolistic market structures, and overlaps in demand that lead to multiple billing practices. Efforts to decentralize the healthcare system have been numerous but generally unsuccessful to date, in large part because implementation has been conducted in a vertical and undemocratic manner. To attend to the issue of decentralization, redistribution of the decision-making power and an increased health budget are necessary. Still, reform efforts continue with a focus on decentralizing the healthcare system, improving healthcare access to the country's self-employed and informal sector workers, and improving the quality and efficiency of Mexico's healthcare delivery network. (World Bank Group 2000).

REFERENCES

Bronfman, M., and López, S. 1999. "Health and Inequality: Accounts Still Pending." *Demos. Demographic Chart of Mexico* 12: 13–14.

Calva, J. L. 2000. "The Alimentary Crisis, Accounts Still Pending." *Demos. Demographic Chart of Mexico* 3: 27–28. arch 2002.

Carrillo, A. M. (in press). "Physicians 'Who Know' and Midwives Who 'Need to Learn.'" In *Midwives in México: Controversy and Change*, edited by F. R. Davis, M. Good-Mauste, and M. Güemez. Austin, TX: University of Texas Press.

———. 2000. "Pioneers of Social Security in Mexico." *The Mexican Journal of the History and Philosophy of Medicine* 3 (2): 26–32.

Centers for Disease Control and Prevention (CDC). 2000. "Rubella Among Hispanic Adults—Kansas, 1998, and Nebraska, 1999." *Morbidity and Mortality Weekly Report* 49 (11): 225–28.

Economic Commission for Latin America and the Caribbean (CEPAL). 2000. "Statistical Yearbook for Latin America and the Caribbean 1999: Mexico." Retrieved 23 June 2000 from www.eclac.cl.

Fleury, S. 2000. "Chapter 1: Reforming Health Care in Latin America: Challenges and Options." In *Reshaping Health Care in Latin America*, edited by S. Fleury, S. Belmartino, and E. Baris. Ottawa: International Development Research Center.

Fleury, S., Belmartino, S., de Vasconcelos Costa Lobato, L., and Tamez, S. 1998. *Policy Brief: Reshaping Health Care in Latin America; A Comparative Analysis of Health Care Reform in Argentina, Brazil and México.* Ottawa: International Development Research Center.

Frenk, J. (ed.). 1997. *The Health Observatory: Needs, Services, Politics, 1st Edition.* Mexico City: The Mexican Health Foundation (Funsalud).

Frenk, J., Bobadilla J. L., and Sepúlveda, J. 1988. "The Transition of the Health in Mexico: The Country's Own Model, Accounts Still Pending." *Demos. Demographic Chart of Mexico* 1: 28–29.

García, J. J. 2000. "An Epidemiological Panorama of the Elderly Adult." *Archives of Geriatric Medicine* 3 (3): 79–83.

Guiscafre, H., Martínez, H., Reyes, H., Perez Cuevas, R., Castro, R., Muñoz, O., and Gutiérrez, G. 1995. "From Research to Public Health Interventions. I. Impact of an Educational Strategy for Physicians to Improve Treatment Practices of Common Diseases." *Archives of Medical Research* 26: S31–S39.

Ham Chande, R. 1993. "México: A Country in the Process of Aging." In *Health of the Aged Population in México,* pp. 688–96, edited by J. Sepúlveda and M. Bronfman. Ottawa: International Development Research Center.

Inter-American Development Bank (IADB). 2000. "Economic and Social Progress in Latin America: Development Beyond Economics: 2000 Report," pp. 2–9. Washington, DC: Johns Hopkins University Press for the Inter-American Development Bank.

Lara-Rodríguez, M. A., Benítez-Martínez, M. G., Fernández-Gárate, I. H., and Zárate-Aguilar, A. 1996. "Epidemiologic Aspects of the Aged at the Mexican Institute of Social Security." *México Public Health* 38 (6): 448–57.

Laurell, A. S. 1999. "The Mexican Social Security Counter Reform: Pensions for Profit." *International Journal of Health Services* 29: 371–91.

Lezana, M. S. 2000. "The Resources of Private." In *Health in Mexico at the Turn of the Century,* edited by J. Sepúlveda. Cuernavaca, Morelos: Instituto Nacional de Salud Publica.

Library of Congress. 1996. "Country Studies: México." Retrieved 17 May 2000 from www.lcweb2.loc.gov.

Londoño, J. L., and Frenk, J. 1997. "Pluralistic Structure: Innovative Reform for the Health Systems of Latin America. In *Needs, Services, and Politics,* pp. 307–46, edited by J. Frenk. Mexico City: Mexican Health Foundation (Funsalud).

López, O., and Blanco, J. 1993. "La Modernización Neoliberal en Salud:

México en los Ochenta. Universidad Autónoma Metropolitana, México, DF, México." In *The Context and Process of Health Care: Reform in México. Reshaping Health Care in Latin America,* edited by S. Tamez and N. Molina. Ottawa: International Development Research Center.

López-Obrador, A. M. 1999. *FOBAPROA: An Open File.* Barcelona: Grijalbo.

Magis-Rodríguez, C., Bravo-García, E., Anaya-López, L., and Uribe-Zúñiga, P. 1998. "The Situation of AIDS in México at the End of 1998." *Substance Abuse and Dependency* 18 (6): 236–44.

Martínez-González, L., Reyes-Frausto, S., and García-Peña, M. D. 1996. "Adequate Utilization of Prenatal Care at the Mexican Institute of Social Security." *Salud Publica México* 38 (5): 341–51.

Medina, E. 2000. "Substance Abuse and Dependence." In *Health in Mexico at the Turn of the Century: Challenges, Instruments, and Responses,* pp. 59–68, edited by J. Sepúlveda. Cuernavaca, Morelos: National Institute of Public Health.

Morelos, J. B. 1999. "Health, Disease, and Death: Accounts Still Pending." *Demos. Demographic Map of México* 12: 9–11.

Morissette, B. 1997. "A Mexican Approach to Health Priorities." *International Development Research Center Report* 22 (1).

National Institute of Statistics, Geography, and Informatics (INEGI). 1984. World Health Statistics Annual. Retrieved 08 August 2000 from www.inegi.gob.mx.

———. 2000. "About Mexico." Retrieved 08 August 2000 from www.inegi.gob.mx.

———. 1998. "Social and Demographic Statistics: Deaths Structure by Main Cause of General Mortality—Selected Countries." Retrieved 06 March 2002 from www.inegi.gob.mx.

Organization for Economic Cooperation and Development (OECD). 2000. "OECD Health Data 1999: Mexico." Retrieved 23 June 2000 from www.oecd.org.

Pan-American Health Organization (PAHO). 1997. "Third Evaluation of the Implementation of the Strategies for Health for All by the Year 2000: Region of the Americas." *Epidemiological Bulletin* 18 (4). Retrieved 23 April 2000 from www.paho.org.

———. 1999. "Basic Country Health Profiles for the Americas: México." Retrieved 08 August 2000 from www.paho.org.

Reyes, H., Tome, P., Gutiérrez, G., Rodríguez, L., Orozco, M., and Guiscafre, H. 1998. "Mortality for Diarrheic Disease in México: Problem of Accessibility or Quality of Care?" *Salud Publica México* 40 (4): 316–23.

Saad Sotomayor, P. 1990. "México's Air Kills 100,000 Children in México." *Excelsior* 6 (1): 69.

Secretaría de Salud (SSA) (Ministry of Health). 1998. "National Survey on Addictions, 1988 and 1998, México: SSA." Retrieved 23 April 2000 from www.ssa.gob.mx.

———. 1998b. "Main Causes of Death for the United States of Mexico." Retrieved 23 April 2000 from www.ssa.gob.mx.

———. 1999. "Epidemiological Information on Morbidity, 1998." Retrieved 23 April 2000 from www.ssa.gob.mx.

————. 2000. "México: SSA." Retrieved 23 April 2000 from www.ssa.gob.mx.

Sepúlveda, J., and Gómez Dantés, H. 1997. *Origin, Direction and Destination of the Health Transition in México and Latin America*. Ottawa: International Development Research Center.

Sepúlveda, J. (ed.) 1993. *The Health of the Indigenous People of México*. México City: Ministry of Health.

Sullivan, K., and Jordan, M. 2000. "México Pulses with Proud Satisfaction." *Washington Post Foreign Services* July 14: A01.

Tamez, S., and Molina, N. 2000. "Program Reform of the Health Sector, 1995–2000." *Diario Oficial de la Federación*, pp. 2–64. México City: Ministry of Health and Assistance.

————. 2000a. "The Context and Process of Health Care: Reform in México." In *Reshaping Health Care in Latin America*, edited by S. Fleury, S. Belmartino, and E. Baris. Ottawa: International Development Research Center.

United Nations Children's Fund (UNICEF). 2000. "Statistical Data: Mexico." Retrieved 17 May 2000 from www.who.int/whosis.

United Nations Educational, Scientific, and Cultural Organization (UNESCO). 1999. "UNESCO's Education Indicators: Country Tables: México." Retrieved 17 May 2000 from www.unesco.org.

United Nations Population Fund. 2002. "National Program on Reproductive Health: Regional Programs: Latin America and the Caribean: Mexico." United Nations Population Fund (UNFPA). Retrieved 13 March 2002 from www.unfpa.org.

U.S. Central Intelligence Agency (CIA). 2000. *The World Factbook 1999*. Retrieved 17 May 2000 from www.odci.gov/cia.

Valenzuela, J. C. 1992. "The Neoliberal Style and the Mexican State." In *The State and Social Policies of Neoliberalism*, pp. 9–42, edited by A. C. Laurell. Fundación Fredrich Ebert Stiftung.

Villarreal-Ríos, E., Montalvo-Almaguer, G., Salinas-Martínez, M., Guzmán Padilla, J. E., Tovar Castillo, N. H., and Garza Elizondo, M. E. 1996. "Cost at the First Level of Care." *Salud Pública México* 38 (5): 332–40.

World Bank Group. 1998a. "México Health System Reform—Mexican Social Security Institute (IMSS) Adjustment Loan." Retrieved 23 June 2000 from www.worldbank.org.

————. 1998b. "World Bank Approves 700 USD for Health System Reform in México." News Release No. 98/1866/LAC. Retrieved 23 June 2000 from www.worldbank.org.

————. 2000. "México: Country Brief." Retrieved 23 June 2000 from www.worldbank.org.

World Health Organization Statistical Information System (WHOSIS). 2000. "WHO Statistical Information System (WHOSIS)." Retrieved 17 May 2000 from www.who.int/whosis.

The World Paper. 1999. "Observatory: The High Price of Low Pay." Retrieved 18 March 2002 from www.worldpaper.com/Observe/thenews.html.

CUBA

Kate C. E. Macintyre and Jorge Hadad Hadad

Background Information

The Cuban health system is frequently seen as one of the outstanding achievements of the 1959 Cuban Revolution. Cubans are justly proud of their system, although they are sensitive to the limits imposed on it by the current economic situation. Designed to provide basic preventive and curative healthcare to the entire population, the health system is based on two fundamental principles: equity and free access to healthcare for all. Since the 1950s, major reforms in healthcare delivery have been implemented in two periods. The first set of reforms, designed to remedy the uneven distribution of healthcare that prevailed in pre-Revolutionary Cuba, occurred in the 1960s following the dislocation caused by the Revolution and the departure of many medical personnel in the early waves of emigration to the United States. The second period of reforms, initiated in the 1990s, has been in response to the serious economic crisis on the island triggered by the dual effects of the collapse of the Soviet Union and the tightening of the U.S. embargo. The strength of leadership in the health system from the president, Fidel Castro, is perhaps unique to Cuba; this earned Castro, at one time, the title of Minister of Health.

Reforms were vital in the 1960s because the existing system, although relatively sophisticated in terms of the type of care it could offer to those who could pay, was highly skewed toward the urban middle and upper classes. For example, there was only one rural hospital in a nation that was still largely agrarian. The reforms addressed many aspects of the health system, from the construction of facilities in underserved areas to human resource development at all levels, medical education reform, and the creation of nutrition, child, and reproductive health programs and support systems for the rapidly aging Cuban population. In general, the reforms constituted a systematic effort to ensure that all Cubans could obtain health services, that access to health services in poorly served areas (such as rural areas) improved, and that healthcare was essentially free for all at the point of service. Overt policies were implemented in an attempt to ensure that no socially manufactured factors (e.g., economic, geographic, racial, or other social barriers) could inhibit any Cuban from having the best care possible. The Cuban health system metamorphosed in a relatively short period of time from a fragmented, urban- and elite-driven, top-down system into a high-quality, preventive-care-oriented, bottom-up system that guarantees access to all.

The economic and political situation since 1990 has required reforms that were not foreseen by the original designers of the health system. Changes have been implemented to offset the acute crisis caused by the collapse of the economy and to protect those most vulnerable to the impact of this crisis. Measures taken at the national level have affected the whole system. These measures include increased popular participation and involvement of grassroots councils and committees in decisions that affect health priorities at the local level; the focus of resources on vulnerable groups (e.g., women, children under seven, the elderly); emphasis on the manufacture of essential drugs in Cuba; and the integration of traditional medical treatments into the Westernized medical system.

The limitations of the health system are neither inconsiderable nor temporary. They arise from two major external constraints and from internal policy decisions that have historically affected the management and resources of the system. For example, the emphasis on human resource development has moved the system toward a huge pool of human resources that cannot be matched by the other resources necessary to run an efficient system. In other words, the system has created a large healthcare work force, but other elements such as facilities and technology have not kept up. The external constraints are due partly to Cuba's unique relationship with the United States and partly to its former relationship with the Soviet Union. The U.S. economic and political embargo has periodically affected the ability of Cuba to import medicines and medical equipment from the United States and has kept Cuba isolated from much of the information and resource flow that might otherwise have influenced the growth and development of its health systems.

The limitations to Cuba's health system—its chronic drug shortages, poorly maintained equipment, low salary structure for health personnel, and poor state of much of its physical plant—also reflect the country's ongoing economic crisis, precipitated mainly by the collapse of the Soviet Union. The loss of subsidies and trading opportunities provided by the link with the Soviets has meant a large decrease in the government's health spending.

Cuba's government is run on a socialist and republican model, which has been led from its inception by Fidel Castro as president. The country is governed by a parliament of elected members from the 14 provinces and 169 municipalities. Cuba held its first general election in 1998; citizens voted by secret ballot for delegates to the municipal and provincial assemblies and to the National People's Assembly. Cuba's parliament is re-elected every five years, but Cuba has only one official party: the Communist party. Those in public office are not required to be members of the Communist party, although many of the most senior officials are indeed members. Two other large, national groups are the Federation of Cuban Women and the Committee for the Defense of the Revolution.

The island of Cuba, which is about 1,000 kilometers long and 100 kilometers wide, lies in an arc about 150 miles off the coast of the United States. It is the largest of the Caribbean islands, with a rich cultural mix of Spanish, European, native Indian (who were ultimately eradicated by the Spanish), and African (who were imported and died in huge numbers) peoples. The history of the island is a fascinating blend of beauty and horror, with all of the horrors attendant on a slave-owning and slave-selling agricultural society (up to the 1880s) alongside remarkable cultural and scientific achievements. Cuba's music, drama, cinema, and fine arts are internationally famous, as are its biotechnological developments in such areas as vaccine development, pharmaceutical advances, and genetically modified crops.

Cuba's population is about 11.1 million (1999). This figure is projected from the last census (1981) and current population registers, which are maintained in every community on the island. Population density is about 100 people per square kilometer, with an urban population that accounts for 75.2 percent of the total. Cuba's population pyramid is shown in Figure 26.1, and it reveals the classic demographic profile of a country with an aging population. This has important ramifications for the future priorities of the health system. Cuba has, in fact, one of the oldest populations in the Caribbean, with 12.7 percent of citizens age 60 years old and older; the proportion of the population in this age group is projected to rise to 21 percent by 2025. It should be noted that Cuban statistics no longer maintain separate racial categories and have not done so for 40 years, and individual socioeconomic indicators are not kept, either. Other general sociodemographic statistics are summarized in Table 26.1.

The birth rate in Cuba has declined steadily since the 1960s, reaching a low of 13.6 per 1,000 in 1998. Fertility has also declined from a general fertility rate of 66.1 per 1,000 women between the ages of 15 and 49 years in 1986 to a mere 46.7 per 1,000 in 1996. The total fertility rate is now below replacement fertility at 1.6, a drop from 2.0 in 1980. The proportion of young people in the population also reflects the aging of the Cuban population; people 15 years old and younger currently make up only 22 percent of the population.

Infant mortality had decreased to 7.1 per 1,000 live births by 1998, which places it among the lowest in the world. The urban/rural distribution of death rates ranges from 6.5 per 1,000 in urban areas to 4.9 per 1,000 in rural areas. This feature of lower rural mortality is a unique fact of modern life on the island and most likely reflects the higher rates of environmental problems and chronic noncommunicable diseases such as respiratory illness and diabetes in urban areas.

Projected life expectancy at birth is 75.5 years (73.6 years for men and 77.5 years for women). Cuba boasts the highest life expectancy and

FIGURE 26.1

Population Structure by Age and Gender

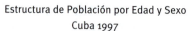

Estructura de Población por Edad y Sexo
Cuba 1997

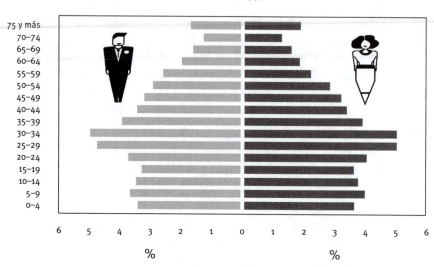

Fuente: Oficina Nacional de Estadistica

the lowest mortality rate among the Caribbean nations. Noting the generally low economic status and high proportion of deaths from noncommunicable diseases, one Cuban wit has observed, "We live like the poor, but die like the rich."

The island's economy remains founded on agricultural exports, principally sugar and tobacco, although tourism is rapidly expanding. The main industries include nickel mining, cement, fertilizer, steel production, fishing, and petroleum extraction. Several relatively new sectors such as biotechnology and electronic industries are being encouraged for their potential to assist Cuba's recovery from the economic collapse of the past decade.

TABLE 26.1

General Demographics

Population	11,122,308
Infant mortality per 1,000 live births	7.1
Under-five mortality per 1,000 live births	9.4
Life expectancy at birth (projection for 1995 to 2000), years	75.5
General fertility rate	46.7
Total fertility rate	1.6
Percent urbanized	75.2

Cuba's economy has slowly begun to grow again during the past few years after a period of deep depression during the early 1990s; the gross national product fell every year from 1989 to 1994, and it has only slowly begun to return to the 1989 level. The rate of increase of the gross domestic product has averaged 0.7 percent per year at 1981's constant prices, with only 1996 reporting a large increase of 7.5 percent. Additional economic data are provided in Table 26.2.

Education statistics reflect another achievement of the past decades, as shown in Table 26.3. Illiteracy was high relative to Cuba's wealth in the 1950s, when about three-quarters of the population 15 years old or older were illiterate and had only a few years of primary education. Today illiteracy has been nearly eliminated, and official statistics report that 98 percent of children attended school to the end of secondary school. In addition, higher education has also undergone a transformation, and the number of university centers has increased from 3 in 1959 to 40 in 1990.

Context: Health Needs

Cuba's health profile is now one of a nation that has passed through the epidemiological transition to a society in which chronic noncommunicable causes of death dominate. Infectious and parasitic diseases are no longer the main causes of disease and death, although some environmentally caused problems such as diarrhea and other intestinal diseases have increased. Hepatitis A, for example, has increased from 24.5 cases per 100,000 in 1989 to 189 per 100,000 in 1996; the incidence of tuberculosis has also increased from its low in the 1980s. These changes may reflect increased surveillance and case detection. Most of the common tropical diseases that plagued Cuba at the beginning of the twentieth century (e.g., malaria, yellow fever) have been eradicated, although a few cases of imported malaria are treated every year. Only dengue and the more deadly version, dengue hemorrhagic fever, occasionally make an appearance, most recently in 1997, when 2,946 cases were reported in the eastern province of Santiago de Cuba. Children in Cuba are vaccinated against all the WHO-recommended diseases, and the success of the immunization program is shown in Table

		TABLE 26.2
GNP per capita (U.S.$)	728.6	Economic and
Real GDP per capita (U.S.$), 1997	1,317	Social
Human Development Index score, 1996	0.726	Indicators
Percent of GDP to health in 1997	9.5	
Percent of health budget in public sector	100	

TABLE 26.3
Education
Indicators

	Male	Female
Adult literacy rate (total)	98.2%	
Primary school enrollment	521,837	494,060
Secondary school enrollment	223,615	225,299

26.4. A current effort to vaccinate the entire nation against hepatitis B is underway.

Noncommunicable diseases and injuries are currently Cuba's main health problems and account for the majority of deaths. Table 26.5 shows the leading causes of death for all ages, including heart disease, malignant neoplasms (lung, prostate, breast, and colon), cerebrovascular diseases, and accidents; these leading causes represent 65 percent of all deaths. In terms of relative trends, however, mortality from heart disease, stroke, and suicide appear to have recently begun to fall, whereas rates of death from cancer, accidents, and diabetes have remained stable over the past five years. Deaths from cirrhosis, chronic/bronchial asthma, homicide, and AIDS have all increased during this same period.

Cardiovascular illnesses are the leading cause of death, with myocardial infarction the major culprit within this group. The mortality rate for these diseases is 205.9 per 100,000, with the rate distributed unevenly between men (222 per 100,000) and women (189 per 200,000). Cuba also had a relatively high rate of death from strokes (72.7 per 100,000) in 1996,

TABLE 26.4
Access to
Health and
General
Immunization
Indicators

	Urban	Rural
Percent access to health services	100	100
Percent access to safe water, 1998	96	69
Percent access to sanitation, 1996	93.6	82.8
Immunization coverage		
Diphtheria-pertussis-tetanus up to 1 year	99.0%	
Diphtheria-pertussis-tetanus at 1 to 8 years	97.6%	
Poliomyelitis	95.2%	
Measles-mumps-rubella	99.0%	

SOURCE: Fuente (1997).

Communicable diseases	1.4	**TABLE 26.5**
Noncommunicable diseases	88.9	Percentages
Injuries (accidents, intentional)	9.7	of Deaths by Type

although this has decreased during the last few years. The crude death rate from any form of cancer has increased in the 1990s to a recent high of about 140 per 100,000, making it the second leading cause of death.

Accidents and injuries represent the fourth leading cause of death in Cuba and the leading cause of death for Cubans between the ages of 1 and 49 years. The crude death rate is 39 per 100,000. Traffic accidents involving cars and bicycles account for a high proportion of these deaths, but suicide and other forms of self-inflicted injuries are also relatively common. See Table 26.6 for further mortality data.

Respiratory problems such as asthma are the leading cause of morbidity. One estimate places the total number of visits for acute asthma at 5 million for 1996, with the majority of these cases involving children. Deteriorating and crowded housing conditions, air pollution, and a shortage of drugs all contribute to this problem.

Diabetes, asthma, and hypertension are also extremely common causes of medical visits, and they account for approximately one-tenth of

TABLE 26.6
Causes of Death

Cause of Death	1970	1975	1980	1985	1990	1998
Heart disease	205.4	185.0	174.4	182.3	170.2	142.6
Malignant tumors	122.4	114.4	111.1	113.9	112.8	111.0
Cerebrovascular diseases	84.6	63.1	57.7	59.7	55.6	52.9
Accidents	38.8	36.1	38.6	41.1	44.5	39.0
Influenza and pneumonia	45.3	44.6	40.1	42.0	23.7	31.3
Diseases of the arteries	36.0	33.9	24.9	22.9	24.1	21.9
Diabetes mellitus	13.3	11.8	11.6	15.2	18.8	12.1
Suicides and self-inflicted injuries	13.5	19.1	22.0	20.9	18.2	15.3
Cirrhosis and other liver disease	8.2	6.4	6.0	6.4	7.7	7.1
Homicide	4.4	4.2	3.5	3.6	6.0	6.4

NOTE: Rates per 100,000 population for 1970 through 1998 (figures for 1998 are provisional).

all visits. The details of the growing problem of these diseases are illustrated in Table 26.7, which shows the prevalence as reported at all medical facilities for these three diseases in the 12-month period from January 1999 to December 1999.

The incidence of AIDS cases (1,486 cases of HIV have been diagnosed, with 381 deaths reported by 1996) remains very low, although it is increasing as Cuba opens more to tourism and external contacts. The incidence of AIDS is also increasing as a result of internal transmission from existing cases. Cuba's policy of quarantining all HIV-positive cases in sanatoria throughout the country has been documented in the healthcare literature (Bayer and Healton 1989; Granich et al. 1995; Perez-Stable 1991). In brief, Cuba's reaction to HIV/AIDS was to initiate a stringent policy of permanent quarantine for all identified cases of the virus. Thirteen sanatoria, distributed evenly throughout the island, were equipped with clinical and nonclinical staff and all necessary additional amenities, including sports facilities, special living quarters (e.g., for homosexual couples), and occupational/enterprise centers (e.g., jewelry making and other craft centers). The idea of this policy was to isolate all HIV-positive individuals from the rest of the population for the rest of their lives. Following considerable pressure from international bodies such as the United Nations and many large nongovernmental agencies, the Cuban policy now officially rests on voluntary quarantine in the sanatoria after a medically recommended stay of eight weeks.

All newly identified persons with HIV are also expected to spend at least eight weeks in a sanatorium. During this time, the HIV-positive per-

TABLE 26.7

Morbidity Data by Age Group, Rates per 1,000 Population

Age groups	Diabetes Mellitus			Hypertension			Asthma		
	Male	Female	Total	Male	Female	Total	Male	Female	Total
Less than 1 year	0.0	—	0.0	—	—	—	20.1	15.9	18.1
1 to 4 years	0.0	0.0	0.0	0.0	0.0	0.0	81.8	66.3	74.3
5 to 9 years	0.2	0.2	0.2	0.1	0.1	0.1	103.6	88.1	96.1
10 to 14 years	0.6	0.6	0.6	0.3	0.3	0.3	121.5	106.0	113.9
15 to 24 years	2.8	3.6	3.2	18.8	19.3	19.0	81.6	79.0	80.3
25 to 59 years	12.4	20.5	16.5	91.3	121.6	106.6	44.5	58.1	51.4
60 to 64 years	89.6	138.3	114.1	424.8	528.5	476.9	98.6	114.4	106.6
65 years and older	43.9	101.0	73.5	220.7	303.0	263.4	39.8	46.7	43.4
Total	13.7	25.7	19.7	82.9	112.4	97.6	64.1	67.8	66.0

son is educated about the disease, counseled about options for care in the community, and given information about how to prevent the disease's spread. At the end of the eight-week educational period, the person is offered the choice of remaining in the sanatorium, where nutrition needs are provided and the patient receives a very small income and an occupation. Some people who are HIV-positive or who have AIDS reportedly choose to remain permanently in the sanatoria.

The prevalence of other sexually transmitted diseases (e.g., gonorrhea, syphilis) also increased from 86.1 per 100,000 to 143.3 per 100,000 between 1990 and 1997, although the rate may have dropped recently due to increased surveillance and contact-tracing efforts.

Organization and Management of the Health System

Because health is considered a strategic objective in the development of society, the Cuban government assumes full responsibility for the healthcare of its citizens. Traditionally, Cuba's health system has been a highly centralized system with a high degree of control concentrated at the highest levels of the ministry. Before the reforms of the 1980s, the Ministry of Public Health dictated how resources were to be spent, what diseases took priority, and which public health strategies should be implemented. Several initiatives have decentralized this system, and priorities and health promotion strategies are now identified at more local levels. The current intent is to operate a system where prioritization decisions are made at the community level, even if resource allocation decisions are made at the central level.

The Public Health Law (1983) was the first important reform of the 1980s, laying out the general activities and responsibilities of the state to protect the health of Cubans; it also established the organization of the health sector. The introduction of the Family Doctor Program in 1984, which aimed at placing a general practitioner in each community, has been compared with the ideal primary healthcare system as envisioned at Alma-Ata (WHO 1979).

The administration of the national health system is organized on three levels: national, provincial, and municipal. The Ministry of Public Health represents the national level. It serves as the lead agency and performs regulatory, coordination, and control functions. Programs such as the Regulatory Bureau for Health Protection and the National Drugs Program have been established to enable the more rigorous collection of data on health trends and the regulation and quality of commonly prescribed drugs. Programs such as these and the pharmaceutical and biotechnological institutes are also managed at the national level. In addition, the ministry coordinates with other ministries that have a role in improving health within the Cuban society, such as the ministries of Agriculture, Education, Science, Environment, and Technology.

The provincial and municipal public health offices are under the financial and administrative authority of the provincial and municipal administrative councils. At these levels, a health representative sits on the local council (committee popular); he or she often holds a senior office such as the vice presidency of the local council. These local councils are responsible for proposing and identifying the priorities and needs for their communities. Responsibilities of the provincial health office include supervision of the major hospitals, the epidemiological monitoring systems, the blood banks, and all training and medical education facilities.

At the municipal level, the public health offices are directly responsible for the polyclinics (community hospitals); rural specialist hospitals; maternity homes; specialized clinics or centers for the elderly, mental health, and oral health; and epidemiological units at the local level. At the municipal level, the popular councils participate actively in the decision-making process.

Figure 26.2 shows a system intended to identify needs at the lowest level, which is the family doctor and municipal level; activity on this level initiates action at the next highest level. The top three boxes in this figure refer to the national level, and the next two represent the provincial and municipal levels; the local level includes the polyclinic and the family doctor.

Assessing the extent to which non-Cubans have influenced the development of the Cuban health system is difficult. Undoubtedly, the model of the family doctor at the community or neighborhood level has some ancestry in the Alma-Ata Conference on Primary Health Care, although elements of this program were already in place in Cuba in the early 1970s. The influence of Soviet architects can be seen in the 1970s and 1980s infrastructure of the medical system. More recently, Cuba has collaborated with several international bodies (e.g., universities in Europe and Latin America) and worked with officials of the World Health Organization, the Pan-American Health Organization, the Food and Agriculture Organization (FAO), the United Nations Children's Fund, and the United Nations Population Fund (UNFPA) on a variety of programs and studies to ease the impact of the economic crisis on health status.

Although some foreign expertise has been used in Cuba in recent years, especially following the unusual outbreak of neuropathy from 1991 to 1994, much medical and public health expertise has flowed in the other direction: from Cuba to other parts of the world. Through a policy called Medical Diplomacy, which gave the Cuban government a political and humanitarian justification especially significant during the Cold War era, Cuba has sent more than 3,000 doctors to over 30 countries in the past ten years. The number of doctors going overseas has decreased since 1989, although Cuba still exports doctors provided their travel, salaries, board, and lodging are paid for by the receiving country. South Africa is currently

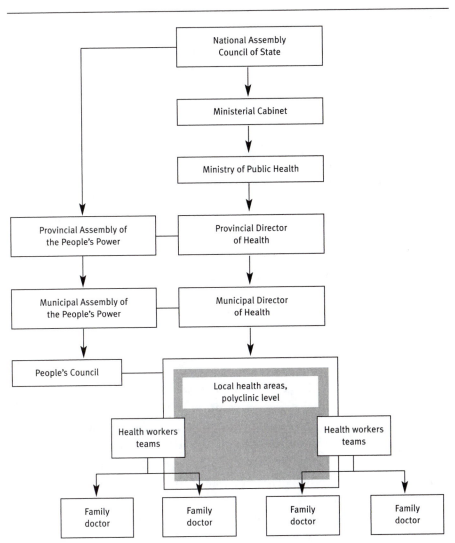

FIGURE 26.2

The Cuban
Health System
Management
Structure

hosting 300 Cuban doctors who are assisting in that country's reorganization of healthcare delivery.

Financing

Cuba's health system is funded primarily by the national budget through
indirect taxation and duties. The government aims to provide free preventive and curative care and rehabilitation, whereas all essential diagnostic tests and drugs are provided free to certain vulnerable groups, including children less than eight years old and pregnant women. These services
are paid for via two separate funding mechanisms and two separate currency systems. Cuban pesos provide the largest share (80 percent of the

total budget), but funding also comes directly to the health budget from foreign currency earned through tourism and exports such as sugar and tobacco. Since 1993, all supplies imported by the Ministry of Public Health must be financed out of the foreign currency budget allocated by the government for this purpose. Salaries, national currency financing, and administration of all resources (including human resources) are managed at the provincial and municipal level.

The 1998 fiscal year health budget was reported at U.S.$826 million; this represents about 5.7 percent of the gross national product and more than 18 percent of all public spending. This suggests that Cuba spends approximately U.S.$750 per capita on health. The financing mechanisms are calculated through population-based estimates on a need basis. One internal Ministry of Public Health report estimates that 90 percent of the Cuban health budget is allocated at the local (provincial or municipal) level and that only 10 percent of disbursement is decided at the national level (Hadad, personal communication, May 2000). More than half of the health budget goes toward wages, and a considerable proportion of the remainder goes toward medications. A fraction of the budget is spent on equipment and facilities.

In terms of individual, out-of-pocket expenditures, Cubans are expected to pay for all drugs for outpatient treatment and material support items such as wheelchairs, hearing aids, and eyeglasses. Prices for these goods are dependent on government subsidies. Vulnerable families can make a case for waiving these costs due to hardship.

Before 1990, the government was heavily dependent on Soviet subsidies for its health budget. However, since the economic crisis, Cuba has sought bilateral grants in aid from various European and Latin American nations. A few international nongovernmental organizations also donate drugs, equipment, spare parts, and other goods. Currently, an estimated U.S.$20 million is provided through these channels each year, which makes up about 2 percent of the health budget. However, this does not include materials and donated drugs that come from Cuban friends and relatives in North America. Because data on these donations cannot be gathered from either the United States or the Cuban authorities, no estimates are available.

Health Resources

Human Resources

Cuba is rich in human resources for healthcare delivery and currently has one of the highest ratios of physicians to population in the world: approximately one doctor for every 175 people. In 1998, there were 63,483 physicians (57.1 per 10,000 inhabitants) and 9,873 dentists (8.9 per 10,000 inhabitants). Details about the healthcare work force are provided in Table 26.8. Cuba currently has 29,924 family doctors and 82,527 nursing personnel (74.2 per 10,000 inhabitants). This is an area of changing policy, as plans have been made to increase the number of nurses in Cuba relative to doctors and move the system to a focus on the medical doctor and the paramedical personnel working in teams at the local level. Special emphasis will be placed on the development of more university-trained nurses.

A policy to integrate traditional medicine into the mainstream health system was first designed in 1993, at the peak of the economic crisis, when traditional medical treatments were seen as a cheap and acceptable method of filling the gap left by the absence of Western medicines. The system now includes a range of healing approaches, most of which existed in Cuba before the crisis but which have been incorporated and adapted much more rigorously since 1993. Alternative therapies offered include many of Asian origin such as acupuncture, shaisu (Japanese massage), tui-na massage, cupping (heat suction), facial massage, mud treatments, and a wide range of herbal medicines (known as green or natural medicine). Other therapies included are electric acupuncture, magnetic and laser therapy, infrared light and color treatment, music therapy, floral essence therapy, and hypnosis.

Although the original justification for integrating traditional medical beliefs with Western medicine was largely economic, other factors have ensured its continuation. The popularity of the traditional healing methods and their claimed efficacy in treating chronic, noncommunicable diseases have ensured that these methods are further developed, tested, and implemented by many doctors in their daily practice, as well as by specialized clinics. Acupuncture is used regularly in place of anesthetics for minor and even major surgery, and chronic pain is treated almost entirely with traditional methods. Several of these methods are still controversial, and some doctors in Cuba are reluctant to use them. An emphasis on testing each procedure and intervention is being proposed at higher policymaking levels.

Although the vast majority of doctors work in the national health system, a few remain in private practice. An estimated 100 private practice doctors are concentrated in Havana and other major cities. At the other extreme on the healing continuum, many practitioners of the ancient healing cult of Santeria remain. These practitioners can be found in most community centers in Cuba, but no form of licensing is in place, nor are their

Physicians	56.8	**TABLE 26.8** Human Resources per 1,000 Population by Type
Nurses	73.7	
Administrators	0.2	
Dentists	8.9	
Technicians	51.0	

practices regarded as legal by the government. The government practices
a policy of distant tolerance for Santeria, recognizing its popularity but dis-
trusting its methods.

Health Facilities

The infrastructure of Cuba's health system is extensive and widely distributed in both rural and urban areas. It is a strongly hierarchical system that
emphasizes primary care but that, at least in theory, has a highly sophisticated and highly technical capacity at the tertiary level. Table 26.9 provides a summary of all of the physical facilities currently open in Cuba. The
facilities are distributed fairly evenly throughout the island, with central
hospitals and polyclinics in all densely populated areas and with family doctors, each with approximately 120 families to care for, also distributed
throughout rural and urban Cuba. The following section further describes
the different health system levels.

Commodities

Because Cuba's system is currently under considerable strain, both drug
and equipment shortages will continue until more resources are available
at the national level to subsidize them. One estimate suggests that Cuba
currently has a shortfall of about one-half of its "needed" drugs. Of the
list of essential drugs drawn up by the World Health Organization, health
authorities try to guarantee availability of about 1,000 drugs, although as
of 1998 only 700 could be provided through imports from overseas or
through domestic production (Hadad, personal communication, May 2000).
Cuba has been steadily increasing its domestic production of pharmaceutical goods, partly as a means to supply the health system with the required
basics that have not been easily available due to the U.S. embargo, and
partly to increase export earnings in foreign currency. Other biotechnological goods, especially vaccines for hepatitis A and B and meningitis, have
also provided much-needed foreign exchange.

TABLE 26.9
Number and
Types of
Health
Services
Facilities and
by Population

	Number	Population
Hospitals	283	389,966
Polyclinics	442	25,081
Institutes	12	919,666
Dental clinics	166	66,481
Maternity homes	220	50,163
Elderly homes	196	56,306
Blood banks	26	424,461

Service Delivery

Family doctors deliver the majority of personal healthcare in Cuba. Official estimates report that family doctors provide 75 percent of all outpatient care given in Cuba, including office and home visits. Cubans use their health system extensively. In 1996, they made 77 million visits to a medical practitioner, of which about 57 million were to family doctors; this was an average of 5.2 visits per person to any medical practitioner and 1.8 per person to an emergency room. The ratio of outpatient to emergency room visits was 2.9. Additional service usage data are provided in Table 26.10.

The referral system works in a typical pyramidal fashion, with family doctors referring patients to a community hospital or polyclinic. The polyclinic staff can then refer patients to a more sophisticated, provincial hospital, and then upward if necessary to the training/referral hospitals in the main urban centers in Cuba. The Hermanos Ameijeiras Hospital in Havana is the central referral hospital in the country.

The polyclinic is a key component of the Cuban system. The combination of the family doctor and the polyclinic is called the primary level of care. Cuba has 442 of these small community hospitals or health centers. As the first medical treatment centers after the family doctor and the coordinating units for the family doctors, the polyclinics are staffed by a small team of specialists; this team serves approximately 25,000 individuals. The team at the polyclinic consists of a pediatrician, an obstetrician/gynecologist, an orthopedic surgeon, nurses, paramedics, technical staff, and a driver for transporting patients in emergencies. These large clinics have the capacity to provide support and rehabilitation for minor surgeries and basic radiology and to do some laboratory work for common diagnoses. Any illness that requires further attention is referred to the municipal or provincial hospital. In addition, senior staff at the polyclinics is responsible for collecting epidemiological and relevant environmental data. This information is processed by a highly sophisticated and comprehensive health information system that is used at the municipal and provincial levels to make policy decisions.

	Number	Per 1,000 Population
Hospital admissions	1,441,896	131
Hospital days	1,417, 213	1,284
Outpatient visits	57,738,302	5,232
Clinic visits	98,198,882	8,898

TABLE 26.10
Service Use and Rates

The secondary level of care is provided at municipal hospitals that have more equipment and technicians. These hospitals are expected to handle the majority of pediatric and elderly specialty care for their communities and all but the most complicated births. All pregnant women are expected to give birth in hospitals or in the specialized obstetric or maternity hospitals because most polyclinics are unable to support maternity units. Less than one percent of births occur outside of a medical setting.

Tertiary care is provided at provincial hospitals equipped with more sophisticated technology and more highly skilled workers than is found at the lower-level facilities. This level of care takes place in the national hospitals, which are linked to the biomedical research institutes. The Hermanos Ameijeiras Hospital in Havana is the largest in the country, with 1,000 beds and more than 30 separate specialized medical services. Here treatments are carried out for visitors from many countries in Latin and Central America who come specifically to seek treatment under the Cuban system. This service has become a considerable source of foreign currency for the government in recent years.

Prospects for the Future

Poverty in general and poor housing in particular have probably been responsible for the increase in environmentally linked illnesses such as asthma. In addition, the housing shortage in Havana is a critical problem, as crowding in unsanitary conditions in many areas is creating potential health hazards on several levels.

Maintaining the quality and quantity of water supplied to most Cubans and improving trash collection and disposal are two additional public health priorities. Water supply in urban areas, particularly in Havana, may approach critically low levels of quality and quantity soon if the infrastructure of the system is not upgraded. Although enough water is theoretically available for domestic and industrial needs in Cuba, the system that delivers water to households and businesses is decidedly inadequate; it is both aged and under stress. The small borehole size and age of water pipes cause them to break under the pressure and the quantity demanded of them. Pump technology is old and often deficient because of lack of spare parts. Storage sites are scarce and have not kept pace with population growth. In addition, the economic crisis has led to shortages of chlorine and other means of treating stored water.

Official statistics show that, as of 1998, 96 percent of urban and 69 percent of rural areas had access to potable water. Thus, most urban neighborhoods are without water for part of every day. An urgent priority for the Cuban government is to rectify the aging water supply system in urban areas before the poor quality of water affects the health status of large numbers of Cubans.

An additional challenge for Cuban health authorities is the rapidly aging population. The combination of older people, the high rates of smoking in the adult population (approximately 28 percent of all Cubans smoke), and the traditional diet, which is relatively high in cholesterol and sugar, means that the incidence of chronic diseases may rise. Simultaneously, communicable diseases may resurface if the water and sanitation situations in urban Cuba are not rectified soon.

Despite these grave circumstances, Cubans retain the advantage of a sophisticated and equitable system with a large, experienced, and well-trained human resource pool; all of these qualities indicate that Cuba's leadership cares about the islanders' health. As described above, Cuba's health system is entirely the responsibility of the state. The government retains the stated priority of guarding the citizens' health through the provision of the best care possible. Clearly, given the current economic conditions, this is somewhat idealistic. At present, providing the level of care to which the government aspires is not possible. What cannot be denied, however, are the tremendous gains that have already been made and the fact that the most vulnerable Cubans have been protected even during the tremendous economic difficulties of the 1990s.

REFERENCES

Bayer, R., and Healton, C. 1988. "Controlling AIDS in Cuba: The Logic of Quarantine." *New England Journal of Medicine* 320 (15): 1022–24.

Fuente, J. B. 1997. *Informe de la Marcha del Programa Nacional de Acción a Favor de la Infancia.* Havana: Statistics Office, Government of Cuba.

Granich, R., Jacobs, B., Mermin, J., and Pont, A. 1995. "Cuba's National AIDS Program: The First Decade." *Western Journal of Medicine* 163 (2): 139–44.

Perez-Stable, E. 1991. "Cuba's Response to the HIV Epidemic." *American Journal of Public Health* 81 (5): 563–67.

World Health Organization (WHO). 1979. "Primary Health Care and Health for All by Year 2000. Alma-Ata Conference. Geneva: World Health Organization.

27

COSTA RICA

William H. Dow and Luis B. Sáenz

Introduction

Costa Rica is frequently called the Switzerland of Latin America. Unlike its Central American neighbors, the country has enjoyed remarkable political stability since peacefully gaining independence from Spain in 1821. The current republican constitution adopted in 1949 has largely been respected with democratic elections, a fact that is often linked with Costa Rica's abolition of its military during the same year. Another remarkable feature of the country is its life expectancy of 77 years at birth, which is equivalent to that of OECD countries despite its per capita income, which lags at only about one-fifth (by P.P.P.) of that found in the United States. In part, this high life expectancy is the result of the high levels of educational and public health investments during the past century in both urban and poorer rural areas.

Historically the country has had a more even wealth and land distribution than many of its neighbors. Costa Rica was relatively isolated during the colonial period, and it was settled largely by small landholders with a less dominant aristocracy than other areas. Little remains of the small indigenous population, leaving an extremely homogeneous ethnic composition that is currently 96 percent white and mestizo.

Agriculture commodity exports such as bananas and coffee have traditionally been the largest sector of the Costa Rican economy, but the growth of the tourism industry is contributing to economic diversification. "Ecological tourism" has been a particular recent focus, as 25 percent of the country is protected in public park land that ranges from rain forests on the coastal plains to the rugged volcanic mountains that separate the coasts. Transportation and marketing of crops are aided by the small size of the country and its narrow shape, with most areas being located within a few hours' drive of either a port or the capital city of San Jose. About 60 percent of the population of just over 3.4 million lives in the central valley around San Jose, which is centrally located and sits at a temperate elevation of more than 1,000 meters. Additional demographic information is provided in Table 27.1.

Costa Rica prides itself on its social and human capital investments, and equity of access to healthcare services is a long-held goal toward which

TABLE 27.1
General
Demographics

Population	3,464,170
Infant mortality (per 1,000 live births)	11.83
Under-five mortality (per 10,000)	5
Life expectancy at birth (years)	76.8
Fertility rate (percent)	2.94
Percent urbanized	44

SOURCE: Direccion General de Estadistica y Censos (various years).

much progress has been made. Literacy is 95 percent for both men and women over the age of 15 years; 4.5 percent of the gross domestic product goes to education, 90 percent of men and 91 percent of women obtain four years or more of schooling, and the average education for current youth is ten years for men and nine years for women. Women's education has been a government priority since the late 19th century, and literacy was already estimated at more than 70 percent in the 1940s when the government began a concerted effort to further increase social expenditures.

Demographic indicators changed dramatically during the twentieth century: infant mortality fell from more than 200 per 1,000 live births in 1920 to 74 in 1960 and to 19 by 1980, and total fertility dropped precipitously from 7.6 in 1960 to under 4 by 1973. In the 1970s, public health expenditures were further increased from 5.1 percent of GDP in 1970 to about 7.6 percent by 1980. During this same time, the public sector expanded social security health coverage from about 40 to more than 70 percent of the population and simultaneously implemented large primary healthcare programs. This level of social expenditure was later scaled back during the debt crisis of the early 1980s. Since the late 1980s, progress in social and health investment has again resumed, although debates and experiments aimed at improving the efficiency of the large public sector are ongoing. Currently 89 percent of the population is enrolled in social insurance, although by law all people are eligible for access to healthcare through the universal health insurance system. Sociodemographic information is provided in Tables 27.2, 27.3 and 27.4.

Context: Health Needs

Costa Rica is well along in its epidemiological transition. Infant mortality and life expectancy are at developed-country levels, and the fall in total fertility has contributed to a rapidly aging population. The leading causes of death are cardiovascular diseases, cancer, and accidents.

TABLE 27.2
Economic
and Social
Indicators

GNP per capita (U.S.$), 1997	2,640
Real GDP per capita (P.P.P.$), 1997	6,410
Human Development Index score, 2001	0.82 (position 41)
Percent of GNP to health	10.7% (7.7% public, 3% private)

SOURCE: Direccion General de Estadistica y Censos (various years); Proyecto Estado de la Nacion (various years).

Great strides have been made toward eliminating vaccine-preventable diseases, and wide access to primary care, safe water, and sanitation—along with increased education—have decreased the incidence of many infectious diseases. Polio was certified as eradicated in 1994, the last neonatal tetanus death was reported in 1988, and the last diphtheria death occurred in 1974. Nevertheless, reaching the remaining portion of the population vulnerable to infectious disease remains an important priority. Recent years have seen increases in the incidence of diseases previously under control, such as malaria, measles, cholera, dengue, and tuberculosis, and in the 1990s some child vaccination rates, such as those for diptheria-pertussis-tetanus, have fallen back to less than 90 percent. Acute respiratory infections and diarrhea still represent the third and fourth most common causes of childhood death, and they are among the most frequent causes of healthcare resource use. AIDS is also a growing problem, with more than 1,000 reported cases in the country through 1996, primarily among urban young men. Additional mortality data are provided in Table 27.5.

The prominence of chronic and degenerative diseases reflects the increasingly modern lifestyle characterized by rising obesity from poor diet and insufficient exercise and the problems that result from tobacco use and alcohol abuse. Despite the growing proportion of deaths caused by these diseases, death rates have been falling rapidly, and since the 1960s, adult men in Costa Rica have had lower age-specific death rates than those in the United States. This decline was especially fast among young adults in the 1950s and older adults in the 1980s, despite the economic recession

TABLE 27.3
Education
Indicators

Adult literacy rate (15 years or older), 1995 (percent)	95
Primary school enrollment rate, 1995 (percent)	92
Secondary school enrollment rate, 1995 (percent)	43

SOURCE: World Bank (1998).

TABLE 27.4

Percentages of Population with Access to Health-Enhancing Factors

Access to health services	100
Access to safe water	87.13
Access to sanitation	96.25
Immunization levels	More than 90

SOURCE: Proyecto Estado de la Nacion (various years).

and declining health spending during the 1980s. Rosero (1994) reports that lower heart disease and lung cancer death rates account for much of the differences with the United States, although these differences are counterbalanced by Costa Rica's higher death rates for stomach cancer, stroke, diabetes, accidents, and cervical cancer. In comparison with other Latin American countries (e.g., Chile, Argentina) death rates are also somewhat lower, with especially important differences in infectious and parasitic disease rates.

Important public health issues for the future include lowering accident rates, keeping infectious diseases under control, improving health behaviors such as diet and smoking, and increasing healthcare access to the 11 percent of the population that is currently uninsured. Access to care is no longer a problem primarily of financial insurance but rather one of healthcare administration, with long waiting times to receive general medical services and poorly managed waiting lists for specialists.

Organization and Management of the Health System

The Costa Rican health system is highly socialized, with the federal government currently controlling most health sector activities. The Caja

TABLE 27.5

Leading Causes of Mortality

Cause of Death	Percent of Deaths
Cardiovascular diseases	30.8
Tumors	20.7
Injuries and poisoning	11.2
Respiratory diseases	10.6
Digestive diseases	6.3

SOURCE: Ministerio de Salud (1998).

Costarricense de Seguro Social (Costa Rican Social Security Administration [CCSS]) administers the public social security health insurance, which is mandatory among formal sector workers and covers 89 percent of the population. Since the 1970s, the CCSS has also owned and administered most hospitals and inpatient services, with only about 225 private hospital beds existing in the country out of more than 6,000 total beds.

More than two-thirds of doctors are also employed in the public sector, although most have private offices as well. This has led to accusations of physician absenteeism from public jobs to attend wealthier patients who are attracted to private office hours to avoid ubiquitous queues. The CCSS has recently begun to contract out nonphysician services; Figure 27.1 illustrates some of the areas that have recently begun to be privatized, such as auxiliary services like laboratory tests. Managed care experimentation is also occurring, with four urban Areas de Salud (Health Areas) being run as HMO-like "Cooperativas" that can contract private medical services. Efficiency gains in the Cooperativas have been limited, however. They are still publicly run, and each services only a limited geographic area, with consumers still unable to choose among Cooperativas. These private-sector experiments are likely to continue expanding only slowly in the near future.

After hospital services were consolidated within CCSS during the 1970s, the Ministry of Health became primarily responsible for public health programs. During the last ten years, further attempts have been made to eliminate the duplication of effort between the CCSS and the Ministry of Health. Currently the administration of many primary health services is being transferred to the CCSS in an attempt to rationalize resource use, and in the future the Ministry of Health will focus mainly on regulatory and monitoring functions.

Since 1995, the CCSS has embarked on a major reform to decentralize primary healthcare to 800 Integrated Health Care Basic Teams (EBAIS) in 90 Health Areas. Whether significant changes have occurred at the level of resource allocation decision making is not yet clear, but anecdotal accounts indicate changes in employee motivation, in the delimitation of management decisions, and in community participation in quality control. In 1998, the Legislative Assembly approved a decentralization law for CCSS facilities that included increased community participation in management, budgetary flexibility, and equipment-purchasing autonomy. Human resource contracting, however, remains centrally controlled.

Medical training activities are under only slightly less central government control. Although both public and private universities offer degrees in medicine, nursing, dentistry, and other medical professions, all specialty training takes place in the government's CCSS hospitals and clinics. The CCSS also regulates specialty training and oversees both clinical and administrative certification processes.

FIGURE 27.1

Sources and Uses of National Health Financing

Financing Source	Provider Type		Percent of Health Financing
	Public	Private	
Federal budget	State pays matching contributions of 0.25% of payrolls into CCSS		9
Mandatory contributions to CCSS and INS	Outpatient and inpatient visits at CCSS facilities	1. CCSS contracting of (a) high-technology diagnostic and treatment services, (b) specialty doctors and surgeons to ameliorate long waiting lists, and (c) medicine transportation	67
		2. Primary care Cooperativas (about 5% of the population); INS purchase of private services for patients with transportation and occupational accidents	
Voluntary insurance		Voluntary public and private insurance contracts to prepay private healthcare within the country and abroad	1.5
Out-of-pocket user fees	Uninsured patients at CCSS facilities pay according to set outpatient and inpatient fee schedules		22
Mixed		1. "Enterprise medicine," in which employers contract a mix of private providers and CCSS services for employees	0.5
		2. "Mixed medicine program," in which patients pay private providers and CCSS covers certain diagnostics and medicine	
		3. "Physician choice program," in which the CCSS pays 60% of private provider service costs for childbirth and specialty services	

NOTE: CCSS = Caja Costarricense de Seguro Social (Costa Rican Social Security Administration); INS = National Insurance Institute.
SOURCE: Castro Valverde and Bernardo Saénz (1998).

Financing

Federal government programs account for most health spending; the remaining 20 to 25 percent of private spending is out-of-pocket because little private health insurance is available (Figure 27.1). The CCSS revenues are derived from wage taxes and federal general budget revenues. For the main sickness and maternity insurance, salaried workers pay 5.5 percent of their salaries, employers pay an additional 9.25 percent, and the government contributes 0.25 percent of the payroll level. Pensioners pay 5 percent, whereas their pension fund pays 8.75 percent, and voluntary (nonformal sector workers) subscribers pay 15.25 percent for combined sickness and pension insurance. Any residual budgetary shortfall or surplus becomes part of the overall federal budget.

Insured users have few copayments, with some exceptions such as for eyeglasses. Generally no use of private services is reimbursed, although the CCSS will pay a portion of certain high-technology procedures that are not available at government facilities, including magnetic resonance imaging. Individuals are responsible for expenses above the basic approved services (e.g., nonapproved medications, elective tests). In practice, many patients pay out-of-pocket to use private facilities even for basic services to avoid the extensive queues at CCSS facilities.

Most immediate family members of the primary insured are also covered by CCSS. Legally, all uninsured individuals have access to CCSS facilities for emergency services, and they are charged according to income for other services. The uninsured typically use private facilities for routine healthcare and enroll in CCSS only in case of the need for high-cost care.

Monitoring of financial flows is poor. Evasion and underpayment of wage taxes is considered to be widespread, and enforcement has been difficult. Within the CCSS, unit budgeting controls are not currently well-developed. Hospital expenses account for about 70 percent of CCSS expenditures, and their share has been growing. CCSS and Ministry of Health workers are currently civil service employees on direct salary, with few pecuniary incentives for delivering efficient, high-quality care.

The other agency involved in the health-financing system is the National Insurance Institute (INS), which collects premiums and administers insurance for claims related to occupational health (obligatory for employers) and automobile accidents (obligatory for licensed drivers). The INS also sells supplemental health insurance policies that reimburse private healthcare expenses, but few people buy the policies, and they only account for one percent of total healthcare financing in the country.

Health Resources

Since hospitals were nationalized during the 1970s, the state has controlled the vast majority of health resources. As of 1997, Costa Rica had 29 public CCSS hospitals in the country, which provided 5,924 hospital beds; only 225 private beds were available in the entire country. According to a 1995 PAHO study of hospital equipment, only 1.6 percent was idle, with 93.4 percent being used appropriately (Proyecto Modernizacion 1997). The CCSS had a total of 170 facilities including hospitals, and in 1997 the Ministry of Health administered 1,428 facilities, primarily health centers and health posts.

In 1997, the CCSS had 28,907 employees, of which 5,704 were medical professionals. This number included 3,021 physicians, 1,817 professional nurses, 211 dentists, 249 pharmacists, 379 microbiologists, and 27 psychologists. Other employees included 4,024 nurses' aides and 97 nutritionists. A large number of private physicians practice in the country, although no reliable data exist on the exact number. Other human resources data available for Costa Rica found 168 midwives, 460 malaria volunteers, 6,000 community health educators, 600 nutrition committees, and 157 dentistry committees in health centers. See Table 27.6 for additional information on healthcare human resources.

As of 1992, Costa Rica had 175 publicly run pharmacies and 352 private pharmacies. A small number of private laboratories manufacture pharmaceutical products, but public production infrastructure is limited.

Service Delivery

Primary care has been an important emphasis of the health system, particularly with the start of the Rural Health Program in 1973 and the Community Health Program in 1976, which aimed to provide primary healthcare to underserved populations. By 1980, 60 percent of the pop-

TABLE 27.6
Human Resources, Facilities, and Utilization

Physicians (per 10,000)	8.7
Professional nurses (per 10,000)	5.2
Nurses' aides (per 10,000)	11.6
Midwives (total)	168
Hospitals (total)	29
Hospital beds (per 1,000)	1.7
Hospital admissions (per 1,000)	87.7
Hospital days (per 1,000)	518.5

SOURCE: Ministerio de Salud (1998); Caja Costarricense de Seguro Social (various years).

ulation was covered by these programs, which included the establishment of hundreds of new Health Posts and Nutritional Education Centers as well as trimonthly home visits. Recently the Rural and Community Health Programs have been phased out, and their responsibilities are being taken over by staff of each Health Area, which include the EBAIS teams and other support personnel in pharmacies, clinic laboratories, family medicine, and social work. Each EBAIS is designed to serve 4,000 people on average and consists of a nonspecialist physician, a nurse practitioner, and a community health worker. Each Health Area encompasses nine EBAISs on average and provides additional support including a pharmacy, a laboratory, a nurse, and a social worker. The EBAIS is responsible for the administration of programs in six general areas of health: child, adolescent, women's, adult, elderly, and environmental. Between 1995 and 1998, 548 EBAISs in 66 Health Areas were established, which covered about two-thirds of the population.

In 1994, the CCSS determined that the "neediest" cantons, according to a range of social indicators, were also those that received the lowest per capita primary healthcare spending. As a result, the EBAISs have been phased in earliest in the neediest areas, and the CCSS reports that much of that discrepancy in spending has now been eliminated. As one indicator of the degree of equity in outcomes, infant mortality in the 81 cantons from 1993 to 1995 ranged from a low of 5.8 to a high of 23.6 per 1,000 live births.

Primary care spending makes up only about 20 to 30 percent of CCSS expenditures, with the hospitals consuming the large part of health resources. Legally, equity in hospital access exists because virtually all hospitals are run by the CCSS, and health insurance is in principle universal. Furthermore, the small size of the country, along with the existence of a network of regional hospitals, means that much of the population has physical access to at least a low-level rural hospital, although many specialty procedures are only available in urban centers. More than 10 percent of the population choose not to join CCSS, despite the sliding scale premiums for informal sector workers who join voluntarily.

The quality of CCSS services is a frequent source of dissatisfaction to users. Long queues and poor motivation among the civil service workers lead many enrollees to use private doctor services instead, paying out-of-pocket despite having the right to free CCSS care. Alleged favoritism and corruption by employees may also be a source of differences across socioeconomic groups in the quality of care within the CCSS system. The expense of private hospitals leads all but a few to rely on the CCSS for inpatient services, however, and overall the access to such services is considered substantially more equitable than in many other countries at similar levels of economic development.

Prospects for the Future

The health system is currently in the middle of a major reform and modernization project, with three basic components. First, primary care delivery is receiving renewed attention and resources through the EBAIS system, which aims to decentralize decisions and strengthen the preventive and public health aspects of the healthcare system. Although EBAIS teams are now in place in much of the country, decisions are still largely centralized, and several more years may pass before the new high-priority programs are functioning. Whether the EBAIS will receive sufficient resources and have the expertise and motivation to substantially affect health outcomes remains to be seen.

Second, an effort is being made to eliminate the duplication of services by consolidating the administration of all healthcare programs within the CCSS and refocusing the Ministry of Health to concentrate on monitoring, regulation, and planning activities. This reform has been taking place slowly for several years and is not likely to be fully completed for at least several more.

Third, the CCSS has outlined an ambitious reform of its management and resource allocation activities. In the first phase, the current lack of financial accounting will be addressed with modernized management and bookkeeping procedures, and a system of internal budgets will be established to improve transparency. A second phase will then introduce a system of "performance contracts" for each unit, which will be intended to provide budgetary incentives for increased efficiency. After a detailed monitoring system has been put into place, the budgets and contracts will be linked to measurable outcomes using a system of hospital production units, with adjustments for case mix by diagnosis-related groups. These reforms are still in an early phase, however, and their eventual shape is still the subject of some debate. Many details have yet to be made legally feasible, such as allowing civil service employees to potentially receive salary bonuses tied to the performance contracts, and adequate information and monitoring systems for the measurement of hospital production units and diagnosis-related groups will not be established for some time.

The eventual impact of these reforms on the root problems that underlie health sector inefficiency, such as poor worker motivation and the absence of competitive market discipline, is not clear. Without individual financial bonuses or threats of unemployment for poor performance, meaningful supply-side incentives for improving individual productivity are not assured. Current plans do not involve the significant privatization or contracting out of services, so competitive forces are also unlikely to play a role. Likewise, copayments are not being considered, so demand-side disciplines on inefficient expenditures arising from moral hazard will not play a role either. Thus, although management reforms may correct some of the most egregious misallocations, CCSS costs may nevertheless continue their rapid growth. Many uncertainties remain about how best to address inefficient service delivery and health financing problems, and continued experimentation with reforms is to be expected in the coming years.

REFERENCES

Castro Valverde, C., and Bernardo Saénz, L. 1998. *La Reforma del Sistema Nacional de Salud.* San Jose: Ministerio de Planificacion Nacional y Politica Economica.

Direccion General de Estadistica y Censos. Various years. *Anuario Estadístico.* San Jose: Direccion General de Estadistica y Censos.

Ministerio de Salud. 1998. *Memoria 1997.* San Jose: Ministerio de Salud.

Proyecto Estado de la Nacion. Various years. *Estado de la Nacion.* San Jose: Editorama.

Proyecto Modernizacion. 1997. *Hacia un Nuevo Sistema de Asignacion de Recursos.* San Jose: Caja Costarricense de Seguro Social.

Rosero, L. 1994. "Adult Mortality Decline in Costa Rica." *Notas de Poblacion* 22 (60): 103–39.

World Bank. 1998. *World Development Report.* Washington, DC: World Bank.

JAMAICA

Wadia Joseph Hanna and Marjorie Holding-Cobham

Background

Jamaica is a Caribbean island nation located approximately 90 miles south of Cuba and 100 miles west of Haiti. The island was originally inhabited by a peaceful tribe of Amerindians who are thought to have migrated up the Caribbean island chain from South America. Jamaica was discovered in 1494 by Christopher Columbus and remained a colony of Spain until 1655, when it was conquered by the British; it was a British colony until it gained independence in 1962. Jamaica is the largest of the English-speaking Commonwealth Caribbean Islands and the third largest island in the region, with only Cuba and Hispaniola (shared by the Dominican Republic and Haiti) being larger. The island is strategically located along the main sea-lanes for the Panama Canal.

Jamaica is divided into 14 parishes with two major urban centers. The capital city of Kingston is situated on the south coast, and the second-largest city of Montego Bay is on the northwest coast. Approximately 50 percent of the population is urban. The island covers a total area of 10,990 square kilometers, which makes it slightly smaller than the U.S. state of Connecticut; Jamaica has 1,022 kilometers of coastline. The climate is tropical, hot, and humid, with a temperate interior. The terrain is mostly mountainous, with a narrow, discontinuous coastal plain. Its highest point is the Blue Mountain Peak at 2,256 meters. Of environmental concern are matters of deforestation; pollution of coastal waters by industrial waste, sewage, and the occasional oil spill; damage to coral reefs; and air pollution resulting from vehicle emissions.

Population Characteristics

As of mid-1998, Jamaica's population was estimated at 2,634,678. The population growth rate was estimated at 0.7 percent and represents a steadily declining figure from 1.2 percent in 1995 and 1 percent in 1996. In keeping with this trend, the proportion of the population under the age of 15 years was 34.3 percent as compared with 38.4 percent in 1982.

The ethnic mix is 90 percent black and 7 percent mixed, with the remaining 3 percent made up of Chinese, Lebanese, and Caucasian. Additional population demographics are provided in Table 28.1.

TABLE 28.1
General
Demographics

Population in millions	2.6
Infant mortality per 1,000 live births	24.5
Under-five mortality per 1,000 live births	Not available
Life expectancy at birth (years)	Male: 72
	Female: 73.2
Fertility rate	2.8
Percent urbanized	50

SOURCE: Planning Institute of Jamaica (1999).

Socioeconomic Overview

Key sectors of Jamaica's economy are bauxite (alumina and bauxite account for more than half of Jamaica's exports) and tourism. During the 1960s, bauxite mining enjoyed great prominence as a source of foreign exchange, eclipsing even the agricultural sector; however, with the decline of aluminum prices worldwide in the 1980s, tourism has replaced the bauxite industry as the chief earner of hard currency. Earnings from the traditional areas of agriculture (sugar, bananas, and citrus) have also been overtaken by tourism. Gross foreign exchange earnings from tourism in 1998 were an estimated U.S.$1.128 billion, up from U.S.$950 million in 1993 and U.S.$1.0695 billion in 1995.

Marked fluctuations have occurred in the exchange rate, and the value of the Jamaican dollar has shown a trend from 24.949 for every U.S. dollar in 1993 to 36.051 in November 1997. In 2000, the exchange rate declined further, and tight monetary and fiscal policies were put in place in an attempt to slow inflation and stabilize the exchange rate. Economic growth has slowed from 1.5 percent in 1992 to 0.5 percent in 1995. Serious problems continue to plague the island's economy, including high interest rates and increased foreign competition in the global market.

Table 28.2 provides further details of social and economic indicators in Jamaica.

Poverty in Jamaica is no longer associated only with unemployment; the new category of working poor has emerged. In 1998, 19.9 percent of the population (13.6 percent of households) lived in poverty. This was more pronounced in rural areas (73 percent) than in the Kingston metropolitan area (KMA), where this figure was only 13.6 percent; the incidence was somewhat lower in other towns throughout the island (13.1 percent). The available workforce was 1,128,600, and the unemployment rate was 15.5 percent, with females having a higher unemployment rate. As com-

		TABLE 28.2
GNP per capita (J$)	66,930*	Economic and
Human Development Index score	.82	Social
Percent of GNP to health	7.4	Indicators
Percent of health budget in public sector (national, regional, local)	35	

* U.S.$1 = J$40.
SOURCE: Planning Institute of Jamaica (1999).

pared with 1996 data, the unemployment rate had decreased in the KMA and townships and increased in the rural areas.

In response to the increasing incidence of poverty, the government has made poverty eradication one of its primary development strategies. This strategy is a part of the broader development framework outlined in the National Industrial Policy, which targets growth with equity. Strategies have included increased access to land by the poor, expansion in educational and training opportunities, and an increase in community-development activities funded by various national social development agencies (e.g., Jamaica Social Investment Fund, Social Development Commission). In addition, the policy is aimed at integration to reduce duplication and waste. Strategies include the following:

- partnership activities with the private sector, nongovernmental organizations, communities, donor and lender agencies, and other government departments
- community-based participation that empowers communities
- ensuring the sustainability of the programs themselves

The target groups of these poverty-eradication strategies include children, residents of economically deprived areas, unemployed youth, the aged, women, and people with disabilities. Seventy programs targeting these groups are currently in place, including the Food Stamps Program (introduced in 1984 and described as one of the "flagships of anti-poverty initiatives"); the School Feeding Program; the Drugs for the Elderly program; Special Education for the Disabled; Assistance to Needy Students and Basic Schools; the Social Investment Fund; and Operation PRIDE, which focuses on making land more accessible and affordable to people who do not own land.

Education

Overall, the population of Jamaica is relatively well educated, with 85 percent of the total population achieving literacy and 70 percent of the total school-aged population enrolled in schools, including near universal enrollment for primary education. Table 28.3 provides further information about educational indicators for the Jamaican population.

Access to Health-Enhancing Factors

The Ministry of Health is aware of the need for intersectoral collaboration in ensuring access to health-enhancing factors and full employment, education, housing, and cultural, sporting, and recreational facilities all form a part of its spectrum of activities. Collaboration with the community is important to ensure a comprehensive national health service that incorporates preventive and curative services. As with other countries, access to health-enhancing factors is better in urban than in rural areas. Although access to piped water is available in the larger rural townships, expansion of the water system has been slow, and safe, piped water accessible to all of the population remains a predominantly metropolitan phenomenon (Table 28.4). Central sewage facilities are only found in the KMA.

Context: Health Needs

Maternal and child health have been identified as priorities of the government of Jamaica since the 1970s, and later in that decade, the primary healthcare approach was adopted. To underscore the importance of this commitment, a very senior technical post, Senior Medical Officer Maternal and Child Health (later upgraded to Principal Medical Officer level) was established, and a detailed manual for this service was developed; this model has since been shared with other Caribbean countries. In the recently reorganized organizational structure of the ministries, this priority of maternal and child health has been highlighted with the employment of a Program Development Officer for Maternal and Child Health.

Health of Children and Adolescents

The health and welfare of children remains a matter of national concern. Programs regarding mental, sexual, and reproductive health for adolescents have assumed very great importance. Some of these programs are funded

TABLE 28.3
Education
Indicators

Adult literacy rate (percent)	Male: 81
	Female: 89
Primary school enrollment (percent)	97
Secondary school enrollment (percent)	81.6

SOURCE: Planning Institute of Jamaica (1999).

Percent access to health services	100	**TABLE 28.4**
Percent access to safe water	81.2	Access to Health-
Percent access to sanitation	99.5	Enhancing Factors
Percent immunized	82 or more	

SOURCE: Planning Institute of Jamaica (1999).

through partnerships between the government and United Nations Population Fund and United States Agency for International Development. Adolescents have been identified as high-risk for many illnesses, particularly those related to sexual and reproductive conditions, nutrition, and accidents and injuries. Sexually transmitted diseases, HIV/AIDS, anemia, and chronic diseases have consistently increased in this age group.

Adolescent girls (10 to 19 years old) have a 2.7 times higher risk of HIV infection than boys in the same age group. Similarly, the Reproductive Health Survey of 1997 identified adolescents as the age group with the highest fertility rate; both could be related to the common practice of young girls having sexual intercourse with older men. An adolescent health project recently funded by USAID aims to improve reproductive health practices among Jamaican adolescents; the project is anticipated to involve collaboration with existing institutions in the health sector as well as with the youth services sector to develop innovative methods to tackle this problem. The expected outcomes of this project are increased use of HIV/sexually transmitted disease services and preventive practices, improved access to quality reproductive health and HIV/sexually transmitted disease services, improved knowledge and skills regarding reproductive health practices, and the implementation of national policies and guidelines for service providers.

In another effort, a pilot project for the prevention of maternal-child transmission of HIV has been implemented in four parishes. Eight thousand pregnant women will benefit from voluntary HIV testing and receive medication as necessary. Medication will include a single dose of an antiretroviral drug for the HIV-positive mother and a breastfeeding substitute for the infant. This program is being conducted by the National HIV/sexually transmitted diseases program of the Ministry of Health in collaboration with PAHO and the World Health Organization, UNICEF, and UNAIDS.

Malnutrition among Children

Various surveys have sought to assess the extent of malnutrition in Jamaica. Table 28.5 presents data from the Ministry of Health's Annual Report 1997 for children between zero and five years of age (this report is compiled from data submitted by government clinics and does not reflect the actual prevalence of malnutrition islandwide).

The 1998 figures show a decrease in both the moderately (4.2 percent) and the severely (0.25 percent) malnourished. A more detailed look at nutritional status for 1998 as related to gender is shown in Table 28.6; the data are drawn from the monthly clinic summary report.

In 1998, 52 percent of babies seen at postnatal clinics were fully breastfed at six weeks, and 47 percent were fully breastfed at 12 weeks. The national target set is for 64 percent at six weeks. As of 1997, Jamaica had nine baby-friendly health facilities.

Immunization

Immunization has always been a priority program for the Jamaican government, and figures for the less-than-one-year-old age group for 1999 show coverage for polio at 83.3 percent, diphtheria-pertussis-tetanus at 83.8 percent, and bacillus Calmette-Guérin at 88.5 percent. Mumps-measles-rubella vaccine coverage for the under-24-month age group was 82 percent. Very serious efforts were being made to improve the coverage to more than 90 percent in 2000.

Hospital and Health Center Visits

Of the 1,887,365 visits to hospitals and health centers during 1998, 16 percent were child health visits. The main causes of hospitalization for children less than one year old in 1998 were conditions related to the perinatal period, which accounted for 47 percent of cases discharged from public hospitals. In the one- to four-year-old age group, accidents and injuries were the leading causes of hospitalization (20 percent) followed by chronic respiratory diseases (18 percent), acute respiratory diseases (15 percent), and diarrheal diseases (10 percent). Such a high incidence of accidents and injuries in this and other age groups in children is a conern, and it may reflect the need for access by working mothers to more childcare facilities as well as increased health promotion and education messages on home safety. Table 28.7 provides further details on pediatric morbidity and hospitalization.

TABLE 28.5
Malnutrition
Data

	1993	1995	1997
Percent moderately malnourished	6	5.2	5.1
Percent severely malnourished	0.4	0.3	0.5

SOURCE: Planning Institute of Jamaica (1998).

Nutritional status	Male	Female
Percent normal	97	94.2
Percent grade 2	2.9	5.6
Percent grade 3	0.2	0.2

TABLE 28.6
1998
Nutritional
Status

SOURCE: Planning Institute of Jamaica (1999).

Social Services for Children

Children in need of protection are the responsibility of the Family Services Division of the Ministry of Health. This division has the responsibility for

Cause of Death	Less than 1 Year Old	1 to 4 Years Old	5 to 9 Years Old	Total
Perinatal conditions	4,292			
Sexually transmitted diseases including HIV	44	25	8	77
Congenital syphilis	26	N/A	N/A	26
HIV	18			18
Diarrheal diseases	672*	908	166	1,746
Septicemia (newborn)	114			114
Anemia	54	208	159	421
Otitis media and other inner-ear infections	107	132	28	267
Acute respiratory disease	1,019*	1,258*	302*	2,579*
Chronic respiratory disease	511*	1,530*	702*	2,743*
Accidents and injuries	453	1,675*	1,346*	3,474*
Total	3,018	5,736	2,711	11,465
Grand total	9,186	8,473	4,546	22,205

TABLE 28.7
Pediatric
Morbidity,
1998

* Most common disease for age group.
NOTE: Data refer to public hospitals and university hospital.
SOURCE: Planning Institute of Jamaica (1999).

providing safe placements for children awaiting investigation and court orders. Eight government and four private institutions provide these services on the island. For the first quarter of 1999, the private institutions were 73 percent occupied, and the government facilities ran an occupancy rate of 97 percent.

Children's homes, 5 government- and 33 privately owned, also exist for children who become wards of the state. Occupancy rates for these institutions were 52 percent and 87 percent, respectively, for the first quarter of 1999. Medical coverage for these institutions is primarily through clinics and other government health institutions. General practitioners may provide coverage for a few facilities, but this is not the norm. Common health problems found in these homes are those that commonly occur with institutional care, such as diarrhea, coughs, and colds. Immunization status of the children is usually up-to-date.

The health and welfare of street children is also a matter of national concern; however, no in-depth research and analysis has been done to determine the scope and nature of the problem. In 1993, the United Nations Children's Fund estimated that Jamaica had approximately 2,500 street children, but an obvious (although not yet counted) increase of street children is now seen in rural towns. Most of them are boys between 6 and 17 years of age.

Street children are categorized in the following manner:

1. children of the street: these children go home at night
2. children on the street: these children live on the street permanently but have families and homes, and poverty, neglect, conflict, abuse, and poor housing are the factors that contribute to their being on the street
3. children who are abandoned and have no biological family

Seven major agencies now provide services for approximately 1,300 street children. Some of these organizations are the Save the Children Fund (United Kingdom), the Learning for Earning Activities Program (LEAP), Children First, the Young Men's Christian Association (YMCA), and the National Initiative for Street Children. These organizations focus their efforts on areas such as remedial education, skills training, social well-being, and parenting education. Health needs of the children are met either by volunteers or through the government's health institutions.

Plans to improve the current situation for street children include an islandwide census in 2000 with the assistance of both private sector and government agencies, the formation of a committee for the development of a program of basic education and skills training, and the establishment of a 25-bed drop-in center, the site for which has already been identified in downtown Kingston. The National Initiative for Street Children, a voluntary organization, will spearhead this with the involvement of the Kingston Restoration Company, the army, the Ministry of Health, the United Nations

Children's Fund, the YMCA, the Multi Care Foundation, and the Van Leer Foundation. Six nongovernmental organizations and five children's homes will network with the center.

General Population Morbidity

Of the 132,626 inpatients discharged from government hospitals and the University Hospital of the West Indies in 1998, nearly half (52,303) were uncomplicated births. Additional data concerning use of health facilities is provided in Table 28.8.

The major causes of illness in those 65 years old and older are similar to those chronic noncommunicable diseases that occur in developed countries. Major causes for hospitalization in 1998 were related to the cardiovascular and endocrine systems (usually diabetes) followed by neoplasms, usually of the gastrointestinal system. The major cause of death was cardiovascular disease. Table 28.9 further describes leading causes of morbidity and mortality.

Organization and Management of the Health System

The health system in Jamaica comprises private- and public-sector-administered facilities and services, the latter being administered through the Ministry of Health and its related statutory bodies; the private sector is administered by independent persons and entities. The few private hospitals (eight) and clinics are administered by various churches (three) or groups of people with common interests (e.g., Doctors Hospital in Montego Bay). The number of private diagnostic centers continues to grow, and an increasing level of interest is being shown in service areas such as renal dialysis. Planning in the public health sector is done at all levels of the services and is guided by the Corporate and Operational Plans developed centrally by the Planning and Evaluation Unit (1999). Regulation of the private sector has to date been ineffective, but improved regulation in both the

Hospital Discharge Data (percent)	Health Clinic Visits (percent)	**TABLE 28.8** Usage of Health Institutions
Uncomplicated births: 52,303 (39.4)	Dressings (22)	
Accidents and injuries: 14,474 (10.9)	Hypertension (16)	
Respiratory diseases: 9,362 (7.0)	Respiratory tract infections (12)	
Circulatory diseases: 9,061 (6.8)	Skin infections (10)	
Diseases of the digestive system: 8,244 (6.2)	Diabetes (7)	

SOURCE: Planning Institute of Jamaica (1999).

TABLE 28.9

Leading
Causes of
Morbidity
and Mortality

	Percent of Deaths	Percent of Discharges (morbidity)
Cardiovascular diseases	72.1	7.5
Perinatal	12.2	3
Vaccine-preventable diseases*	See note	See note
Respiratory infections	27.2	8
Diarrheal diseases	8.7	6.2
Tuberculosis*	See note	See note

* 1999 provisional data for vaccine-preventable diseases: 90 cases of tuberculosis, 10 cases of flaccid paralysis, 60 suspected cases of measles (none confirmed), 17 cases of pertussis-like syndrome, and 6 cases of tetanus (none neonatal).
SOURCE: Planning Institute of Jamaica (1999).

public and private sectors is anticipated with the recent establishment of the Standards and Regulation Division in the Ministry. This division will be responsible for updating laws and developing standards. The administration of health services is influenced greatly by the availability of resources. Recently, efforts have been made to strengthen the management of services at all levels; this has been accomplished through funding from both USAID and the Inter-American Development Bank.

Despite the fact that the majority of hospitals and clinics in Jamaica are government-owned, in 1998, an estimated 57 percent of ambulatory care was delivered within the private sector as compared with 38 percent in the public sector; the remaining percentage used both sectors. In the KMA, 64 percent used private facilities; 55 to 57 percent used private facilities in other regions of the country. In this area, the differences in use of public and private sectors were marked when related to consumption quintiles; use of the private sector was lowest in the poorest quintile and highest among the more affluent. Most hospital and preventive care are traditionally delivered through the public sector.

Health Insurance

Private health insurance coverage is low throughout Jamaica; at present, only three health insurance companies operate on the island, and these cover an estimated 12.1 percent of the population. In the KMA, 21 percent of the population is covered by these companies, whereas 7 percent is covered in the rural areas.

The Bismarkian model of social insurance, in which insurance is supported by contributions from both workers and employers based on the worker's wages, has not met with the same level of success in the Caribbean as it has in Europe. This is primarily because of differences in the worker populations of the two regions. In Europe, most of the labor force consists of wage-earning urban workers employed in industries that employ large numbers of workers. In the Caribbean, the workforce is made up mainly of agricultural and fishery workers (19.2 percent), craft and related trade workers (16.4 percent), elementary occupations (16.4 percent), and plant and machine operators and assemblers (6.8 percent). Professionals, senior officials, technicians, clerks, and shop and market sales workers make up approximately 40 percent of the working population.

In Jamaica, a system of national insurance and social security exists, but coverage is uneven, and the payments from this insurance are often inadequate for basic needs and health costs. Contributions are compulsory and involve both employee and employer obligations. However, only those workers who are on the "pay as you earn" system make regular contributions. If the informal employer were forced to fulfill his or her obligation, the small profit he or she currently earns would be so diminished that some businesses would have to close, thus worsening the already unacceptable unemployment level.

The highest rates of insurance coverage are, therefore, in the formal, salaried sector of the population. A large percentage of the informal (self-employed) sector does not contribute and therefore cannot derive benefits from this system.

Financing

The health service delivery system in the country for both public and private sectors is funded by the following sources:

- the government of Jamaica, which often purchases specialized services (e.g., laboratory, radiology) that may not be available in the public-sector institutions
- fees collected from users of the public services (these are becoming increasingly important)
- the private sector
- charitable nongovernmental organizations
- official assistance from donors and lending agencies

This level of diverse contributions represents the partnership approach to healthcare funding. In 1998, the Jamaican government spent 7.4 percent of its recurrent budget on healthcare; this represented 3.3 percent of the gross domestic product, or J$8.9 billion (on average, U.S.$1 = J$40) for the budget year April 1999 to March 2000. The Ministry spent approximately $J6.3 billion on recurrent expenditure and J$713.1 million on capital expenditure; this is in addition to fees for that year collected by hospitals and health centers, which totaled J$474,975,301.

Recently, the proportion of the Ministry of Health's budget spent on primary care has been increasing. This, however, has been coupled with an overall decline in public health sector financing from the Ministry of Finance. A reduction in capital expenditure, an increase in user fees collected, and an increase in employee compensation have also been seen.

Public expenditures are estimated to represent 35 percent of total health expenditures. Over the past decade, this has represented a shift to more private sector involvement and, as mentioned above, is most applicable to ambulatory care. Jamaica has been successful in developing ongoing relationships with donor agencies for financial and technical cooperation. A number of international agencies and foreign governments have been active in the Jamaican health sector, including the Inter-American Development Bank, the Pan-American Health Organization, various United Nations agencies, and the governments of the Netherlands, Japan, Italy, and Germany.

Health Resources

Through the years, a large and complex public network of primary care centers and hospitals has developed around the country. Jamaica currently has 24 hospitals and more than 300 health centers. A varied selection of services is offered, depending on the level and type of hospital:

- *Type A hospitals* (3, including the teaching hospital at the University of the West Indies): Services at these hospitals include surgery; medicine; obstetrics and gynecology; pediatrics; accident and emergency; and some specialties such as ear, nose, and throat; orthopedics; dermatology; ophthalmology; radiology; urology; and plastic surgery. Support services such as physiotherapy, radiology, and full laboratory services are also offered.
- *Type B hospitals* (4): These hospitals include services in medicine, surgery, obstetrics and gynecology, some pediatrics, an accident and emergency/casualty service, and some support services.
- *Type C hospitals* (12): Services at this level include basic medicine, surgery, obstetrics and gynecology, and accident and emergency/casualty.
- *Specialist hospitals:* These hospitals cater exclusively to specialized areas such as obstetrics, pediatrics, chest diseases, mental illness, and hospice care for people with terminal cancer. In many instances, the services are offered at a price that is unrelated to and much lower than the actual cost.

Sustainability of services remains a problem, and the rising costs of healthcare coupled with the devaluation of the Jamaican currency and increasing expectations of the clients have led to a gap between available and required resources. A breakdown of hospital statistics is shown in Tables 28.10, 28.11, and 28.12.

Health Resources

Human Resources

Ministry of Health data for January 2000 indicate that 489 physicians (many of whom work in both the public and private sectors) and 1,957 registered nurses are employed in the public health sector. Of the nurses, 234 are trained public health nurses, 57 are nurse practitioners, and 29 are nurse anesthetists. These numbers represent an increase from 1991 and 1995. Several categories of health personnel remain in short supply: pharmacists are at 52 percent of complement, therapeutic radiologists are at 31 percent, enrolled nurses are at 54 percent, and mental health officers are at 38 percent. In general, the distribution of personnel follows the affluence of the area; that is, better supply is found in areas of high affluence and urban areas.

Table 28.13 further describes the breakdown of human resources for healthcare in Jamaica.

The government is the primary sponsoring and training agency for health workers; some specialized training is provided overseas. Medical training is an area that could benefit greatly from international aid and influence as well-trained professionals are actively recruited by both the private sector within the country and developed countries outside to augment their own health systems. The country also needs to develop innovative incentive programs for healthcare workers that are sustainable.

Equipment and Technology

Most of the sophisticated equipment and technology are located in the regional type A or B hospitals. In the past, a central facility called the Health Facilities Maintenance Unit (HFMU) was designated to maintain and repair the equipment and facilities scattered throughout Jamaica. As a result of health sector reform and decentralization, four regional maintenance units have been established to meet preventive and restorative needs. This decentralization is hoped to make the process more efficient, with the HFMU

		TABLE 28.10
Physicians	2.5	Public Human
Nurses	7.9	Resources per
Midwives	1.2	10,000 Population

SOURCE: Planning Institute of Jamaica (1999).

TABLE 28.11

Hospital Statistics

	Male	Female	Total
Admissions (all hospitals)			
General medicine	16,669	18,650	35,319
General surgery	20,123	18,890	39,013
Pediatrics	14,993	10,629 (includes specialty pediatric hospital)	25,622
Obstetrics		59,137 (includes specialty obstetrics and gynecology hospital)	59,137
Bellevue Psychiatric Hospital	533		533
Total			159,962
Discharges from hospitals			
General medicine	16,578	18,518	25,096
General surgery	20,199	19,136	39,335
Pediatrics	15,038	10,671 (includes Bustamante Hospital for Children)	25,709
Obstetrics		57,792 (includes Victoria Jubilee Hospital)	57,792
Bellevue Psychiatric Hospital	270		270
Total			158,851

SOURCE: Planning Institute of Jamaica (1999).

being the repository of very highly skilled people available to the regions as necessary. The HFMU will also be responsible for regulating and setting standards for maintenance islandwide.

Health Reform

Recent health reform programs have been instituted in response to the changing needs identified in Jamaica. These programs are being realized with the collaboration of several technical cooperation agencies including USAID, the Inter-American Development Bank, and the World Bank. The objectives of the new programs include the institution of measures that are fundamental, sustainable, and purposeful, all with an eye toward improv-

TABLE 28.12
Average Bed
Complement
(all hospitals)

Medicine	909
Surgery	1,121
Pediatrics	738
Obstetrics	594
Bellevue Psychiatric Hospital	1,190
Bustamante Hospital for Children	253
Victoria Jubilee Hospital	197
Total	4,768

ing healthcare delivery. This restructuring process is anticipated to better address the following issues:

- the rising costs of healthcare delivery
- the improved management of facilities and services
- financing
- efficiency, equity, and quality assurance
- human resource needs
- changing epidemiological profile
- client satisfaction with the system
- health promotion and protection (including individual and community responsibility for health)
- the expanding role of public/private partnerships in health
- the information needs of the system

    A major component of health reform in Jamaica has been the decentralization of the management of service delivery to four autonomous Regional Health Authorities (RHA), each with a board of management and a regional director. These authorities were established by the National

TABLE 28.13
Mean Length
of Stay in Days
by Specialty

Specialty	Male	Female
Medicine	8.3	7.2
Surgery	7.3	6.5
Pediatrics	6.2	5.8
Obstetrics		2.6
Victoria Jubilee Hospital		2.4

NOTE: Overall mean is 5.5 days.
SOURCE: Planning Institute of Jamaica (1999).b

Health Services Act 1997 and, through the signing of annual service agreements and other reporting requirements, they accept responsibility for the health of communities within their geographical boundaries as well as any eligible client presenting in their jurisdiction. The RHAs are funded from budgets provided as block grants by the Ministry of Finance and the Ministry of Health. RHA funding is supplemented by fees collected at institutions as well as any funds raised through approved innovative endeavors (e.g., selling specialized health services to the private sector).

The Ministry of Health's head office now has responsibility for strategic corporate planning, policy development, setting and auditing standards and regulations in both public and private health sectors, monitoring and evaluation, and international health (Policy Development Unit of the Planning Institute of Jamaica 2000).

Another major reform program targets human resource development and includes incentives for reducing attrition, the transfer of the training function from the Ministry of Health to the Ministry of Education, an increase in the throughput of training programs, and a review of the skills mix required for optimal service delivery. The last target will follow a strategic review of the health sector carried out in collaboration with the Department for International Development. This review is expected to result in the development of service agreements for the regions as well as benchmarks for service delivery. The service delivery component of health reform includes the areas of quality assurance, health promotion and protection, emergency medical services, mental health, and preventive maintenance of equipment. The Ministry of Health intends to ensure that individuals needed for service delivery are given the opportunity to receive relevant training through scholarships, fellowships, and bursaries.

Prospects for the Future

An increase in the level of dissatisfaction among a demanding public and healthcare providers was the primary catalyst for the reform of the health sector in Jamaica. Reforms undertaken in previous years (e.g., the employment of new cadres of workers and decentralization of primary/community services) have shown that the changing environment requires newer, more innovative approaches. The present program of health reform is expected to make a significant difference in the level of satisfaction of all stakeholders.

Health promotion and protection have been identified as priority programs for which strategic and implementation plans will be developed. These programs will design the framework for necessary research and analysis as well as the behavior-modification programs (e.g., smoking cessation, nutritional counseling) at the level of service delivery; the latter will be integrated with activities and programs planned by other agencies.

In the area of financing, the National Health Insurance Plan will reimburse hospitals and health facilities in both the public and private sectors for a stipulated range of services. Among those being considered are hospital inpatient services as well as all diagnostics and pharmaceuticals, both public and private; this will prove valuable in ameliorating the financial position of these institutions and make available more of those funds supplied to the public sector for primary care services.

The quality assurance program has already resulted in new or updated manuals and protocols for some clinical activities; it has also been responsible for initiating a clinical audit program. The program will continue work in this area and assume a monitoring role to ensure that activities are maintained at the level of service delivery.

A change in mental health service delivery is also planned. The only institution dedicated exclusively to the treatment of the mentally ill, Bellevue Hospital, has seen its inpatient load reduced considerably during the past five years as a result of the further integration of mental health services with primary care. An assessment of services available islandwide in both public and private sectors has been completed. Strategic and implementation plans for service delivery will be developed, and the training of additional mental health officers and the establishment of halfway houses will be undertaken.

Information systems have also been a focus of the reform program. Computerized systems are used to compile information databases across the healthcare spectrum for preventive and corrective maintenance, drugs for the elderly program (which subsidizes drugs used in the treatment of the five most commonly encountered conditions experienced by the elderly), the blood bank, the national public health laboratory, human resource management, and the financial management system. The objective of this reform is to make information more accurate, more available, and more user-friendly for decision making.

The health reform programs are expected to result in a better-regulated and more customer-friendly health service. Customer satisfaction surveys should assume a more significant role in providing feedback for evaluating the effectiveness of the programs. In addition to providing an assessment of client comfort with the services delivered, the results of these surveys will inform the strategic planning process for continuous quality improvement of the programs themselves.

The reform process and the programs involved are expected to improve the health service delivery system and enable the country to better meet the needs of the communities in the face of a constantly changing healthcare paradigm. Improved integration of the delivery system and the alignment of its objectives with national health and social priorities will ultimately result in a healthcare system that is very responsive to changing healthcare needs at all levels.

APPENDIX 28.A

Status of Human Resources— Healthcare Professionals in Jamaica

Category of Personnel	Cadre	In Post	Vacancy
Doctors	544	489	10%
Public health nurses	260	234	10%
Nurse practitioners	77	57	26%
Nurse anesthetists	31	29	6%
Other registered nurses	2,191	1,631	26%
Midwives (single trained)	528	305	42%
Mental health officers	34	13	62%
Enrolled assistant nurses	1,090	586	46%
Community health aides	563	781	39% or more
Psychiatry aides	152	137	10%
Pharmacists	147	76	48%
Pharmacy technicians	105	88	16%
Dentists	68	53	22%
Dental nurses	149	144	3%
Dental assistants	126	110	13%
Prosthetics	4	2	50%
Nutritionists	9	8	11%
Dieticians	15	14	7%
Dietetic assistants	34	23	32%
Assistant dieticians	8	5	38%
Nutrition assistants	15	13	13%
Public health inspectors	449	289	36%
Veterinary public health inspectors	14	11	21%
Health education officers	37	27	27%
Diagnostic radiographers	63	50	21%
Therapeutic radiographers	16	5	69%
Physiotherapists	36	25	31%
Occupational therapists	7	1	86%
Medical technicians	142	103	27%

REFERENCES

Planning and Evaluation Unit Ministry of Health. 1999 "Report on Gender Equity in the Health Sector with Emphasis on Health Reform, Jamaica 1999." Kingston: Planning and Evaluation Unit Ministry of Health.

Planning Institute of Jamaica. 1998. "Economic and Social Survey." Kingston: Planning Institute of Jamaica.

———. 1999. "Economic and Social Survey." Kingston: Planning Institute of Jamaica.

Policy Development Unit of the Planning Institute of Jamaica. 2000. "Survey of Living Conditions." Kingston: Planning Institute of Jamaica.

INDIA

Ojas N. Shah

Background Information

India is the seventh largest country in the world geographically, spanning approximately 3.3 million square kilometers. Its population is estimated to have crossed the one billion mark in 1999, making it the second most populous country in the world after China. Although population growth has slowed considerably during the last decade to 1.58 percent in 2000, it continues to be an issue of significant concern. Overcrowding and insufficient resources to support the rapidly increasing population continue to haunt successive Indian governments.

Table 29.1 shows the demographic characteristics of India's people, 32 percent of whom are less than 15 years old; 64 percent are between the ages 15 and 64 years and 4 percent are 65 years old or older. In 1996, life expectancy at birth for women was 63 years; men lagged slightly behind at 62 years. This represents a dramatic improvement from 1991, when both men and women could expect to live approximately 56 years. The fertility rate among women in 1996 was 3.11 children per woman.

Education

Adult literacy in India stands at about 52 percent, with a significant discrepancy between men and women; the literacy rate for men is 66 percent, whereas that for women is nearly 30 percent lower at 38 percent. Considerable variation is also found among literacy rates by region, with the eastern and northern parts of the country having significantly lower literacy rates than the western and southern regions.

Economic Dimensions

India is the fifth largest economy in the world. Its gross domestic product, estimated at U.S.$1.8 trillion at prices current in 1999, is the second largest among emerging economies on the basis of purchasing power parity. About 31 percent of the GDP originates in the primary sector (mainly agriculture), 28 percent in the secondary sector (mainly manufacturing), and 41 percent in the tertiary sector (mainly services, trade, and commerce). Nearly two-thirds of the working population is employed in the primary sector,

TABLE 29.1
Selected
Demographic
and Education
Data, India,
2000

Total area (in thousands of square kilometers)	3,288
Population in millions	1,014
Population growth rate, 1999 (percent)	1.58
Age structure of population as percent of total population	
0 to 14 years	34
15 to 64 years	62
65 years old and older	4
Life expectancy (years)	Female: 63.13
	Male: 61.89
Infant mortality (per 1,000 live births)	64.9
Total fertility rate	3.11
Literacy rate	Male: 65.5
	Female: 37.7

SOURCE: CIA (2000).

and the secondary and tertiary sectors employ 14.5 percent and 20.5 percent of the workforce, respectively.

With the introduction of liberalization policies in the early 1990s, the economy has recovered from near bankruptcy and grown very quickly. Economic reforms initiated in 1991 by Prime Minister P. V. Narasimha Rao targeted the privatization of certain key government industries, and the reforms also reduced the barriers to entry for international investment in India. The 1999 real growth rate for India's GDP was 5.5 percent, and the inflation rate stabilized at 6.7 percent. The increased economic growth has not, however, translated into large improvements in healthcare spending. Total health spending for 1990 through 1998 amounted to 5.2 percent of the GDP, which was average for most developing countries during that period. Most health spending came from private sources. Table 29.2 offers a more detailed picture of India's economy.

Context: Health Needs

As in many developing countries, the major contributors to morbidity and mortality in India are communicable diseases. Although India has made great strides in reducing the incidence of communicable diseases since becoming an independent nation, they still contribute to 56 percent of India's disability-adjusted life years, whereas noncommunicable diseases and injuries account for 29 percent and 15 percent, respectively. India's

TABLE 29.2

Selected Employment and Economic Indicators, India, 1999

Total labor force in millions	N/A
Number of unemployed in millions	37.2*
Percent of population below the poverty line	35
GDP	
Total in trillions of U.S.$ at current exchange rates	1.805
Per-person in U.S.$ using P.P.P.	1,800
Inflation rate (percent)	6.7
Health spending	
Percentage of total GDP	5.2
Percentage of public share of GDP†	0.6
Percentage of private share of GDP‡	4.1
Health expenditure per capita in U.S.$	133

* This figure is disputed as no national survey has determined the extent of unemployment in India.
† Public health expenditure consists of recurrent and capital spending from government (central and local) budgets, external borrowings and grants (including donations from international organizations and non-governmental agencies), and social (or compulsory) health insurance funds.
‡ Private health expenditure includes direct household spending (out-of-pocket), private insurance, charitable donations, and direct service payments by private corporations.
SOURCE: CIA (2000); WHO (2000).

attempts to reduce the incidence of communicable diseases have been hindered by the emergence in recent years of pathogens like multidrug-resistant mycobacterium tuberculosis, 0139 cholera, and HIV (Kumar 1999). Table 29.3 offers a complete picture of mortality in India.

The low health status of women and the explosive growth of HIV/AIDS are major causes for alarm in India. Currently, nearly 120,000 women (437 per 100,000) die of maternity-related causes every year, a maternal mortality rate that is 50 times higher than in developed countries. Strikingly, the risk of death during pregnancy is much higher, with a rate nearly 200 times that of the developed world. This increased risk is largely because of the higher number of pregnancies in India, but the lack of medical care for women is also a large contributor. Trained personnel do not examine 50 percent of pregnant women at any time during their pregnancy, and about 75 percent of pregnant women are not protected against tetanus or provided with iron and folic acid tablets. As a result, anemia and reproductive tract infections have been found to be responsible for most of the maternal deaths in India. Other factors compounding the low health status of women include the re-emergence of epidemics like malaria, cholera, tuberculosis, and meningitis; increasing incidence of HIV/AIDS; and unsafe abortion practices. Many of the illnesses affecting

TABLE 29.3

Causes of
Mortality in
Percentages,
India, 1990

Communicable diseases	56.4
Infectious and parasitic diseases	28.9
Respiratory infections	11.9
Maternal disorders	2.6
Perinatal disorders	8.8
Nutritional deficiencies	4.2
Noncommunicable diseases	29.0
Malignant neoplasms	11.7
Other neoplasms	0.1
Diabetes	0.8
Endocrine disorders	0
Neuropsychiatric disorders	7.0
Sense organ disorders	1.1
Cardiovascular disorders	8.2
Respiratory disorders	2.7
Digestive disorders	2.2
Genitourinary disorders	0.7
Skin disorders	0
Musculoskeletal disorders	0.5
Congenital anomalies	2.9
Oral disorders	0.4
Injuries	14.6
Unintentional injuries	13
Intentional injuries	1.5

SOURCE: WHO (2000).

maternal health have their origin in poor nutrition, which in turn points to the lack of basic resources available to women (Nath 1998).

The AIDS epidemic is one of the most serious public health concerns to have arisen in India during the last decade. Although the number of officially reported HIV infections and AIDS cases is only in the thousands, conservative estimates indicate that the actual number of HIV infections approaches nearly 11.5 million, which is more than 1.5 percent of the population. Nationwide surveillance data collected in 1998 confirmed that HIV infection is now prevalent in all parts of the country and has spread from urban to rural populations and from individuals involved in high-risk behavior to the general population. About 80 percent of HIV transmission occurs through primarily heterosexual sexual activity, and the remainder occurs through blood transfusions and intravenous drug use. Only 3 to 5 percent of HIV-infected individuals can afford antiretroviral therapy, despite the fact that the drugs are sold at half the international rates. The drug azidothymidine (AZT) has recently been made available free of charge or at subsidized rates in some public hospitals as part of the perinatal HIV intervention program. However, disease treatment and prevention measures are limited, and the country faces a major calamity.

Organization and Management of the Health System

Although all three levels of government (central, state, and local), contribute to public healthcare spending, the Indian Constitution assigns primary responsibility for healthcare to the states (Purohit 2001). The central government assists the state governments in defining policies, providing a national strategic framework, and financing healthcare as well as regulating medical education, drug control, and immunization programs; the Ministry of Health and Family Welfare (MOHFW) oversees these functions. Each state and union territory also has its own MOHFW that is responsible for carrying out the policy directives of the central MOHFW.

Within the state and union territories, districts are the principal units for health administration. A district health officer, who reports to the state health officer at the state headquarters of the MOHFW, oversees all ministry activities in a district (Roemer 1993). Although a major portion of public expenditures (nearly 90 percent) in the healthcare sector comes from the state budgets, the states depend on the central government to some degree for funding.

Health System Planning, Past and Present

Since India's independence in 1947, health planning has largely followed a centralized, Soviet-style planning model. The initial plan for the development of India's health infrastructure in 1946, the Health Survey and Development Committee Report (Bhore Report), called for radical reorganization of the entire health system, with the government taking responsibility for providing complete health services for the entire population. The report's proposals were incorporated into India's First Five Year Plan for the socioeconomic development of the country.

Since that time, a series of five-year plans have served as blueprints for the development of health services. These plans have largely concentrated on implementing large programs for training personnel and constructing health facilities. For many reasons (e.g., overambitious goals, lack of resources, faltering political will), the achievements of each five-year plan have fallen far short of expectations (Roemer 1993).

Because of the failure of its planning policies, India had to introduce corrective reforms in the 1990s under pressure from international organizations. The Ninth (1992–97) and Tenth (1997–2002) Five Year Plans have largely reflected structural adjustment policies based on the recommendations of the International Monetary Fund and the World Bank. These reforms focus on cutting health sector investments, opening medical care service provision to the private sector, introducing user fees, encouraging private investment in public hospitals, and developing technocentric public health interventions (Qadeer 2000).

Financing

India's healthcare system is financed through a mixture of government insurance programs, private insurance, and out-of-pocket payments. As shown in Table 29.4, the majority of health expenditures are out-of-pocket payments, with government expenditures and private insurance accounting for the remainder. The financing method used largely depends on the socioeconomic status of the patient.

Government Insurance Programs

Two major government insurance programs provide medical care for individuals in India. The first program, the Central Government Health Scheme (CGHS), provides healthcare to employees of the central government. The CGHS covers employees, pensioners, and their families, allowing the central government to eliminate cumbersome and expensive reimbursement of medical costs. In 1999, the CGHS covered 948,000 employees and their dependents (nearly 4.3 million people), providing services in its own facilities or through public and private resources under contract. The CGHS presently operates in 20 cities and covers allopathic treatment as well as other traditional forms of treatment (ayurvedic, homeopathic, unani, and siddha); currently 200 private hospitals have been recognized for use by CGHS beneficiaries (Indian Embassy Information Index 2000).

TABLE 29.4
Selected Health Financing Statistics, India, 1997

Per capita expenditure in U.S.$	23
Public expenditure as percent of total health expenditure	13
Private expenditure as percent of total health expenditure	87
Out-of-pocket payment as percent of total health expenditure	84.6

SOURCE: WHO (2000).

The second government program that provides medical care in India is the Employees State Insurance (ESI) scheme. The Employee State Insurance Act, which created ESI, was passed in the interest of state government and private industry employees. The provisions of the Act provide an insured individual and his or her dependents with sickness, maternity, and disability benefits, as well as funeral expenses. ESI beneficiaries receive care from institutions designated as ESI hospitals and dispensaries. The ESI Corporation and state governments have also made arrangements with private medical institutions for the treatment of beneficiaries in specialties and subspecialties for which facilities are not available in ESI hospitals and dispensaries. The state government releases the amount expended for such treatment either in advance or as reimbursement after the treatment.

The ESI Fund is held and administered by the ESI Corporation. The Corporation collects and recovers contributions from employers and pays benefits directly to the employees or their dependents. Participation in the ESI Scheme is compulsory for both employers and employees. Employees whose salaries fall below a financial ceiling (in 2000, less than Rs. 6,500/-pm), which is periodically reviewed by the ESI Corporation, are covered under the Scheme. The employer contributes 4.75 percent of the employee's gross salary to the scheme, and the employee contributes 1.75 percent of gross salary. Compliance with the ESI Act is advantageous to an employer because it allows the employer to cover employees under ESI Health Insurance and absolves the employer of statutory obligations to provide workers' compensation and maternity benefits. Additionally, the employer has a financial incentive in the form of an income tax exemption equal to the amount contributed to the ESI Corporation.

National Illness Assistance Fund

Another recently created government program, the National Illness Assistance Fund, serves as an emergency financial resource for disadvantaged patients. The National Illness Assistance Fund was created by the Ministry of Health and Family Welfare to provide financial assistance to patients living below the poverty line who suffer from life-threatening illnesses; these patients can seek treatment at many of the public and private hospitals throughout the country. Assistance is provided through grants disbursed directly to a hospital in which a needy patient is receiving treatment. The central government has also advised the state governments and union territories to set up similar assistance funds to take care of smaller expenditures for disadvantaged individuals.

Private Healthcare

The portion of the workforce not eligible for ESI (those having a salary higher than the ESI cap) may be provided with health insurance by employers. Several health insurance plans are available, and employers generally select the plan for the employees. The oldest and most prevalent form of private insurance used by employers is the Group Mediclaim Insurance Policy administered by the National Insurance Company. This policy is designed to cover hospitalization expenses for illness or injury sustained by an insured individual. Employees are covered for a specified amount, and the premium is payable annually as a percentage of the sum insured. Maternity benefits are available through the payment of an additional premium. In the event of a claim, the National Insurance Company pays the insured individual on a retrospective basis through fee-for-service reimbursement.

The potential health insurance market is estimated at nearly 135 million people, predominantly individuals in the upper-middle income segment of the population. The current annual health insurance premium market share of Indian insurance companies is a meager 1.6 million individuals. As a result, several international insurance corporations have recently started to compete with Indian insurance organizations by tailoring policies for the Indian population (Purohit 2001).

Many hospitals have introduced health plans that provide comprehensive hospitalization services designed specifically for employers to cover the hospitalization expenses of employees. These managed-care analogues initiated by the Apollo Group (India's largest chain of private hospitals) charge a monthly premium that covers expenses for both outpatient and inpatient services for the length of the contract. The plans differ in the comprehensiveness of services provided and the level of coverage.

Health Resources

An estimated 70 percent of India's health resources is localized in urban regions, whereas 70 percent of the population live in rural areas. As a result, the government of India has focused on the development of a rural health infrastructure through a network of integrated health delivery centers. The network consists of three types of health facilities designed to provide healthcare at the grass-roots level: community health centers, primary health centers, and subcenters.

A community health center offers services to between 80,000 and 120,000 people and is staffed with a medical specialist, a surgical specialist, a child specialist, a gynecologist, and 25 other paramedical and ministerial staff; it has 30 beds, a well-equipped laboratory, and an x-ray facility. A primary health center is staffed with a medical officer, a pharmacist, a staff nurse, a female multipurpose worker, a health educator, a laboratory technician, a female health assistant, a male health assistant, and four or five other ministerial staff; it serves a population of 30,000 in the plains areas and 20,000 in tribal or difficult terrain areas. A subcenter is staffed by one female and one male multipurpose worker covering a population of 5,000 in plains areas and 3,000 in hilly, tribal, or difficult terrain areas.

An examination of India's health system reveals a sizeable disparity between India's health resources and the resources available to developed nations. As shown in Table 29.5, India had 15,097 hospitals, 28,825 dispensaries, 21,802 primary health centers, and 132,285 subcenters in 1995. These resources provided a total of 870,161 beds, which is less than one bed per 1,000 people; the number of physicians and other health professionals is also strikingly low. India had 474,000 practicing physicians in 1996, which resulted in 0.52 physicians per 100,000 people. India's medical colleges offer some hope, augmenting the existing work force with 15,000 highly trained and specialized physicians each year. The number of nurses in 1996 stood at 512,000, which was 0.62 per 1,000 people. The private sector holds a large number of the healthcare resources in India, accounting for nearly 57 percent of hospitals and 80 percent of licensed allopathic physicians (Bhat 1999).

In addition to an overall shortage of physicians, India also faces problems in the distribution of physicians in the rural regions of the country. Every year, thousands of physicians seeking a better livelihood leave the rural areas for urban centers. The central government has recently attempted to remedy this problem by providing financial incentives for graduating medical students and physicians to practice in rural centers.

Alternative health accounts for a significant percentage of India's healthcare resources. Nonphysician providers such as pharmacists and tra-

TABLE 29.5
Health Resources and Use, India, 1995

Inpatient care	
Hospitals*	15,097
Dispensaries	28,825
Primary health centers	21,802
Subcenters	132,285
Beds, total	870,161
Medical colleges	160
Physicians	474,270
Nurses	512,595
Auxiliary nurse-midwives	229,304
Dentists	10,751
Pharmacists	175,000

* These statistics represent the number of licensed facilities and providers; note that many healthcare facilities or providers may not be licensed or may not have been included in the census of health resources by the government.
SOURCE: Government of India (1996, 1996a, 1997).

ditional healers play a major role in providing health services, especially in rural areas. The number of alternative healers in the country is about the same as allopathic physicians, and these healers are widely distributed in cities and rural villages.

Delivery of Health Services

Patterns of health service delivery in India largely depend on socioeconomic and geographic factors. The great number of poor people in India (nearly 350 million) must depend on traditional healers (generally ayurvedic or homeopathic practitioners) or government physicians (allopathic) for ambulatory care services. Traditional healers, located in both urban and rural areas, generally provide herbal medications to the patient along with advice on lifestyle changes. A poor patient in a city or region with government facilities may attempt to see a physician at a government hospital or a health professional at a subcenter, primary health center, or community center. In dire circumstances, the patient may approach a private physician who provides charity care or one who may agree to a discounted or staggered fee schedule.

An individual from the middle socioeconomic level of Indian society may seek services from a physician in a government facility, but in most cases he or she will see a private physician in a clinic as an initial response to illness. In general, these clinics are modest in size and staffed only by physicians. The government insurance programs, private health insurance, or out-of-pocket payments may pay for care for this socioeconomic stratum.

For the upper level of Indian society, health services are obtained almost exclusively through the private sector. In the cities of India, many well-trained and specialized physicians derive their livelihoods from treating upper-income clientele. These physicians usually practice in technologically advanced private clinics with a highly trained staff of nurses. Typically, any type of service—from vaccinations to major surgery—can be provided at these locations. Most patients at these clinics bear the full cost of medical care out of pocket, although payment may be made through a health insurance policy.

The patterns of delivery of hospital care are similar to those for ambulatory care. Nearly three-quarters of India's hospital beds are in government facilities at both the state and central levels. These beds are accessible to everyone regardless of socioeconomic status and are, therefore, extremely crowded. Additionally, government hospitals are generally lacking in amenities, wards are ill-kept, and the sanitary facilities usually leave much to be desired (Roemer 1993).

A large proportion of the remaining hospital beds are found in private facilities under the sponsorship of voluntary agencies or religious organizations. These hospitals generally maintain higher standards in terms of facilities, personnel, and patient care largely because they are better funded (via private donations and patient fees) than are government hospitals. Because fees are higher in these facilities, their patients usually belong to higher socioeconomic groups, although some of the beds may be reserved for the poor as charity beds.

Corporate hospitals have recently begun to emerge as a force in the major cities. These hospitals, which emulate the best in the world, have the latest technological equipment and extremely qualified personnel, and they employ a large number of nurses, specialists, and subspecialists. They are almost exclusively focused on curative medicine, and they seldom engage in preventive or community care. Although these hospitals target the highest socioeconomic groups, many of them have been granted land and tax exemptions with the understanding that they will provide treatment for some poor patients.

Prospects for the Future

Since gaining its independence in 1947, India has shown dramatic improvement in the health status of its population. However, it still lags behind developed nations in health status and availability of health resources. Current foci include improving access to health services for all segments of the population and expanding education about disease prevention; these will continue to be issues in the future and must form the basis of national health policies for the twenty-first century. Additional issues that will likely have an effect in the future include the following:

- improvements of emergency medical services to address deaths due to injuries and catastrophe; currently, nearly 4 percent of all deaths in India can be attributed to lack of emergency medical services
- incentives for medical students aimed at increasing the supply of physicians in the rural regions of the country
- the addition of government health facilities in rural regions of the country in the form of primary health centers, community centers, and subcenters; currently, government health centers are frequently inaccessible to members of rural communities because of geographic distance or difficult terrain
- the further development of private and government aid for future improvements of India's health infrastructure
- the continued development of government programs aimed at eradication or control of communicable diseases and sexually transmitted diseases; a special emphasis must be placed on the impending HIV/AIDS epidemic in India
- increased education efforts aimed at maternal and child health; government and international organizations must continue to focus on maternal diet and health as well as infant disease prevention

- increased education efforts aimed at population control, specifically in rural regions of the country; the development of fiscal incentives for this purpose should be investigated
- the development of additional government aid for segments of the population that do not qualify for health insurance
- increased emphasis on quality at medical facilities
- the continued development of water projects in regions without access to safe drinking water; these projects will reduce communicable diseases due to contaminated well water and improve prospects for agriculture in drought-stricken areas

India will undoubtedly continue the centralized policymaking process that has guided the development of its health system in the past. Taking into account the incremental nature of improvement in India's history, a radical reorganization of health services cannot be expected.

REFERENCES

Bhat, R. 1999. "Characteristics of Private Medical Practice in India: a Provider's Practice." *Health Policy and Planning* 14 (1): 26–37.

Government of India. 1996. "Economic Survey of India." Retrieved 19 May 2000 from http://finmin.nic.in/.

———. 1996a. *Rural Health Statistics of India Bulletin*. Ministry of Health. Retrieved 31 May 2000 from http://mohfw.nic.in/.

———. 1997. "Ninth Five Year Plan." Retrieved 19 May 2000 from http://finmin.nic.in/.

Indian Embassy Information Index. 2000. "India 2000." Retrieved 25 May 2000 from http://www.indianembassy.org/.

Kumar, S. 1999. "Report Spells Out India's Poor Health." *Lancet* 354 (9182): 929.

Nath, I. 1998. "India: Challenges of Transition." *Lancet* 351 (9111): 1265–75.

Purohit, B. C. 2001. "Private Initiatives and Policy Options: Recent Health System Experience in India." *Health Policy and Planning* 16 (1): 87–97.

Qadeer, I. 2000. "Health Care Systems in Transition III. India, Part I. The Indian Experience." *Journal of Public Health Medicine* 22 (1): 25–32.

Roemer, M. 1993. *National Health Systems of the World*. New York: Oxford University Press.

U.S. Central Intelligence Agency (CIA). 2000. *The World Factbook 2000*. Retrieved 17 May 2000 from http://www.cia.gov/.

World Health Organization (WHO). 2000. "World Health Report." Retrieved 03 June 2000 from http://www.who.int/.

NIGERIA

Linda Lacey

Background Information

Located on the Gulf of Guinea in West Africa, Nigeria has a population of 88.5 million people (1991 census) in an area of 355,174 square miles, making it one of the largest countries in sub-Saharan Africa. Nigeria gained its independence from the United Kingdom on October 1, 1960, and it is now a federation of 36 states and the Federal Capital Territory, Abuja. The country's diverse multicultural society comprises approximately 380 different ethnic groups. Like most sub-Saharan African countries, Nigeria is experiencing rapid urban population growth, with about 42 percent of the population currently residing in urban areas.

Nigeria's economy is based on oil revenues, local industries, and agriculture. Although much of the nation's income is derived from the export of petroleum, the agricultural sector provides employment to most Nigerian citizens, primarily in the form of small-scale farming and informal sector trading. Nigeria has a small, capital-intensive urban sector concentrated primarily in cities and towns. Urban economies generally consist of local industries, a few multinational firms, and a large number of government conglomerates (World Bank 1996).

Nigeria ranks among the 13 poorest countries in the world (World Bank 2001), with a per capita gross national product of U.S.$300; close to 70 percent of the population lives in poverty. The World Bank estimated that, in 1997, 70 percent of the population lived on one dollar a day and that 90 percent subsisted on two dollars a day (World Bank 2000). Nigeria's complex political history, widespread corruption, and heavy dependence on oil revenues are largely responsible for the very low standard of living. Additional economic data are provided in Table 30.1

Because educational attainment is closely linked to the economy, Nigeria's literacy levels remain fairly low, although the implementation of a policy of free universal primary education seems to have brought about some improvement, especially among young people. As indicated in Table 30.2, 50 percent of adult males and 78 percent of females were illiterate in 1980. More recent data indicate some improvement. In 1998, the male and female illiteracy rates had declined to 30 percent and 48 percent, respectively. Government and private schools are helping the majority of children

TABLE 30.1
Economic and
Social
Indicators,
1998

GNP per capita (U.S.$)	300
Real GDP per capita (P.P.P.$)	740
Human Development Index score, 1999	.455
Percent of GDP spent on healthcare	.7
Percent of GDP spent in public sector	.2
Health expenditure per capita (U.S.$)	9

SOURCE: UNDP (2001); World Bank (2000).

and young adults receive a basic education. In 1998, only 12 percent of males between the ages of 15 and 24 years and 19 percent of females in the same age cohorts were illiterate.

Context: Health Needs

Infant and childhood mortality rates are important measures of the effectiveness of the healthcare system and of the overall level of welfare in a country. Although poverty levels are high in Nigeria, infant mortality and under-five mortality rates have declined during the past ten years. Based on the Nigeria Demographic and Health Survey (DHS) of 1999, infant mortality is 70.8 per 1,000 live births, and under-five mortality is 140 per 1,000 live births (see Table 30.3). Regional differences, however, are significant; infant mortality is 115 per 1,000 live births in the northwest but only 50 per 1,000 live births in the central region. Similarly, under-five mortality rates are 188 per 1,000 live births in the northwest and 84 per 1,000 live births in the central region. These variations are closely linked to regional inequities in access to healthcare services.

TABLE 30.2
Adult and
Youth
Illiteracy
Percentages

	Male	Female
Adult illiteracy rate, 1980	50	78
Adult illiteracy percentage, 1998	30	48
Illiteracy rate for ages 15 to 24 years, 1998	12	19

SOURCE: World Bank (2000).

TABLE 30.3
General
Demographics

Population (1991 census of 88.5 million)	121 million
Infant mortality per 1,000 live births, 1999	70.8
Under-five mortality per 1,000 live births, 1999	140
Maternal mortality per 100,000 births	1,000
Life expectancy at birth (years)	53.0
Total fertility rate	5.3
Percent urbanized	42.0

SOURCE: National Population Commission (2000).

The decline in infant and child mortality does not reflect increases in immunization levels. The percentage of children between the ages of 12 and 23 months who are fully immunized actually declined between 1990 and 1999 (National Population Commission 2000), with 38 percent of children unvaccinated in 1999 as compared to 37 percent in the 1990 study. Among those children receiving vaccines, about 41 percent received a measles vaccine, and 53 percent received a bacillus Calmette Guérin vaccination for protection against tuberculosis (National Population Commission 2000). About 50 percent of those vaccinated received the first dose of diphtheria and polio; a lower percentage received the second and third doses of these vaccines. The authors of the 1999 Nigeria DHS report major shortages of these two vaccines from 1996 to 1998, which could account for the decline in immunization coverage. Additional information concerning access to health-enhancing factors may be found in Table 30.4.

Leading Causes of Mortality

Information about the leading causes of death in Nigeria is limited. Although mortality statistics are collected at government health facilities, facility data are not complete because a limited number of Nigerians use government health services; an estimated 60 percent of Nigerians use private sector

TABLE 30.4
Percent Access
to Health-
Enhancing
Factors

Access to health services, 1995	51
Access to safe water	39
Access to sanitation	36
Immunization for diphtheria	45

SOURCE: Kaul and Tomaselli-Moschovitis (1999); World Bank (2000).

rather than government health services (World Bank 2001). That being said, Egunjobi's (1993) analysis of mortality statistics collected by state ministries of health does provide some insight into the most common causes of deaths in the country. His examination shows that the six leading causes of death are infectious, parasitic, and diarrheal diseases; 85 percent of all deaths in Nigeria are accounted for by measles, pneumonia, malaria, dysentery, tetanus, and tuberculosis (Egunjobi 1993).

Although diseases such as malaria, measles, and diarrhea continue to account for a large proportion of deaths, other infectious diseases like cerebrospinal meningitis, yellow fever, and lassa fever also occur with increased frequency and often in epidemic proportions (Federal Ministry of Health 2000). Infectious diseases—particularly dysentery, malaria, and measles—account for a large proportion of deaths among infants and children.

The incidence and prevalence of noncommunicable diseases such as hypertension, coronary heart disease, diabetes, cancer, and stress-related illnesses are growing as well. On the basis of a 1989 survey, the Federal Ministry of Health estimates that 3.5 million Nigerians have mild hypertension, 1.2 million have moderate hypertension, and 0.5 million have severe hypertension. The prevalence of hypertension is estimated at 8 to 10 percent in rural areas and at 10 to 12 percent in urban communities (Federal Ministry of Health 2000).

Maternal Mortality

Child bearing is a leading cause of death among Nigerian women in their reproductive years. The Federal Ministry of Health (2000) estimates maternal mortality at 948 per 100,000, ranging from 339 per 100,000 in the southwest to 1,716 per 100,000 in the northeast. Maternal mortality is closely linked with the age of mother, birth spacing practices, and number of prior births. Teen mothers and older mothers are more likely to experience complications that lead to death.

Maternal mortality rates are also influenced by access to medical facilities. According to the 1999 DHS, 37.3 percent of births in that year occurred at a health facility and 58 percent occurred at home; 33.7 percent of births were delivered by a nurse-midwife, 20.7 percent by a traditional birth attendant, 7.9 percent by a doctor, and 23.7 percent by a relative or friend. In most cases, women received some form of prenatal care. About 47 percent received four or more visits, and about 9 percent received two or three visits.

According to the 1999 DHS, the fertility rate is 111 per 1,000 among women between the ages of 15 and 19 years and 24 per 1,000 among women between the ages of 45 and 49 years (National Population Commission 2000). Close to 13 percent of women between 15 and 19 years old have given birth to at least one child, and 4.6 percent of women in this age group have given birth to two children.

Complications from unsafe abortions also contribute substantially to maternal mortality, claiming the lives of both unwed teens and married women in high numbers.

HIV/AIDS

HIV/AIDS is a leading cause of death in sub-Saharan Africa, especially in southern and eastern African nations. Nigeria has been hit particularly hard by the epidemic, with the prevalence of HIV infection and AIDS-related death rates even higher than those in most neighboring countries (Table 30.5). According to UNAIDS (a division of the United Nations) and the World Health Organization (2000), about 5 percent of Nigerian adults between the ages of 15 and 49 years were infected with HIV in 1999 compared to 4.1 percent in 1997. An estimated 250,000 adults and children died of AIDS during 1999. As a comparison, in nearby Ghana, WHO estimates that 3.6 percent of adults are HIV positive and that 33,000 AIDS deaths occurred in 1999. Similarly, in Niger (Nigeria's northern neighbor), 1.35 percent of adults are infected, and 6,500 AIDS deaths occurred.

Organization and Management of the Health System

Administration

The primary healthcare system is organized into three levels: village, district, and local government. Each level has its own health committee that is established by locally elected councils in consultation with the state Ministry of Health; these committees make decisions about primary healthcare (Olowu and Wunsch 1992). The health committee includes representatives of the council, the State Hospital Management Board, nongovernment organizations, and professional health staff and leaders of the local community. The health committee formulates project proposals, col-

Prevalence of anemia as percent of pregnant women	55	**TABLE 30.5** Leading Causes of Morbidity and Mortality
Low-birth-weight babies as percent of all births	15	
Tuberculosis, incidence per 100,000, 1997	24	
Prevalence of HIV as percent of adults, 1997	4.12	
Prevalence of HIV as percent of adults, 1999	5.06	
Prevalence of HIV, people infected all ages, 1997	2,300,000	
Prevalence of HIV, people infected all ages, 1999	2,700,000	

SOURCE: World Bank (2000); Kaul and Tomaselli-Moschovitis (1999); WHO (2000).

lects basic health data, and mobilizes resources for healthcare; it is also responsible for service delivery and intersectoral coordination (Federal Ministry of Health 1988). State ministries are slowly transferring responsibilities to health committees.

The health staff of the local government authority consists of a varied skill mix that may include a chief medical officer, physicians, community health supervisors, public health nurses, midwives, nurses, a community health superintendent, laboratory technicians, dispensary/pharmacy technicians, record officers, community health assistants, and a family planning manager (typically a nurse). As part of the ongoing impetus toward decentralization, health staff members have begun to report to the health committee chairpersons rather than to the state Ministry of Health.

Health Services Planning

Public health services in Nigeria originated from the colonial medical services provided as early as the late 1800s by the British government and missionaries (Schram 1971). Since achieving independence, the Nigerian government has incrementally expanded healthcare services. The first effort to establish a national healthcare system infrastructure was introduced in Nigeria's Third National Development Plan, 1975–80 (WHO 1992). This plan introduced the Basic Health Service Scheme as a means of attempting to accomplish the following goals:

- increasing the proportion of the population receiving healthcare from 25 to 40 percent
- correcting imbalances in the location and distribution of health institutions and between preventive and curative medicine
- providing the infrastructure for all preventive health programs (control of communicable diseases, family health, environmental health, and nutrition)
- establishing a healthcare system to meet local conditions

To these ends, the Basic Health Service Scheme advocated the creation of a Basic Health Unit in each local government area that would include a 60-bed comprehensive healthcare center serving as the health headquarters, four primary health centers each serving about 40,000 patients, and community-based clinics. Under the scheme, each primary health center would meet the referral needs of five surrounding health clinics, which were to be the first point of contact for preventive and curative care within the community. The Basic Health Unit would serve a population of 150,000 (Adeokun 1981).

This first plan was not fully implemented, because the resources needed to construct the 25 healthcare facilities for each local government authority were simply unavailable (WHO 1992); the few healthcare facilities that were built were not well maintained. One positive outcome of the Basic Health

Services Scheme has been the establishment of training facilities (Ayo et al. 1993); schools of health technology continue to train community health workers who work primarily in local government health facilities.

The health sector plan in the Fourth National Development Plan of 1980–85 also focused on providing basic healthcare services and facilities at the local government level. However, revenues from the sale of petroleum declined drastically in the early 1980s, which greatly reduced the government's ability to implement national health planning efforts.

Another major attempt to develop a national healthcare system began with the development of Nigeria's National Health Policy in the 1980s. A national committee established between 1983 and 1985 sought widespread participation of health leaders, institutions, and Ministry of Health staff throughout the country. Ransome-Kuti (1998) states that the principal aim of the policy was "to provide the Federal, State and Local Government health institutions and their functionaries, other health related organizations including international agencies, and non-government organizations with a formal framework for an appropriate national direction in health development in Nigeria."

The policy emerged during a period when most healthcare services were offered in urban areas, where only 30 percent of the population resided. An estimated 35 percent of the population had no access at all to modern healthcare services at the time (Ayo et al. 1993), and basic infrastructure and logistical support were grossly inadequate to meet the needs of the rural population.

Nigeria's current national health policy, The National Health Policy and Strategy to Achieve Health for All Nigerians, was officially implemented in 1988. The foundation of the policy is the guaranteed provision of primary healthcare as defined in the Alma-Ata Declaration. Primary healthcare services include the following:

- health education
- promotion of adequate food supply and proper nutrition
- an adequate supply of safe water and basic sanitation
- maternal and child healthcare, including family planning
- immunizations
- prevention and control of locally endemic and epidemic diseases
- appropriate treatment of common diseases and injuries
- provision of essential drugs and supplies

The policy sets out four main strategies for implementation:

1. the involvement of nongovernment agencies, private practitioners, and employer clinics in the provision of healthcare
2. the coordination of federal, state, and local governments and among volunteer and private-sector healthcare providers

3. the development of mechanisms to involve communities in the planning and implementation of health services
4. the integration of primary, secondary, and tertiary care in a three-tier structure

Under the policy, primary healthcare is the jurisdiction of local governments; secondary healthcare, including services at general hospitals, is placed under state control; and tertiary healthcare, which consists of teaching-hospital services, is the responsibility of the federal government.

The policy defines the roles and functions of each level of government within the health system. In addition to physician training, the provision and maintenance of tertiary curative health services, and communicable-disease control, the Federal Ministry of Health is responsible for a number of policy and planning activities, including developing a national implementation plan and seeking its adoption by the government, formulating the necessary legislation, monitoring and evaluating the policy implementation effort, and coordinating implementation efforts among the governmental levels and nongovernment providers. The Ministry of Health also supports state Ministries of Health in their coordination with local government authorities; the state ministries of health are primarily responsible for providing secondary and nonspecialized tertiary health facilities. They also coordinate healthcare services among local governments and with other development sectors within the state and are responsible for helping mobilize political and financial support for the healthcare policy. Other roles include developing a logistics system to ensure regular and timely distribution of supplies and equipment, coordinating the availability of transportation, ensuring the provision of training and health manpower, and developing plans for healthcare facilities. Local governments are primarily responsible for planning, providing, and evaluating the delivery of primary healthcare at the community level.

Ransome-Kuti (1998) indicates that implementation of the policy began before its official approval. In 1986, 52 local governments were paired with a college of medicine and a school of health technology (designated to provide planning assistance) to develop models for primary healthcare services. During that period, village health services were also established within the model government areas. Each model government was divided into health districts of populations of 30,000 to 50,000 people. Village health district centers were established to handle problems that could not be managed at the village level; village development committees were also formed to develop and manage services.

Because of the limited government resources devoted to healthcare, the policy of 1988 has never been fully implemented. A key contribution of the policy, however, is its role in providing a framework for decentralized primary healthcare.

Decentralization Policies

In 1989, the Nigerian Federal Military Government directed the states to give responsibility for development efforts, including primary healthcare, to the local governments. This decision was part of Nigeria's decentralization efforts, an outcome of major reforms introduced by the military government in 1976 as a reaction to the centralized powers of President Gowen's administration. After Gowen was overthrown, the new military government institutionalized a system of power sharing among the three levels of government in the belief that a representative local government system was essential for developing a national democratic system of governance and that a local system of administration would be more responsive to local needs and conditions (Gboyega 1985).

In 1994, 589 local governments oversaw population segments ranging in size from 150,000 to 500,000 people. At present, there are 774 local government authorities, and more are likely to be formed as a result of community pressure on federal and state government officials. By becoming a local government authority, communities are eligible for federal funding for community-development programs.

Financing

Healthcare expenditures in Nigeria are influenced by petroleum sales. During the country's oil boom (1973 to 1979), the government invested heavily in the Basic Health Service Scheme as part of the National Development Plan of 1975–80. During the period of the Plan, the number of physicians per capita increased fourfold and the number of nurses increased sevenfold to meet the staffing needs of new hospitals and medical centers (World Bank 1996). After oil revenues collapsed in 1980, investments in the health sector declined.

Although oil exports continue to be a major part of the economy, government revenues used to support the health sector are limited. Only 0.7 percent of the nation's gross domestic product is spent on healthcare, and 0.2 percent of the GDP is used for public healthcare services and facilities. The government spends an estimated U.S.$5 per individual on health services (Kaul and Tomaselli-Moschovitis 1999).

To implement decentralized primary healthcare, local government authorities can receive financial support from six sources: (1) the Federation Account, (2) the model local government authority grant program, (3) the state budget, (4) local taxes, (5) donor organizations, and (6) community members and their migrant offspring (Ayo et al. 1993). The majority of funding comes from the Federation Account.

The Federation Account is the basis for sharing national revenues among the three tiers of government. About 75 percent of the Federation

Account comes from the sale of oil; therefore, even local budgets are influenced by conditions in the international oil market. In 1989, the states received about 32 percent of the Federation Account; local government authorities received about 10 percent (Ayo et al. 1993). In 1990, the intergovernmental transfer system was restructured, and local government authorities began receiving 20 percent of the Federation Account.

The amount of the Federation Account allocated to local government authorities is based on the same formula used to allocate resources among the states. The 1990 revenue-sharing formula for states was based on a number of factors, including equity among states (40 percent), population (30 percent), internal revenue efforts (10 percent), land mass/terrain (10 percent), and a social development factor (10 percent), which includes the geographic distribution of the population, primary school enrollment, the number of health institutions and hospital beds, water supply, and rainfall (Ayo et al. 1993). States typically develop their own formulas for revenue sharing with local authorities.

Each tier of government can generate revenues through taxation. Local government authorities generate revenue from property taxes, market and trading fees and licenses, motor park dues, canoe park dues, entertainment taxes, motor vehicle taxes, driver license fees, land registration fees, and license fees on television and radio stations. However, about 90 to 95 percent of local government funding comes from transfer payments from the federal and state governments. Transfer payments are reduced if local government authorities generate income locally, resulting in a disincentive for taxation (Olowu and Wunsch 1992). More importantly, this system does not take into account the actual costs of delivering healthcare services at the community level.

Within each local government authority, the elected council determines how government revenues are allocated to development programs. The council collects and reviews all development budgets, including that of the health committee. In an urban local government authority (such as mainland Lagos), the council reviews five major budgets: (1) works and housing, (2) education, (3) agriculture and rural development, (4) community development and welfare, and (5) health. Most of the health budget is for staff salaries; little money is budgeted for drugs and medicine.

Health Resources

Nigerians have limited access to modern healthcare services. Nigeria has an estimated 0.2 physicians per 1,000 population, 1.7 hospital beds per 1,000 population, and 142 nurses per 100,000 population. Data on the distribution of healthcare facilities show that there are 12,384 health service facilities including 2,545 hospitals, 2,846 health centers, 4,406 clinics, and 2,587 maternity centers (Kiragu, Chapman, and Lewis 1995).

Healthcare services are more widely available in the southwest and eastern regions than in other regions. Additional information on healthcare human resources and facilities is provided in Table 30.6.

Service Delivery

Primary Healthcare

As part of the decentralization policy of 1989, local government authorities were given responsibility for local development efforts, including the provision of primary healthcare. The Constitution of the Federal Republic of Nigeria Decree of 1989 states that the functions of local government include the following (Federal Republic of Nigeria 1989):

1. the provision and maintenance of primary, adult, and vocational education
2. the development of agricultural and natural resources
3. the provision and maintenance of health services

The state administers the state healthcare system and trains nurses, midwives, and auxiliary staff. Secondary and nonspecialized tertiary hospitals and some primary healthcare facilities are also operated at the state level. The state ministries of health coordinate primary healthcare efforts among the local government authorities under their jurisdiction.

The Hospital Management Board manages the state's hospitals. The Board also manages healthcare personnel and the financing and management of logistical support systems including drugs, supplies, equipment, and facilities maintenance. In some states, the chairman of the Hospital Management Board reports to the State Commissioner of Health (World Bank 2001).

Local government authorities are responsible for the operation of health facilities within their areas, including the provision of basic outpatient, community health, hygiene, and sanitation services. Local governments must also mobilize community support for the health plan and provide and maintain the healthcare infrastructure within their jurisdictions (Olowu and Wunsch 1992). The primary health system includes village

		TABLE 30.6
Physicians per 1,000 population	.2	Human
Hospital beds per 1,000 population	1.7	Resources and
Nurses per 100,000 population	142.0	Facilities for
Percent of births attended by skilled staff	31	Healthcare

SOURCE: World Bank (2000); Kaul and Tomaselli-Moschovitis (1999).

health posts (serving about 500 people), dispensaries (serving 10,000), health clinics (serving 20,000 to 50,000), and primary healthcare centers (serving 20,000 to 80,000 people).

Primary healthcare is a fairly new responsibility for local government authorities. As would be expected, numerous problems have emerged as the authorities adapt to their new responsibilities. Local governments often lack adequate staff and health committees that can solve problems, develop priorities, collect and use data for strategic planning, and develop realistic budgets. Similarly, supervisory mechanisms are largely nonexistent. Local government authorities will take several years to build the capabilities to effectively operate, coordinate, maintain, and expand primary healthcare services, including family planning.

The Private Sector

The private sector, which includes the traditional medical system, private clinics and hospitals, chemist stores, and health services provided by non-government organizations, provides an estimated 60 percent of healthcare services in the country (World Bank 2001). The traditional medical system includes traditional midwives, bonesetters, herbalists, and mental illness care providers. In isolated rural areas, the traditional medical system meets the majority of needs. Data from the 1999 DHS show that 20 percent of births are supervised by traditional birth attendants (National Population Commission 2000).

Nongovernment Organizations

Nongovernment organizations are very active in the Nigerian healthcare sector. The largest organization is the Christian Health Association of Nigeria (CHAN), which functions as a coordinating body for all church-sponsored healthcare in the country. Founded by the Catholic Secretariat of Nigeria, it works in collaboration with the Federal Ministry of Health. CHAN provides care through 3,851 affiliated health facilities including 94 hospitals, 820 health clinics, 180 clinics, 446 maternity centers, 1,139 mobile clinics, and 164 primary healthcare centers. Almost 85 percent of CHAN-affiliated health facilities are located in urban slum and poor rural areas of the country (World Bank 1996).

Prospects for the Future

Decentralization can play a major role in strengthening the healthcare system in Nigeria. In a country with numerous ethnic groups and languages, decentralization can help adapt service delivery to suit local needs and reduce the amount of time and resources required to respond to problems or changes because local staff and health committees can address problems and constraints as they emerge. Given that local government authorities can generate and retain financial resources, this new approach may encourage staff to mobilize resources within local communities to expand health services. Decentralized services may also increase the capabilities of regional and local organizations to plan, implement, and coordinate projects and programs.

Nigeria's proper implementation of a decentralized healthcare system throughout the country will take years. Presently, the system is plagued by problems at the local government level such as understaffing (especially in rural local government authorities), a scarcity of equipment, an inadequate logistics system for delivering essential drugs and medicine, and poor incentives for government workers. Other problems include limited planning, budgeting, management, and evaluation skills at the local level (Federal Ministry of Health 2000).

However, hope is renewed for a decentralized healthcare system in the country: President Obasanjo has made health a national priority. In September 2000, the Federal Ministry of Health introduced a new plan to implement Nigeria's Health Policy of 1988. The new plan is called the Health Sector Reform Medium Term Plan of Action, 2001–2003. The Plan's objectives focus on expanding and strengthening primary healthcare; eradicating childhood diseases; expanding reproductive health services; improving secondary and tertiary healthcare hospitals; providing essential drugs and vaccines; and coordinating the provision of healthcare among donors, the government, and nongovernment agencies. The government is also exploring ways to introduce a national health insurance program. More importantly, it has introduced a strategic plan to strengthen the capacity of local government authorities to plan, manage, and provide primary healthcare services. A great deal of effort will focus on training local staff to provide high-quality services to communities and getting locally produced drugs and medicine to communities (Federal Ministry of Health 2000).

REFERENCES

Adeokun, L. A. 1981. "Local Government Responsibility for Basic Health, A Demographic Analysis." In *The Administration of Social Services in Nigeria: The Challenge to Local Governments,* pp. 79–91, edited by D. Olowu. Ille-Ife: Local Government Training Programme, University of Ife.

Ayo, D., Hubbell, K., Olowu, D., Ostrom, E., and West, T. 1993. *The Experience in Nigeria with Decentralization Approaches to Local Delivery of Primary Education and Primary Health Services.* Burlington: Associates in Rural Development.

Egunjobi, L. 1993. "Spatial Distribution of Mortality from Leading Notifiable Diseases in Nigeria." *Social Science Medicine* 36 (10): 1267–72.

Federal Republic of Nigeria. 1989. *The Constitution of the Federal Republic of Nigeria.* Lagos: Federal Republic of Nigeria.

Federal Ministry of Health. 2000. *Health Sector Reform, Medium Term Plan of Action, 2001–2003.* Abuja: Federal Ministry of Health, Government of Nigeria.

Gboyega, A. 1985. "Local Government Reform in Nigeria." In *Local Government in the Third World,* pp. 225–248, edited by P. Mawhood. Chichester: John Wiley & Sons.

Kaul, C., and Tomaselli-Moschovitis, V. 1999. *Statistical Handbook on Poverty in the Developing World.* Phoenix: Oryx Press.

Kiragu, K., Chapman, S., and Lewis, G. L. 1995. *The Nigeria Family Planning Census.* Baltimore, MD: The Johns Hopkins School of Public Health.

National Population Commission. 2000. *Nigeria Demographic and Health Survey 1999.* Abuja: National Population Commission.

Olowu, D., and Wunsch, J. 1992. *Local Governance and USAID Health Projects in Nigeria.* Lagos: United States Agency for International Development.

Ransome-Kuti, O. 1998. "Who Cares for the Health of Africans? The Nigerian Case." *International Lecture Series on Population Issues.* John D. and Catherine T. MacArthur Foundation. Retrieved March 2002 from http://macfound.org/speeches/population_lecture_series/index.htm.

Schram, R. 1971. *A History of the Nigerian Health Services.* Ibadan: Ibadan University Press.

United Nations Development Programme (UNDP). 2001. *Human Development Report 2001.* New York: Oxford University Press.

World Bank. 1996. *Nigeria: Poverty in the Midst of Plenty, The Challenge of Growth with Inclusion.* Washington, DC: The World Bank.

———. 2000. *World Development Indicators.* Washington, DC: The World Bank.

———. 2001. *Health Systems Development Project—II: Government of Nigeria.* Washington, DC: The World Bank.

World Health Organization (WHO). 1992. *Local Government Focused Acceleration of Primary Health Care: The Nigerian Experience.* Lagos: The World Health Organization.

———. 2000. "Epidemiological Fact Sheet: Nigeria, on HIV/AIDS and Sexually Transmitted Infections." Retrieved 18 March 2002 from http://www.who.int/emc-hiv/fact_sheets/.

THE DEMOCRATIC REPUBLIC OF THE CONGO

Malikwisha Meni, Mbadu Muanda, Kwilu Nappa Fulbert,

Lina M. Piripiri, and Jane T. Bertrand

Background Information

The Democratic Republic of the Congo (DRC) is a vast country of 2,345,000 square kilometers in the center of the African continent. It shares its 9,000-kilometer border with ten countries: the Central African Republic and the Sudan to the north; Uganda, Rwanda, Burundi, Tanzania, and Zambia to the east; Zambia and Angola to the south; and the Republic of Congo–Brazzaville to the west. Kinshasa is the capital of the DRC.

The DRC is dominated by plains surrounding a central basin that comprises 48 percent of the country. This area, largely covered by virgin tropical forests, is crossed by the 4,700-kilometer-long Congo River. A large number of tributaries, navigable and well-stocked with fish, feed the Congo. In the mountainous east of the country, lakes Albert, Edward, and Tanganyika are nestled within the Graben Mountains. The equator crosses the DRC, and the country benefits from a high level of rainfall (2,200 millimeters per year). Some areas have a tropical climate with rainy and dry seasons. The east has a temperate climate, which supports the cultivation of a number of Mediterranean and temperate European vegetables.

Its large size, fertile soils, wealth of minerals, and wide variety of flora and fauna combine to make the DRC an object of desire and aggression. Since the first years of independence, the country has struggled with Mulelist rebellions, secessions, interethnic war, and other forms of violence. These conflicts—particularly the ongoing war of occupation ravaging the east—have destroyed flora and fauna in the ecosystems of the Virunga, Kahuzi-Biega, Garamba, and Maiko parks. Natural disasters such as floods, erosion, and earthquakes have also taken their toll on the country in recent years.

The DRC's 11 provinces are divided into 35 districts, which are further divided into 178 territories. Governors manage the provinces, and district commissaries, territory administrators, and burgomasters (mayors) manage districts, territories, and communes, respectively. The national government established in May 1997 is moving toward a presidential regime, but it has not yet achieved this goal. At this time, the head of state serves as both president of the Republic and head of the government, which is made up of the president, ministers, and vice ministers.

Sociodemographic Characteristics

Bantus constitute the major ethnic group, followed by Sudanese (tribes), Nilotics, Pygmies, and Hamites. More than 70 percent of the population lives in rural areas. The four most common religions, in descending order of prevalence, are Roman Catholicism, Protestantism, Kimbanguism, and Islam. Many smaller religious groups have become active since the beginning of the socioeconomic crisis in 1980, and especially since 1990.

From the time of its independence to the advent of the Third Republic, the official language of the DRC (used in official documents, the administration, and national education) has been French. At the time that the Third Republic was established, English and Swahili have also been introduced as official languages. The national languages (used in the media) are Swahili, Lingala, Kikongo, and Tshiluba. Swahili is an international African language recognized by the Organization of African Unity and is spoken in Eastern Africa from southern Somalia through the north of Mozambique, including all of the eastern provinces of the DRC (Eastern Province, North Kivu, South Kivu, Maniema, and Katanga).

In 1958, the population of the DRC was estimated to be 13.5 million. By 1984, the year of the first and only scientific census, the population had grown to 30.73 million. Currently, the population is estimated to be between 53 and 59 million (INS 1993; Ngondo 1998; Baer 2002), making it the third most populated country in Africa, exceeded only by Nigeria and Ethiopia. The population is very young; 56 percent are less than 20 years old. This is the result of a high crude birth rate (48 per 1,000) and a decreasing mortality rate (16.8 per 1,000). Fertility remains high; each woman has an average of 6.7 children in her lifetime. The growth rate is 3.1 percent, which will result in a doubling of the population in 22.6 years (INS 1984). This population growth began after independence and is not matched by economic growth, which creates a great challenge for the country.

Infant and child mortality rates are high (148 and 220 per 1,000 live births, respectively). Life expectancy at birth is 47 years, which is one of the lowest levels in the world. This can largely be attributed to the economic crisis that has been gripping the country for the past 30 years, which has weakened socioeconomic infrastructures and caused deterioration in living conditions, leading to the reemergence of some previously eradicated diseases, the growth of the HIV/AIDS epidemic, and the lack of adequate vaccination coverage. Additional demographic data are provided in Table 31.1.

Urbanization is proceeding at a staggering pace, and this is expected to continue. In 1945, barely 3 percent of the population lived in cities. This percentage increased to 5 percent by 1950, 12 percent by 1958, and 28 percent by 1984. Currently, 10 percent of the population lives in the capital city of Kinshasa alone. The precariousness of life in rural areas has resulted in an exodus from rural to urban centers, and high rural fertility

		TABLE 31.1
Population in millions	59	Demographic
Infant mortality per 1,000 live births	148	Indicators
Under-five mortality per 1,000 live births	220	
Life expectancy at birth (years)	47	
Fertility rate	6.7	
Percent urbanized	28	

SOURCE: INS (1993); UNICEF (1996); Ngondo (1998).

contributes to urban growth (DDK 1998). The population of the country by province is shown in Table 31.2.

Socioeconomic Characteristics

Since 1990, the DRC has faced a devastating economic situation. The gross domestic product is actually shrinking at a rate of 14.7 percent (Ministère du Plan 1998), whereas population growth is increasing rapidly.

From 1998 to 2000, the annual government budget of the DRC had barely reached U.S.$500 million. The tax system does not function to generate revenues, and the government faces ongoing war and mounting

Province	Population	Percent of Total	TABLE 31.2
Kinshasa	5,356,000	11%	Estimated Population by Province, 1997
Lower Congo	2,771,000	6%	
Bandundu	5,272,000	11%	
Equateur	5,224,000	11%	
Eastern Province	5,821,000	13%	
Kivu*	8,500,000	18%	
Katanga	6,175,000	13%	
East Kasaï	3,354,000	7%	
West Kasaï	4,291,000	9%	
Total	46,674,000	100%	

* Includes North Kivu, South Kivu, and Maniema.
SOURCE: Ngondo (1992).

public debt payments. Per capita net income dropped from almost U.S.$350 in 1959 to U.S.$240 in 1981 (UNICEF and Ministère du Plan 1996) to U.S.$110 in 1997 (UNDP 1999). Income is unequally distributed along social and provincial lines. Fifty percent of the national revenue is controlled by just 5 percent of the population, and more than half is concentrated in just the two provinces of Kinshasa and Katanga (UNICEF 1996). Disparities also exist between mining and agricultural areas.

The economic infrastructure has been more affected by this unfavorable economic situation than has the social structure. The people of the DRC, because they lack access to healthcare, education, and potable water, have developed survival strategies that have driven the formation of the informal sector. This informal economy, although dynamic, circumvents taxation structures and the bank circuit (UNICEF 1996). Additional economic indicators are provided in Table 31.3.

Macroeconomic mismanagement for 40 years coupled with monetary hyperinflation has exhausted the Congolese economy and impoverished the population. Measures taken to deter the inflation of the Congolese franc (CF) have not had their intended effect. Put into circulation in 1998 with an exchange rate of CF3 per U.S.$1, the Congolese franc is now exchanged at CF90 per U.S.$1 in the parallel market during the year 2000, whereas the government maintains the official exchange rate at CF23.5 per U.S.$1. Commercial import-export transactions were significantly complicated by this double exchange rate structure. Currently, substantial efforts are being made by the government to maintain both the official and the parallel exchange rates at about CF330 per U.S.$1.

The rivers that irrigate the country from both sides of the equator provide both transportation and hydrologic potential. The DRC possesses 50 percent of the hydrologic power capacity of the entire continent. The country also has 13,000 kilometers of navigable waters, although this length is interrupted by rapids. In addition to this fluvial network, the nation has 148 kilometers of maritime canals and 13,000 kilometers of lake connections. A lack of dredging and insufficiencies in the beaconing system have greatly reduced the functionality of this network. The authority responsible for this work, La Regie des Voies Fluviales (the River/Water Routes Authority), lacks the necessary resources to do so.

TABLE 31.3

Economic and Social Indicators

GNP per capita (U.S.$)	110
Human Development Index score	0.479
Percent of GNP to health	1

SOURCE: UNDP (1999).

Until the mid-1980s, the DRC had a railroad system that covered 5,138 kilometers. Lack of maintenance has made a large portion of this system unusable or obsolete. In addition, the country has 145,100 kilometers of roads, 2,400 kilometers of which are paved. Again, because of the lack of upkeep, only a small portion of this system is currently viable. The country's supply of manufactured products is negatively affected by the lack of motor fuel and spare parts, even though the DRC is a producer of motor fuel.

Education

The DRC is fighting an ever-widening gap between the supply of and demand for education. The Congolese State is no longer capable of financing national education, which has resulted in an inability to accommodate new students. Nor is the government capable of building or improving education infrastructure. Classes are overcrowded, and payment of teachers is modest and irregular. Many private schools have appeared to accommodate the growing school-age population. Unfortunately, these schools put more of an emphasis on finances than on the quality of education; this has led to a worrisome decrease in school attendance, especially among girls.

Several factors explain the limited access to education, including acute poverty, which makes payment of school fees by parents impossible; lack of engagement in the education sector by the government; the priority given to military needs over the needs of the education infrastructure; and increasing pressure of more immediate social needs.

In spite of moderate literacy levels (82.5 percent for men and 56.8 percent for women), the crisis in the education sector has meant that a large proportion of children never attend school. In 1995, 28.6 percent of children between the ages of 6 and 14 (25.7 percent of boys and 31.5 percent of girls) had never been to school. In the same year, 86 percent of boys and 59 percent of girls were enrolled in primary school. As a result, illiteracy is on the rise in the DRC. A study by Lututala and colleagues (1996) found that 67.8 percent of boys and 68 percent of girls between the ages of 6 and 14 years in the capital of Kinshasa could not read or write; the same study also found that one woman in three above the age of 26 years was illiterate. Educational data are provided in Table 31.4.

Context: Health Needs

Development activities including health promotion, investment, income generation, and environmental protection are impossible in the DRC while the country is in a state of war. A number of public health problems require immediate attention, including the deterioration of the health infrastructure, the lack of medical and pharmaceutical products, the shortages of qualified personnel, and the low morale among health service providers.

TABLE 31.4
Education
Indicators
(percent)

	Male	Female
Adult literacy rate	82.3	56.8
Primary school enrollment	86	59
Secondary school enrollment	32	19

SOURCE: Ministère de la Santé Publique (1999a).

The interior of the country is especially hard hit in terms of human, material, and financial resources. The following are the DRC's most pressing health needs at present:

- rehabilitation of damaged and destroyed medical and health infrastructures, construction of new facilities with adequate equipment for medical training, and provision of basic supplies such as essential medications
- improvement of general health conditions, principally access to safe drinking water and sanitary facilities
- training, continuing education, and equitable geographic redistribution of healthcare personnel
- establishment of a health information system with adequate communication resources for emergency management
- augmentation of health coverage in nonfunctional health zones through financial support and technical assistance
- legislation governing the operation of health zones and partnerships
- good government in a participatory democracy (created through decentralization) without external interference
- promotion of traditional medicine and scientific research

The accomplishment of these goals will not be possible until the macroeconomic balance is restored, which in turn must be accompanied by the reestablishment of all channels of communication. Only an improvement in economic conditions will increase the population's purchasing power and consequently its use of health services.

Because of the numerous conflicts, macroeconomic deterioration and its corollaries (i.e., hyperinflation, damaged or destroyed infrastructure, breakdown of international cooperation), and the longest, most tumultuous political transition in Africa, the interventions of exterior partners have been limited to humanitarian efforts. The DRC has not yet ratified a law governing the intervention of outside organizations (partners) in the health sector, which leaves an absence of aid in some sectors and an over-

concentration in others. The majority of these partners distrusts the polit-
ical-administrative structures of the state and bypasses them by working
with local, nongovernmental organizations. By doing so, these partners
dismiss the state's experts in favor of expatriate colleagues who often lack
expertise.

Since the implementation of the Structural Adjustment Program
financed by the World Bank, the Congolese people, who are rarely consulted regarding programs that concern them, have harbored a strong
distrust of it. This population, as represented by their leaders, does not
believe in the sincerity of the fight against poverty; they see much money
being spent on the comforts of the exterior partners at the expense of
the intended beneficiaries. Although good management is recommended,
local and international nongovernmental organizations have not yet shown
financial accountability through financial reporting to the representatives
of the beneficiaries.

During the past ten years, the country has seen several epidemics in
addition to the reemergence of a number of infectious diseases and para-
sites. Accurate estimates of the extent of these diseases are unavailable
because of the lack of reliable information. The principle causes of morbidity as reported by health organizations are malaria, acute respiratory
infections, helminth infections, diarrhea, sexually transmitted diseases,
tuberculosis, measles, cholera, meningitis, and typhoid fever (Ministère de
la Santé Publique 1999). The lack of available safe water for a majority of
the population, poor individual and community hygiene, and an unhealthy
environment have resulted in the emergence of diarrheal diseases such as
cholera, bacterial dysentery, and typhoid fever. Data regarding access to
health-enhancing factors are provided in Table 31.5.

In 1996, 190 deaths from cholera were reported in the Eastern
Province, and 65 were reported in Katanga. Poliomyelitis caused 37 deaths
in the Eastern Kasaï, and 1,025 deaths occurred from measles in Katanga
(Ministère de la Santé Publique 1997a). Malaria remains the primary cause
of death, especially in children. Children under five have, on average, ten
episodes of malaria per year. Childhood diseases (particularly measles,
poliomyelitis, and neonatal tetanus), continue to threaten the lives of chil-

Access to health services	26	**TABLE 31.5** Access to Health- Enhancing Factors (percent)
Access to safe water	46.7	
Access to sanitation	17.4	
Immunization levels	29	

SOURCE: Ministère de la Santé Publique (1999a).

dren in the DRC. Sickle-cell anemia, which is endemic in the DRC, and other parasitic diseases such as trypanosomiasis (sleeping sickness), onchocerciasis (river blindness), and schistosomiasis also constitute major public health problems. The prevalence of leprosy is 2 per every 1,000 population and the annual risk of tuberculosis infection is 3 percent.

Examples of infectious and viral epidemics occurring in the past five years include the following:

- monkey pox (East Kasaï, Equateur, Eastern Province, and some cases in Kinshasa)
- Hemorrhagic fever caused by the Ebola virus (near the equator in 1976, in Bandundu in 1995, and in Durba-Watsa in 1999)
- cerebrospinal meningitis (Kivu, Katanga, Maniema, Equateur, Bandundu, and Kasaï)
- plague (Eastern Province at Ituri)
- poliomyelitis (1,000 cases in Mbuji-Mayi and its surroundings in 1995)

HIV/AIDS is a growing concern, although the observed prevalence in the general population seems to have stabilized at 5 percent. Incomplete information from war-torn provinces in the east indicate the likelihood of a large increase in HIV/AIDS cases in the near future; population movement and the presence of large foreign armies in the country may explain this increase. In addition to the war, the practice of certain risky sexual behaviors, unsafe blood transfusions, lack of educational materials and medicines, and the apathy of the community in fighting HIV/AIDS constitute major obstacles to controlling its spread. More than 42,000 AIDS cases have been reported since 1983.

In spite of efforts made with regard to reproductive health, maternal mortality was reported as 870 per 100,000 live births until 1999, when an inventory by the government found a much higher figure: 1,837 maternal deaths per 100,000 live births. Modern contraceptive usage is low (5 percent), and the abortion rate is believed to be high, especially among teenagers and unmarried young women.

Organization and Management of the Health System

During the first years of the First Republic, the DRC, with the help of international cooperation, administered a health system considered by many as a model for the African countries. This system has made possible the implementation of a primary healthcare strategy that provided both acceptable coverage and quality care.

The harsh changes that occurred from 1986 through 1990 halted this progress. A structural readjustment program instigated by the International Monetary Fund and the World Bank resulted in the government's abandonment of nearly all social sectors. Left on their own, the Congolese people were forced to develop coping mechanisms that permitted them to meet minimal survival needs in the face of continuing catastrophes, war, and epidemics.

Programs to promote health and combat disease have suffered since the breakdown of international cooperation in the 1990s; some of these programs have ceased to exist. This breakdown has resulted in the frequent occurrence of epidemics, the resurgence of certain diseases long ago brought under control (e.g., trypanosomiasis), and the appearance of deadly new entities, the most serious of which is Ebola hemorrhagic fever. This epidemic, which ravaged Kikwit in 1995, served as the impetus for national and international partners in the field of humanitarian assistance to enact a plan of action for the mobilization and coordination of health resources called the Interagency Committee. This committee forms part of a World Health Organization initiative and has since carried out several humanitarian interventions.

Organization of the Health System

The Congolese health system has three levels: the central (strategic) level, the intermediate (logistic) level, and the peripheral (operational) level. As the strategic administrator of the DRC's health system, the central level plays an important role in the conception and orientation of national health policy and relevant strategies; decision making, coordination, and evaluation; the compilation and analysis of information from intermediate and peripheral levels; and communication with different health partners. The intermediate level is responsible for the logistics involved in the training and coordination of health zones. This level comprises 11 provincial and 47 district medical inspectors, each one managing 7 to 20 health zones where they coordinate and supervise activities. Three provinces, North Kivu, South Kivu, and Maniema, as well as the capital of Kinshasa, do not have intermediary district structures. See Figure 31.1 for a depiction of the organization of the Ministry of Health.

The peripheral level, comprised of health zones, is responsible for the operations of the health system and thus is its foundation. A health zone is a medical-health entity located within a well-defined geographic area; each health zone is led by a head doctor (Médecin Chef de Zone) who elaborates or adopts operational plans, supervises health activities, and collects surveillance information.

Each health zone provides care for 100,000 inhabitants in rural areas and 150,000 citizens in urban areas. Each health zone is subdivided into smaller areas, each of which is served by a health center. In theory, the health center serves 5,000 people in rural areas or 10,000 in urban areas and covers a radius of 5 to 8 kilometers. Each health zone has a general referral hospital, and certain health zones also have intermediate health facilities such as referral health centers (health complexes in urban areas)

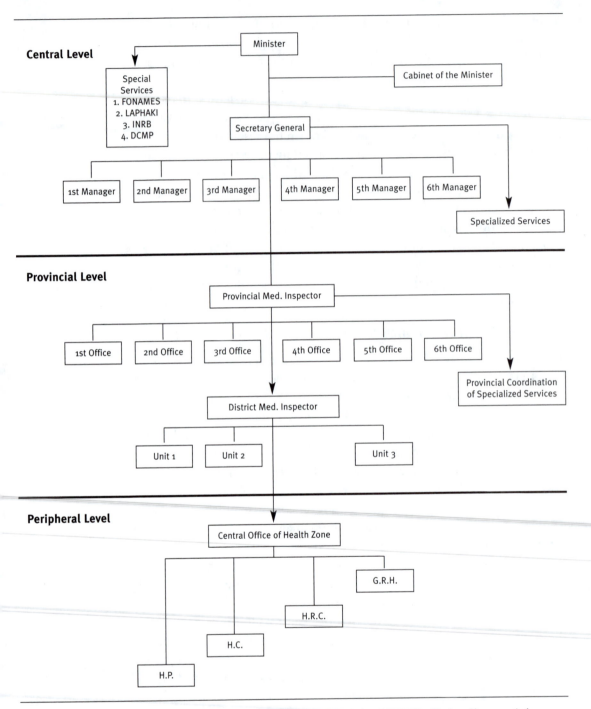

Central Level

Minister

Special Services
1. FONAMES
2. LAPHAKI
3. INRB
4. DCMP

Cabinet of the Minister

Secretary General

1st Manager | 2nd Manager | 3rd Manager | 4th Manager | 5th Manager | 6th Manager

Specialized Services

Provincial Level

Provincial Med. Inspector

1st Office | 2nd Office | 3rd Office | 4th Office | 5th Office | 6th Office

Provincial Coordination of Specialized Services

District Med. Inspector

Unit 1 | Unit 2 | Unit 3

Peripheral Level

Central Office of Health Zone

G.R.H.

H.R.C.

H.C.

H.P.

FIGURE 31.1

Organization of the Ministry of Health

NOTE: FONAMES = National Medical/Health Foundation; LAPHAKI = Kinshasa Pharmaceutical Laboratory; INRB = Biomedical National Research Institute; DCMP = Central Medical-Pharmaceutical Warehouse; H.P. = health post; H.C. = health center; H.R.C. = health referral center; G.R.H = general referral hospital.

1st Manager = of general services and personnel; 2nd Manager = of hospitals; 3rd Manager = of pharmacies and laboratories; 4th Manager = of epidemiology, large endemics, preventive medicine, hygiene, and sanitation; 5th Manager = of primary healthcare; 6th Manager = of teaching and training.

Specialized services are Central Bureau of Coordination of the Fight against HIV/AIDS, National Program of Tripanosomiasis, National Program of Onchocerciasis, National Nutrition Program, Expanded Program of Immunizations, Family Planning Program, Malaria National Program, Basic Rural Health, and Health for All–Kinshasa.

and health posts. Health zones have no legal status and function informally without any statutory law supervision.

In 1985, the DRC was divided into 306 health zones,[1] 30 percent of which were functional in 1998. To be designated as "functional," a health zone must have the following:

1. a head doctor specializing in public health
2. one general referral hospital with five basic services: internal medicine, pediatrics, surgery, gynecology/obstetrics, and diagnostic services including laboratory and radiology
3. at least three functional supervised health centers

The central office of the health zone is made up of a head doctor, an administrator/manager, a nursing supervisor, a pharmacy assistant, a sanitation specialist, and a community leader. In addition to this organizational structure, certain emergency situations, such as catastrophes and epidemics, are managed by intersectoral partners (the Ministry of the Interior, the Ministry of Plan, and the Ministry of Social Affairs). In reality, the Ministers centralize all of the power at the expense of the other structures. The proper functioning of the DRC's health system essentially depends on the partnership system described below.

Partnership in the Health System of the DRC

The term "partner" is used for all parties that contribute (individuals and organizations) to supporting the development of a health system. They may be active in any of the following areas: financing activities; training personnel; rehabilitating equipment or infrastructure; or organizing curative, preventive, and promotional care and expertise. These fall under four types of partners:

1. *International organizations:* the World Health Organization, United Nations Children's Fund, United Nations Population Fund, United Nations Development Programme, the World Bank, the European Union, and the African Development Bank
2. *Bilateral aid agencies:* the United States Agency for International Development, the Governmental Agency of Cooperation and Development (Belgium), Oxford Committee for Famine Relief (OXFAM) (Great Britain), and the Canadian International Development Agency
3. *National and international nongovernmental organizations:* the Diocese Bureau of Medical Works (Catholic); the Protestant medical network; the Kimbanguist Medical Department; the Père Damien Foundation; Doctors Without Borders; World Vision; A Better Future for AIDS Orphans (Congo); Support to Health, Parcels Service, and Information Processing; Society for Women against AIDS in Africa; and Horizon Santé

4.   *Private medical services:* General Mining Company, National Electricity Company, National Water Distribution Company, and Mining Company of Kivu

Functioning of the Healthcare System

At the Central-Strategic Level

The different institutions working at the central level often find themselves in competitive roles, which can lead to conflicts. For example, the National Medical/Health Foundation, the 5th Manager (5e Direction), and the Expanded Program of Immunization all have mission statements that call for intervening in epidemics of endemic diseases (e.g., malaria).

With the ongoing state of crisis in the DRC, the government administration does not have the capability to supervise, control, or evaluate health programs and activities. This lack of regulation allows poor service providers to continue unchecked while successful programs are not expanded. Criteria for hiring, promotion, sanctions, and salary scale depend on the supervisor, the agent, or both.

No legislation exists to govern the actions of outside organizations in the DRC. As a result, organizations have concentrated their resources in one area while other health zones are left without services. This concentration creates an overlap in activities, which leads to an increase in tension among the groups.

The percentage of the state budget allocated to health is insignificant (approximately 1 percent in 1997, although the current government has shown its goodwill by increasing this to 5 percent). Moreover, these rare human, material, and financial resources are poorly allocated, and communication among the agencies concerned is totally deficient.

At the Intermediate-Logistical Level

Program managers at the intermediate level are technically under the authority of the provincial medical inspector. However, given the lack of legal regulations, program managers (who in general have better logistical and managerial skills) often disregard this authority.

The health district is composed of three units working under the supervision of six provincial offices; no regulations exist to define the hierarchical relations between these provincial and district inspectors. At this level as at the central level, legislation is lacking for the governing of the activities of different partners.

At the Peripheral-Operational Level

Many of the doctors serving as hospital directors do not receive continuing education or training in the management of a health zone; this is also true of a number of medical chiefs of health zones. This lack of knowledge has caused numerous problems and conflicts.

Because the health zones lack legal status, the primary healthcare strategy has been applied unofficially since 1985. Likewise, no rules exist for the governing of the action of partners.

Application of Institutional Regulation (Social Security)

The DRC has had a national health insurance system since colonization. This system has evolved over time with the advent of new systems or plans. The word "plan" is used to describe a group of legal measures that govern the social protection of certain groups. The following three plans operate in the DRC:

1. the general plan, which through the National Institute of Social Security theoretically covers all workers in the private and semipublic sectors, students in professional schools, trainees, and unpaid apprentices
2. special plans, which cover a number of groups including state workers, specialty educators, scientific researchers, magistrates, parliamentarians, and members of the revenue court
3. complementary or supplementary plans, which are voluntarily organized associations that cover the risk of illness, such as mutuals, social assistance, commercial health insurance, and collective conventions in private firms

Of the services required by the World Labor Organization in Convention No. 102 (medical care, compensation for illness, unemployment, services for the elderly, services in case of work-related accidents and professional illnesses, services for families, services for disability, services for the survivor), the National Institute of Social Security in the DRC covers only two: those concerning professional risks (work-related accidents and illnesses) and pensions for the elderly or the family of the deceased.

The social security system is ineffective because of inadequate financing and mismanagement, and it covers only a minimum fraction of Congolese workers in the formal sector. The DRC economy currently functions primarily in the informal sector; although this has been true for some time, the shift to the informal economy has accelerated in recent years. According to one study, "Informal Economy of Zaire" (De Herdt and Marysse 1996), the percentage of workers in the formal sector is decreasing. In 1955, 39.9 percent of the working population was in the formal sector; in 1961, 29 percent still had formal employment. By 1990, only 5 percent of workers remained in the formal sector, leaving 95 percent of workers in the informal economy, known locally as the underground market.

In addition, between 1990 and 2000 a number of disruptive events (pillages in 1991, 1992, and 1993; interethnic conflicts; the liberation war of 1997; and the war of aggression, which has been going on since 1998) finished the already weakened economy by destroying the remaining socioeconomic infrastructure. No more than an estimated one percent of urban workers remained in the formal sector in 2000; this leaves 99 percent of Congolese workers without any legal social protection. The International

Office of Work, with its pilot health insurance system in Kinshasa, has been working since 1999 to mitigate the effects of informal sector work.

Health committees of private and semipublic enterprises have never been put into operation. Workers have had access to medical care only through existing collective agreements and only while working. The National Institute of Social Security is in breach of the law because of its inability to ensure medical care to the retired. A very few companies do provide medical care for their pensioners, including the National Office of Transport, General Mining Company, Mining Company of Kivu, Congo Petroluem Company, and the Office of Kilo-Moto.

The Training of Health Professionals in the DRC

The training of health professionals depends on their level in the health-care structure. Low-level health professionals (nurses) are trained by the Ministry of Health, where they are taught primary healthcare concepts, policies, and strategies. Doctors are trained by the Ministry of Education, where this primary healthcare philosophy is not taught.

This divergence in training objectives limits the effectiveness of the country's primary healthcare strategy. For this reason, the Ministry of Health, with the aid of partner organizations, provides specialized on-the-job training for doctors. In addition, since 1986, the School of Public Health of the University of Kinshasa, with the support of certain partners, has trained specialists in public health to ensure the successful application of the public healthcare strategy.

Financing

The health sector of the DRC is financed by international organizations (the World Health Organization, the United Nations Children's Fund, and the United Nations Population Fund), foreign nongovernmental organizations (Doctors Without Borders [France and Belgium], the Père Damien Foundation, the Medice Missie Saenwerking, and the Tropical Medicine Foundation), bilateral aid (Belgium, France, Italy, Germany, the United States, Japan, China), churches (Catholic, Protestant, Kimbanguist), households, and other local associations, as well as the Congolese State, in spite of its current difficulties.

The percentage that each of these sources contributes to the total financing has not been assessed. However, the public-sector contribution is negligible in comparison with other sources; in fact, the Congolese government dedicates only 1 to 2 percent of the national budget to the health sector (Ministère de la Santé Publique 1997). Patients must pay for all health services in both the public and private sectors. The price scale is unregulated; the price-fixing rules that exist are not applied (with some exceptions).

Modes of Payment

In practice, five modes of payment for healthcare are used or have been used by the population—no legislation governs their use:

1. Payment by episode of sickness, including the cost of medications and laboratory expenses: this mode is not currently used because of the difficulty of financing an inventory of medical supplies.
2. Payment by episode of sickness, not including the cost of medications: this is the mode of payment used most widely in health centers, especially those of religious missions; its intended objective is to encourage the use of health services and follow-up care with one payment covering one week of healthcare.
3. Payment by service given in hospitals, polyclinics, and private dispensaries.
4. Payment by a third party: this mode of payment benefits employees and their families. Notably this scheme is rarely followed in reality because of difficulties within the economic climate, and for this reason enlisting financing by private and public businesses (companies, which provided 142 million dollars of financing in 1989, were able to provide health services to 27 percent of the Congolese population) is necessary. This coverage has deteriorated considerably because of two pillages (1991 and 1993) that damaged a large part of the production equipment.
5. Prepayment: this is rarely seen in health zones.

Payment by any of these methods does not always mean an exchange of currency. Leaving something of value as a "deposit" (e.g., a chicken, a goat, a basket of manioc) until funds become available to make a payment or to make a payment in kind is common. These practices make managing a health center difficult.

Health resources are unequally distributed within the state. Provinces are not informed of their allocation, and they receive virtually nothing. Each province has strategies and investment plans that are neither implemented nor monitored because of a lack of finances. The implementation of all of these plans depends primarily on external aid, followed by payment of services by families, and lastly by the government. The Ministry of Health takes charge of epidemics, occasional emergencies due to increases in the internally displaced population (due to war), malnutrition, and vaccination, but it does not take responsibility for all components of primary healthcare.

Regarding insurance, social legislation theoretically protects employees in the private and public sector. However, the government has no budget to cover healthcare, and within companies, the right to medical care is not legally protected because of the National Institute of Social Security's limited ability to intervene.

Individuals have organized themselves to collect a certain amount of money each month to provide for the "emergency" needs of the group (e.g., travel, school fees). Because of the economic crisis gripping the country, these collectives are shifting toward health insurance purposes, although this was not their intended objective. These collectives attempt to cover many risks without substantial knowledge of financing schemes for these services, and they often fail from a lack of managerial experience. They also suffer because people are not familiar with the concept of paying in advance for anticipated risks. The national legislation regarding these organizations does not include protection for the abused beneficiary.

Health Resources

Human Resources

A severe shortage of all medical personnel exists in the DRC, as demonstrated in Table 31.6.

Health Facilities

The DRC has 258 general referral hospitals, 684 referral health centers, 4,555 health centers, 32 specialized clinics, 73 nonspecialized hospitals, 155 hospitals, 1,146 maternity hospitals, 3,473 community clinics, 237 medical laboratories, and 266 pharmaceutical warehouses in the DRC (Ministère de la Santé Publique 1999a). The majority of these health facilities are located in urban areas, with the exception of some rural facilities managed by private organizations and religious missions.

Products

The provision of essential medications by health centers, especially those of the government, is very irregular. Local production of medication is insufficient, and its use is erratic; self-medication has become a popular practice. Medications of doubtful quality are constantly circulating in the population. The recourse to traditional medication is substantial, driven by the extreme poverty of the population and the unavailability of alternatives; studies show that in some areas of Kinshasa, 70 percent of the population has used medicinal plants (Paulus 1995).

The medication provision and distribution system of the government, the Central Medical-Pharmaceutical Warehouse, is no longer functional, and the DRC currently has only one distribution service, the Regional Association for the Supply of Essential Medicines, which has been in the Nord-Kivu since 1994. Accessibility to essential medications is 37 percent (Ministère de la Santé Publique 1999a). Pharmacies are not equitably distributed, and their hours are often unpredictable. Medical facilities are dilapidated, and their equipment is in a state of disrepair because of wear,

Category	Number of Personnel	Ratio	WHO Norms
Doctors	3,801	0.808	1 per 10,000
Pharmacists	800	0.850	1 per 50,000
Dentists	500	0.319	1 per 30,000
Nurses A1	1,286	0.136	1 per 5,000
Nurses A2	6,457	0.274	1 per 2,000
Nurses A3	19,858	0.845	1 per 2,000
Physiotherapists	66	0.007	1 per 5,000
Laboratory technicians	93	0.016	1 per 5,000
Radio technicians	155	0.029	1 per 15,000
Sanitation technicians	105	0.033	1 per 15,000
Pharmaceutical assistants	600	0.063	1 per 5,000
Anesthesiologists	90	0.028	1 per 15,000
Traditional practitioners	25,000	N/A	N/A

TABLE 31.6
Distribution of Medical Personnel by Category

NOTE: Total estimated 1997 population of 47 million. Private sector not included.
SOURCE: Ministère de la Santé Publique (1997).

a lack of spare parts, and the absence of trained and competent maintenance workers and user manuals.

The central and provincial administrations do not have the means to effectively control the quality of medications sold in pharmacies. This is especially a problem in times of hardship or war, when a permanent danger of the sale of false or outdated medications exists. Only one pharmacy school exists in the entire country, and as a result, the DRC has very few pharmacists; the qualified few are primarily concentrated in Kinshasa. In light of the lack of a national pharmacology system, the Belgian system, which is inappropriate for the tropical Congo, is still being used. The wild liberalization of the economy during the Second Republic resulted in the deregulation of medication prices, which are now exorbitant, making these medications financially inaccessible to the population. In addition, the list of essential medications has never been publicized. The traditional sector, which meets the healthcare needs of the majority of the population, lacks scientific and administrative training. Pharmaceutical policies addressing these issues were created in 1997, but they still have not been implemented.

TABLE 31.7
Number and
Types of
Health
Services
Facilities and
by Population

	Number	Per 1,000 Population
Hospitals	258	0.005
Health centers	4,555	0.096
General clinics	73	0.0015
Specialty clinics	32	0.00068

SOURCE: Ministère de la Santé Publique (1999a).

Service Delivery

A large disparity exists between rural and urban areas and between the rich
and the poor with regard to healthcare accessibility. In general, the highest quality and greatest number of services are concentrated in urban areas
(70 percent of doctors practice in urban areas.)

The majority of the Congolese people do not have access to quality care. Distant healthcare facilities are inaccessible because of poorly
maintained or nonexistent roads and the high price of transportation. The
high cost of healthcare puts it out of reach of most of the population,
whose purchasing power is weak (the United Nations Development
Programme classifies the DRC among the least-developed countries in the
world with a gross national product around U.S.$100 per capita, despite
the country's enormous potential). In addition, many people, especially
in rural areas, prefer traditional practitioners and self-medication or distrust Western medicine.

The third level of the healthcare system responsible for treating more
serious illnesses is accessible only to a rare few: the wealthy, politicians,
expatriates, and high-level executives of the administration and public and
private enterprises.

The first level of care corresponds to the peripheral level. Sick individuals may go to the health center or hospital of their choice, depending
on their financial and geographic situation. Many people arrive too late for
effective treatment at the health center and lack the means to support a
transfer to a referral hospital; an unfortunate consequence of this is that
many sick people die after their first contact with the health center. This
explains a large part of the high infant and maternal mortality rates.

Health centers offer a vast range of curative services, from basic treatment of parasitic and infectious diseases to ambulatory surgery. They also
provide essential preventive services. Health centers are in charge of vaccination and encourage children and pregnant women to participate in
their preschool and prenatal preventative programs. In rural areas, health

centers generally include a maternity ward of 5 to 15 beds and several beds for minor surgery, and they may also offer a variety of health education activities. They often own a microscope for simple diagnostic laboratory tests and some, particularly those belonging to religious missions, have basic stocks of medications and the minimum laboratory kit.

Referral health centers offer, in addition to the services provided by the health center, numerous hospital services similar to those offered by the main hospitals, including a maternity ward and surgical services.

A general referral hospital has about 100 beds and offers hospital services in obstetrics, surgery, general medicine, pediatrics, nutrition, prenatal observation, laboratory tests, and radiology. Each general referral hospital has a maternity ward and sometimes a blood bank.

The second level of the healthcare system corresponds to the intermediate level and is made up of provincial and district hospitals, which are reputed to be better-equipped. These facilities receive only well-to-do patients because of their higher price scales.

The third level corresponds to the central level and is composed of specialized medical facilities such as university clinics or large research laboratories. Because of the exorbitant costs, only a small number of executives, businessmen, and very wealthy families have access to these facilities; a poor person suffering from a cardiac problem or cancer would have no chance of receiving the necessary care.

Because of inadequate salaries, medical personnel are unmotivated, lack respect for ethics, misuse public funds, and are forced to take multiple jobs to ensure their own survival. As a consequence, patients do not receive quality care. This is another reason for the recourse to traditional medicine. Traditional practitioners are numerous and active in the cities, although they are not legally authorized to practice. Health education activities (e.g., vaccination, family planning) are handicapped by the fact that radio and television programs do not reach rural areas. At several kilometers outside the city, health messages by radio and television routes cannot be transmitted.

Prospects for the Future

Since the structural readjustment program instigated by the IMF and the World Bank in 1986, the DRC has been faced with a severe health crisis. This crisis compromises human capital—the first and most important resource of all nations—and is the result of the progressive reduction of national resources allocated to health. It poses an obstacle to development efforts and will continue to do so if the war persists. Health indicators are poor, despite the application of primary healthcare strategies since the 1980s. In theory, health services should meet the needs of local communities, which are the supposed beneficiaries of the primary healthcare strategy; this is not currently the situation. The Congolese people have long complained about this inadequate system, and the current government has begun to seriously consider healthcare reform.

As a result, a situational analysis was carried out in 1998 and 1999. The report of this analysis is now available and illustrates the miserable state of health in the DRC. Because of these results, numerous seminars, workshops, and meetings were held to discuss the restructuring of the entire health system, including establishing national strategies and legislation, mobilizing national resources, and attracting outside partners to aid in local efforts. The proposed changes are as follows:

- Rehabilitate and maintain health infrastructures, medical-health facilities, and social establishments (e.g., health centers, hospitals, training establishments, sports centers, gymnasiums).
- Ensure that a majority of the Congolese people has access to quality healthcare by making essential medications both available and accessible and by encouraging the local pharmaceutical industry.
- Protect poor and vulnerable populations, including children, women, the physically and mentally handicapped, the elderly, beggars, delinquents, street children, sexual perverts, and drug addicts (including alcoholics and those addicted to tobacco products).
- Organize an emergency management system for endemic epidemics and natural or human catastrophes according to national health standards.
- Promote traditional medicine and scientific research.
- Increase sanitation and accelerate the provision of potable water and nutrition.
- Increase the effectiveness of the health system through the efficient and rational management of human, material, and financial resources, which will involve greater participation among the population in designing programs that concern them as well as their participation within management.

The crisis in the DRC is an opportunity for the Congolese people to rethink public health; many of the objectives of the Health for All by the Year 2000 program have not been achieved. Serious evaluation is needed to determine the best strategies to catch up and accelerate these programs to meet the pressing demands of the Congolese population, especially in light of rapid population growth.

The current national political legislation, seen by many as a positive step, should be enacted quickly to address the challenges faced by political and administrative authorities as well as healthcare providers in meeting the needs of the population. It is crucial to include an evaluation plan to ensure that all problems found in the execution are corrected as quickly as possible.

Finally, the Congolese people are scrutinizing the Inter-Congolese Dialogue held in Sun City, South Africa in March 2002 and hope to go back to normal life in the coming years.

Note

1. The DRC health map is currently under reorganization to move from 306 health zones to about 500 health zones in an effort to improve geographic access to health services.

Acknowledgments

The authors wish to acknowledge Allison Tetler and Kristina Lantis for the translation and editing of this chapter.

REFERENCES

Baer, F. 2002 "Coordination of Health Zones and Their Partners in the Democratic Republic of Congo." SANRU III Project, Kinshasa. Retrieved February 2002 from http://sanru.net.

De Herdt, T., and Marysse, S. 1996. *Economie Informelle au Zaire: Survie et Pauvrete dans la Periode de Transition*. Paris: Ed. L'Harmattan, Centre for Development Studies, Universitaire Faculteiten St Ignatius; Belgium: Universiteit Antwerpen.

Department of Demography of the University of Kinshasa (DDK). 1998. *La Question Demographique en Republique Demographique du Congo*. Kinshasa: DDK.

Institut National de la Statistique (INS). 1984. *Zaïre, Un Aperçu Démographique*. Kinshasa: INS.

———. 1993. *Projections Démographiques au Zaïre et en Régions 1984–2000*. Kinshasa: INS.

Lututala, M., et al. 1996. *La Dynamique des Structures Familiales et Acces des Femmes a l'Education*. Kinshasa: DDK.

Ministère de la Santé Publique. 1997. "OK et Ornanisation Mondiale de la Sante (OMS)." Rapport de la Troisième Évaluation de la Mise en Œuvre de la Stratégie de la Santé pour Tous d'Ici l'An 2000. Kinshasa: Ministère de la Santé Publique.

———. 1997a. *Programme Elargi des Vaccinations (PEV) Evaluation externe du PEV en 1996*. Kinshasa: Ministère de la Santé Publique.

———. 1999. *OK. Plan Directeur de Développement Sanitaire pour la Période 2000–2009*. Kinshasa: Ministère de la Santé Publique.

———. 1999a. *OK et Organisation Mondiale de la Sante Etat des lieux du Secteur de la Santé en 1998*. Kinshasa: Ministère de la Santé Publique.

Ministère du Plan. 1998. *Direction des Études Macro-économiques*. Kinshasa: Rapport.

Ngondo P. 1992. *Perspectives Demographiques du Zaire, 1984–1999 et Population d'Age Electoral en 1993 et 1994.* Kinshasa: CEPAS.

———. 1998. "A Combien Sommes-nous et d'u Viennent ces Chiffres?" In *La Question Démographique en République Démocratique du Congo*, pp. 15–24. Kinshasa: DDK.

Paulus, J. 1995. *Enquête PLAM.* Kinshasa: Faculté des Sciences, Université de Kinshasa.

United Nations Children's Fund (UNICEF) and Ministère du Plan. 1996. *Enquête Nationale sur la Situation des Enfants et des Femmes (ENSEF) au Zaïre en 1995.* Kinshasa: UNICEF.

United Nations Development Programme (UNDP). 1999. *Human Development Report 1999.* New York: Oxford University Press.

GLOSSARY OF TERMS

AIDS	acquired immune deficiency syndrome
EU	European Union
GDP	gross domestic product
GNP	gross national product
HIV	human immunodeficiency virus
IMF	International Monetary Fund
NATO	North American Treaty Organization
OECD	Organization for Economic Cooperation and Development
PAHO	Pan-American Health Organization
P.P.P.	purchasing power parity
UNAIDS	United Nations Programme on HIV/AIDS
UNICEF	United Nations Children's Fund
UNDP	United Nations Development Programme
USAID	United States Agency for International Development
WHO	World Health Organization

INDEX

ABOUT THE EDITORS

Bruce J. Fried, Ph.D., is an associate professor in the Department of Health Policy and Administration in the School of Public Health at the University of North Carolina at Chapel Hill. He is director of the master's degree program in the department and a research fellow at the Cecil G. Sheps Center for Health Services Research. Dr. Fried teaches in the areas of organizational theory and human resources management and work force issues in healthcare. His research interests include mental health services, workforce issues, and interorganizational relationships. He has worked with a variety of organizations nationally and internationally in the areas of strategic planning and human resources management. He received his undergraduate degree from the State University of New York at Buffalo, his master's degree from the University of Chicago, and his doctoral degree from the University of North Carolina at Chapel Hill.

Laura Gaydos is pursuing her Ph.D. in health policy and administration at the University of North Carolina at Chapel Hill. Prior to her doctoral studies, she conducted healthcare research and planning activities for the Health Care Advisory Board, Washington, DC, in the areas of women's health and maternal/child health. Ms. Gaydos has also worked extensively in the field of domestic HIV/AIDS policy, with specific focus on youth education and syringe access policies for intravenous drug users. Her current research interests include reproductive health, HIV/AIDS, and international health systems.

ABOUT THE CONTRIBUTORS

Alexandre Abrantes, Ph.D., D.P.H., is sector manager for human development at the World Bank. Mr. Abrantes previously worked as a health specialist developing projects and providing technical assistance to the governments of Argentina, Brazil, Chile, Paraguay, Peru, South Africa, Uganda, Uruguay, and Venezuela and as a scientific officer of the Commission of the European Union. Mr. Abrantes also practiced medicine in Portugal, was professor of preventive medicine and public health at the Lisbon (Portugal) Medical School and the National School of Public Health, also in Lisbon.

Jane T. Bertrand, Ph.D., M.B.A., is director of the Center for Communication Programs and professor in the Department of Population and Family Health Sciences at the Johns Hopkins University Bloomberg School of Public Health. Formerly a faculty member at Tulane University in New Orleans, Louisiana, she worked from 1980 through 1990 in the Democratic Republic of the Congo (then Zaire) to establish family planning services throughout the country.

Jay Bhattacharya, M.D., Ph.D., is an assistant professor of medicine at the Stanford University School of Medicine's Center for Primary Care and Outcomes Research. Dr. Bhattacharya received his medical degree in 1997 and a doctorate in economics in 2000, both from Stanford University, California. Previously, he was an economist at RAND in Santa Monica, California and a visiting assistant professor at the University of California Los Angeles. His current research focuses on the economics of healthcare for special populations in the United States, including HIV positive individuals, the elderly, the disabled, and the mentally ill.

Gerhard Brenner, Dr. rer. pol., has served on various German national and European project coordination teams and as a temporary adviser of the World Health Organization. Dr. Brenner is the author of more than one hundred scientific publications on a variety of topics in the fields of healthcare and healthcare economics published in national and international publications. He has participated in and helped organize congresses on the German national and international levels and has participated in several projects sponsored by the European Commission. Dr. Brenner is also a member of many healthcare-related boards and organizations.

Eric Buch, M.B.B.Ch., M.Sc.(Med), FFCH(CM)(SA), is a professor of Health Policy and Management in the schools of Health Systems and Public Health and of Public Management and Administration at the University of Pretoria, South Africa. In the 1980s he combined his role as an academic with anti-apartheid health activism and rural and non-governmental organization health project developments. In the 1990s he held executive management positions in the emerging post-apartheid health system. He has written extensively on health and healthcare in South Africa. Dr. Buch is registered as a specialist in community health with the South African government.

Ana María Carrillo is a sociologist pursuing a Ph.D. in history. She is a professor in the Department of Public Health of the Autonomous National University of Mexico. She has published articles and chapters in books on the history of professions and of public health. In 2000, Ms. Carrillo was awarded the National Susana San Juan essay prize for her essay, "Traditional Midwives: Their Contribution to Humanity from Prehistory to the Twenty-first Century."

Andrea Cortinois, B.Sc., M.P.H., is a Ph.D. candidate in the Department of Health Policy, Management and Evaluation at the University of Toronto in Ontario, Canada. Mr. Cortinois also works as a research associate at the Centre for Global eHealth Innovation, a joint initiative of the University of Toronto and the University Health Network. Prior to his doctoral work, Mr Cortinois worked for 10 years as a scientific journalist, specializing in health-related issues, and for 15 years in international health, mainly in Latin America developing research activities, managing health-related interventions, and teaching at the postgraduate level. His most recent research activities focus on the use of health services by recent immigrants to Toronto and on the application of new information and communication technologies to reach underserved populations.

Julia Field Costich, J.D., Ph.D., is on the faculty of the University of Kentucky Center for Health Services Management and Research and School of Public Health, where she teaches health law to public health and health professions students. She administered health insurance programs for the state of Kentucky from 1994 to 1997. Her previous experience includes the private practice of healthcare law, clinical services administration, and teaching French.

Kelly Matthews Deal, M.P.H., is a research associate at the Durham Veterans Administration Medical Center, working on a project to improve patient-provider communication. She recently completed coursework for a Ph.D. in health policy and administration at the University of North Carolina at Chapel Hill and completed her master's of public health degree at the University of Utah, Salt Lake City, in 1996. Ms. Matthews Deal has worked in the areas of international disease prevention, reproductive health, and program evaluation.

William H. Dow, Ph.D., is assistant professor of health policy and administration at the University of North Carolina at Chapel Hill. He has a Ph.D. in economics from Yale University and in 1998 was a Fulbright Scholar at the University of Costa Rica. He received the 1999 Kenneth J. Arrow best paper award from the International Health Economics Association and the 2001 John D. Thompson Prize for Young Investigators from the Association of University Programs in Health Administration.

Teresa Maria Durães, M.H.A., is a hospital administrator working in Amadora/Sintra Hospital, the first privately managed public hospital in Portugal. She received her master's degree from the University of North Carolina at Chapel Hill in 2000, during which time she received a scholarship from Luso-American Development Foundation. She has also worked as a social psychologist, a consultant in the Ministry of Health on a National Clinical Performance Appraisal Project, a coordinator for health training programs with the European Social Fund, and an intensive care nurse with the first Portuguese team to perform a cardiac transplant.

Péter Gaál, M.Sc., works for the Health Services Management Training Centre, Semmelweis University, Budapest, Hungary, where he is a lecturer of health policy and the director of the master of health administration program. He is also working on his Ph.D. concerning informal payment systems in Hungary at the University of London. His professional areas of interest are health policy and health system management.

Juan Jose Garcia Garcia, M.D., is a physician, full-time professor, and epidemiologist in the Department of Public Health at the Faculty of Medicine of the Autonomous National University of Mexico. He has published articles on epidemiologic methods and public health analysis with special focus on pediatric and elderly populations.

Laurie J. Goldsmith, M.Sc., is a research associate at the Cecil G. Sheps Center for Health Services Research and a doctoral candidate in the Department of Health Policy and Administration at the University of North Carolina at Chapel Hill. Her research interests include comparative healthcare systems, the politics of healthcare delivery, access to care, the measurement of underservice, and the use of qualitative methods in health services research. Previously, Ms. Goldsmith was a researcher at the Centre for Health Economics and Policy Analysis at McMaster University in Hamilton, Ontario, Canada.

Revital Gross, Ph.D., is a senior researcher and deputy director of the Health Policy Research Program at the JDC-Brookdale Institute in Jerusalem, Israel. She is also a senior lecturer at the Bar-Ilan University School of Social Work and has been appointed guest editor of the *Social Security Journal of Welfare and Social Security Studies* special edition entitled "The Israeli Health Care System Following Implementation of the National Health Insurance Law." Dr. Gross has been studying Israeli healthcare reform since the enactment of the National Health Insurance law in 1995. Her other research areas include the role of primary care physicians, implementation of guidelines in primary care, quality assurance programs, and women's health.

Jorge Hadad Hadad, M.D., M.P.H., is the former dean of the National School of Public Health in the Faculty of Medicine, Havana, Cuba. He remains a professor at this and several other health training institutes in Cuba. His current major responsibility is as the director of the National Programme for the Hospitalization of International Visitors.

Wade Hanna, M.D., M.P.H., FFARCSI, is a senior service fellow at the Division of Public Health Systems Development and Research at the Centers for Disease Control and Prevention in Atlanta, Georgia. Previously, he was chairman of the Department of Anaesthesia and Intensive Care at the University of the West Indies in Kingston, Jamaica. Dr. Hanna has a wide base of experience with a variety of health systems in different countries. He is currently the deputy director of the World Health Collaborating Center for Public Health Systems and Practice at the Centers for Disease Control and Prevention.

Helena Hnilicová, Ph.D., is assistant professor of the Institute of Social Medicine and Public Health at the First Medical School, Charles University, Prague, Czech Republic. She is also involved in the postgraduate education program in public health organized by the School of Public Health of the Institute of Postgraduate Medical Education in Prague. Her professional interests are in the fields of healthcare systems, human resources management, and organizational behavior. She participates in research projects on patient satisfaction and quality of life.

Maarjorie Holding Cobham, M.D., is director of policy, planning, and develoment for the Ministry of Health in Jamaica. She is a public health–trained physician who has practiced in Jamaica and served as a lecturer at the University of the West Indies, Mona, Jamaica, during the 1980s. She has done consultancies for several international bodies and has managed diverse health projects.

Carel IJsselmuiden, M.D., M.P.H., FFCH, is professor of epidemiology and director of the School of Health Systems and Public Health at the

University of Pretoria in South Africa. He has more than 20 years of experience in rural and urban healthcare provision, assessment, evaluation, and management. He has been involved in healthcare transformation in various roles: currently he is a member of the Essential National Health Research Committee and the National Ethics Committee appointed by the Minister of Health. His present focus is on high-level personnel education for the health sector, health research ethics, and environmental health and epidemiology.

Zhou Jian, M.D., M.H.A., was recently appointed the director of the Department of External Relations and Projects Management, the International Health Exchange Center, Ministry of Health, People's Republic of China. He practiced medicine and medical administration for 16 years, including participation in a one-year international exchange program. He earned his medical degree in 1984 at Western China University of Medical Sciences (now merged with Sichuan University) in Chengdu, Sichuan Province, and his M.H.A. in 1994 at the University of New South Wales in Sydney, Australia.

Anna Johnson, M.S.P.H., is a health services researcher at the R. Stuart Dickson Institute for Health Studies in Charlotte, North Carolina. Her research interests include community health, health promotion, and disease prevention.

Hye-Young Kang, Ph.D., is a research assistant professor in the Department of Public Health, the Graduate School of Yonsei University, Seoul, Republic of Korea. Dr. Kang received her master's degree in pharmacy administration and her doctoral degree in health policy and administration from University of North Carolina at Chapel Hill. Her major research areas are quality assessment/assurance of healthcare services and development/analysis of pharmaceutical policy.

Hanjoong Kim, M.D., Ph.D., is a professor in the Medical School and dean of the Graduate School of Health Science and Management of Yonsei University, Seoul, Republic of Korea. Dr. Kim has served as consultant and advisor of the Western Pacific Regional Office in the areas of healthcare financing and health services research. He has also served as a member of the Presidential Commission for Policy and Planning and the National Economic Advisory Council of Korea. He was an editor of *Korean Journal of Health Policy and Administration.*

Linda Lacey, Ph.D., is a professor of city and regional planning and research fellow of the Carolina Population Center at the University of North Carolina at Chapel Hill. She joined the faculty in 1981 and teaches courses on pop-

ulation analysis for planners and international development planning. She
has written a number of articles and chapters in books on population, health,
and housing issues in sub-Saharan African countries. She also has 20 years
of experience providing technical assistance to developing countries, including Nigeria, Ghana, Liberia, Botswana, Uganda, Bangladesh, the Philippines,
and Thailand. She received her master's and doctoral degrees in regional
planning from Cornell University.

Tom Lazenby, M.H.A., is a business consultant for Arthur Andersen in
the healthcare division. He received his degree from the University of North
Carolina at Chapel Hill. Mr. Lazenby currently resides in Atlanta, Georgia.

Peter Lloyd-Sherlock is a lecturer in social development at the University
of East Anglia, United Kingdom. He previously held posts at the London
School of Hygiene and Tropical Medicine and the University of Glasgow.
He has worked extensively on health policy in Latin America and also has
research interests in social policies for older people. Mr. Lloyd-Sherlock is
editor of *Healthcare Reform and Poverty in Latin America* (Institute of
Latin American Studies, London, 2000) and wrote *Old Age and Poverty
in the Developing World. The Shanty Towns of Buenos Aires* (Macmillan,
London, 1997).

Kate Macintyre, Ph.D., is an assistant professor in the Department of
International Health and Development at Tulane University, New Orleans,
Louisiana, where she teaches health policy and comparative health behav-
ior classes. Dr. Macintyre's current research focuses on adolescent health
program evaluation and community-based control of emerging and re-
emerging infectious diseases such as malaria, tuberculosis, and HIV/AIDS.
She conducts health-system-related research in South Africa, Kenya, Cuba,
Eritrea, Ecuador, and Scotland.

Meni Malikwisha, M.D., is a researcher at the Research Institute of
Health Sciences in Kinshasa and is preparing a dissertation in environment management at Kinshasa University, Democratic Republic of the
Congo, where he received his medical degree in 1983. Dr. Malikwisha
has substantial experience in hospital management as well as in health
zones management.

Kwang-ho Meng, M.D., Ph.D., is a professor of preventive medicine at
and former dean of Catholic University of Korea College of Medicine,
Seoul, Republic of Korea, where he received his medical degree in 1968.
He continued his postgraduate training in the field of preventive medicine
and public health there and at the Johns Hopkins University School of
Hygiene and Public Health. From 1979 to 1983, Dr. Meng received a

Ph.D. degree in the field of epidemiology and biostatistics from the University of Hawaii School of Public Health, attending as an East-West Center grantee.

Mbadu Muanda is a demographer from the Economy Department, Kinshasa University, and is currently chief of the operations research division at the National Program of Reproductive Health, Ministry of Health, Democratic Republic of the Congo. He is also a teaching assistant at the Cardinal Malula University, Kinshasa.

Kwilu Nappa Fulbert, M.P.H., is a teaching assistant in the health system management department in the School of Public Health at Kinshasa University, Democratic Republic of the Congo, where he received his master's degree in 1993. Mr. Kwilu Nappa Fulbert has more than ten years of experience as a health manager and administrator in hospitals and health zones.

Lina M. Piripiri, M.P.H., works in the health department of the United Agency for International Development in Kinshasa, Democratic Republic of the Congo. She received her master's degree from the School of Public Health and Tropical Medicine, Tulane University, New Orleans, Louisiana, in 1993 and is now in the process of completing her doctoral dissertation in public health at Tulane. Ms. Piripiri worked at the School of Public Health, Kinshasa University, as a research and teaching assistant for about eight years.

Rui Portugal, M.D., M.Sc., is a Portuguese public health physician. He is currently enrolled in a doctoral program in health policy and administration at the University of North Carolina at Chapel Hill. Previously, he worked as a public health physician and a hospital administrator in Lisbon, Portugal. He taught at the Medical School of the University of Lisbon in the field of public health, where he developed several international programs. He cofounded the Doctors of the World program in Portugal.

Pavel Ratmanov, M.D., is assistant professor of public health and health services management at the Far Eastern State Medical University (Russia) and head of the Sector of Medical Services Price Setting at the Khabarovsk Territory Compulsory Medical Insurance Fund. His medical degree is in internal medicine from Far Eastern State Medical University.

Ana Rico, Ph.D., M.Sc., is a research fellow in the European Observatory on Health Care Systems. Previously, she was assistant professor of public policy at the Pompeu Fabra University of Barcelona, Spain. Her current research interests include the evaluation of healthcare reforms, the governance of primary healthcare services, the decentralization of the state, and the measurement of citizen satisfaction.

Dale Rublee, Ph.D., is director of outcomes research at Aventis Behring in Marburg, Germany, where he conducts economic evaluations of therapeutic proteins for the treatment of immune disorders, hemophilia, blood clotting disorders, and hereditary emphysema. Previously, he has held posts in Europe with Quintiles Transnational and in the United States with the American Medical Association's Center for Health Policy Research. He is an authority on the economics of the German healthcare system and has published extensively in peer-reviewed journals such as *Health Policy, Health Affairs,* and *Journal of the American Medical Association.*

Luis Bernardo Saenz, M.D., is an independent public health consultant. From 1995 through 1998, he was director of the Proyecto Modernizacion at the Caja Costarricense de Seguro Social in Costa Rica, a government commission to reform the social health insurance system.

Jeff Sanders, M.H.A., graduated from the University of North Carolina School of Public Health, Department of Health Policy and Administration, in May 2001. He has experience in healthcare policy through his work with former Senator George Mitchell, the Association of American Medical Colleges, and PricewaterhouseCoopers. He is currently completing a one-year postgraduate fellowship at Intermountain Health Care in Salt Lake City, Utah.

Ojas Shah, M.H.A., is a healthcare consultant within Arthur Andersen's Business Consulting Practice and a member of the American College of Healthcare Executives. He has experience working with health systems in the United States and India, which includes work in strategic sourcing, organizational redesign, and performance measurement. Mr. Shah received his master's degree from the University of North Carolina.

Euichul Shin, M.D., Ph.D., has a joint appointment as an associate professor at the College of Medicine and the Graduate School of Healthcare Management and Policy, The Catholic University of Korea, Seoul, Republic of Korea. He also holds an adjunct faculty position in the Department of Health Policy and Administration, University of North Carolina at Chapel Hill. His areas of research interest are healthcare organizational theory, continuous quality improvement, and public health surveillance.

Arie Shirom, Ph.D., is professor of organizational behavior and healthcare management in the graduate programs of Health Administration and Organizational Behavior of the Faculty of Management, Tel-Aviv University, Israel. He received his doctoral degree from the University of Wisconsin–Madison. The analysis of Israel's healthcare system, as presented in chapter 12 of this book, reflects ideas developed during and after his term of office as a member of the State Commission of Inquiry into the Effectiveness of the Israeli Health Care System (1988–90). His current research interests include theory construction in healthcare management and the effect of work-related stress and burnout on employees' health and performance.

Scott Stewart, M.S.P.H., is currently pursuing a Ph.D. in public health at the University of North Carolina at Chapel Hill. Mr. Stewart worked with food security and reproductive health programs in Botswana from 1986 to 1997.

Aysit Tansel is a professor of economics at the Middle East Technical University in Ankara, Turkey. Her areas of research include applied econometrics, labor economics, health economics, and gender issues. She has written on economic and social issues in Turkey and the West African countries of Cote d'Ivoire (Ivory Coast) and Ghana. Her articles have appeared in leading journals in the United States, the United Kingdom, and Turkey.

Vaughn Upshaw, Ed.D., M.P.H., develops, teaches, and manages residential, executive, and distance-learning courses for doctoral and master's students as a clinical assistant professor in the Department of Health Policy and Administration at the University of North Carolina. She also directs the public health leadership doctoral program in the School of Public Health. She initiates and participates in research and service opportunities related to public health organization, management, governance, change, strategy, and leadership. She serves as vice chair of the Public Health Foundation's board of directors and is past-president of the National Association of Local Boards of Health.

James E. Veney, Ph.D., is professor of health policy and administration at the University of North Carolina at Chapel Hill. He has extensive international experience through work with the World Health Organization and the United States Agency for International Development. This experience includes work in health services planning and evaluation in more than 20 countries of Asia, Africa, and Latin America.

Philip C. Williams, J.D., Ph.D., M.P.H., serves as assistant vice president for academic affairs at Gardner-Webb University in Boiling Springs, North Carolina, where he is also assistant professor of health management and law in Gardner-Webb's Broyhill School of Management. Dr. Williams previously practiced law for 15 years.

Cesar Woldarczek graduated from a doctoral program in law, management, and economics. Dr. Woldarczek is currently a professor of social policy at the InstiJagiellonian University, Poland. He also holds an appointment at the Medical College and Institute of Public Health at the University of Lodz where he is on the Faculty of Law and Administration. Dr. Woldarczek is the author of seven books and many papers on such subjects as healthcare reform in new democracies and specifically in Poland.

Aki Yoshikawa, Ph.D., is chairman of the Global Health Institute, a California-based not-for-profit healthcare research foundation, and is also the managing partner of the GHC, an international healthcare consulting firm. Dr. Yoshikawa founded the Comparative Health Care Policy Research Project at Stanford University, serving as director for seven years since initiating the program in 1990. He is an author of *Health Economics of Japan: Patients, Doctors, and Hospitals under a Universal Health Insurance System* (University of Tokyo Press, 1996) and *Japan's Health System: Efficiency and Effectiveness in Universal Care* (Faulkner & Gray, 1993).

Monika Zajac, M.P.H., M.Sc., received her degree in social sciences at Jagiellonian University, Cracow, Poland, and her degree in public health at Maastricht University, the Netherlands. She was awarded the Dutch Job Cohen Fellowship at Maastricht University and a Soros Fellowship at London School of Hygiene and Tropical Medicine. She also worked for Harvard & Jagiellonian Consortium for Health and the Ministry of Health in Poland.

David Zakus, Ph.D., M.Sc., M.E.S., is director of the Centre for International Health in the Faculty of Medicine at the University of Toronto, Ontario, Canada and he teaches graduate courses, supervises postgraduate students, and coordinates the international health activities for the faculty and university. In 1995 he was appointed director of international affairs, and in 2000 he became director of the international health program for the faculty. His teaching and research focus within the departments of Health Policy, Management and Evaluation and Public Health Sciences is on international health, health systems development and reform, community-based health services, primary healthcare, and community participation. Prior to his full-time appointment at the University of Toronto, he was president and chief executive officer of Canadian Physicians for Aid and Relief and was director of several other international health-related programs in Canada.

Roberto Zanola, Ph.D., M.Sc., is professor of public economics and director of the Centre for Health Economics Research at the University of Eastern Piedmont, Italy. He has written a number of articles and chapters in books on health economics, cultural economics, and taxation issues. His areas of research interest in health economics are healthcare expenditure, pollution, and transplants.